Circulatory Problems in Podiatry

Karger Continuing Education Series

David I. Abramson
Chicago, Ill.

Circulatory Problems in Podiatry

Foreword by Philip R. Brachman

53 figures and 7 tables, 1985

KARGER

Basel · München · Paris · London · New York · Tokyo · Sydney

David I. Abramson, MD, FACP

Emeritus Professor of Medicine and of Physical Medicine and Rehabilitation,
University of Illinois College of Medicine at the Medical Center, Chicago, Ill., USA
Consultant, West Side (Chicago, Ill.) and Hines (Maywood, Ill.) Veterans
Administration Hospitals
Formerly Head of the Department of Physical Medicine and Rehabilitation at the
University of Illinois College of Medicine and Lecturer in Peripheral Vascular
Disorders at the Chicago College of Podiatry, Chicago, Ill., USA

Karger Continuing Education Series, Vol. 7

Topics covered in the Karger Continuing Education Series are selected to help
improve clinical skills and introduce the reader to health-related areas undergoing
exceptional growth. Produced as compact instructive texts, volumes set forth information which serves to heighten the general awareness and command of current
medical procedures and practice. The concise textbook format enhances the value of
these books as convenient teaching and training tools for medical scientists, medical
clinicians, and health professionals.

National Library of Medicine, Cataloging in Publication
    Abramson, David I. (David Irvin), 1905 –
    Circulatory problems in podiatry
    David I. Abramson. – Basel; New York: Karger, 1985
    (Karger continuing education series; v. 7) Includes bibliographies and index
    1. Leg – blood supply   2. Vascular Diseases – diagnosis   3. Vascular Diseases – therapy
    I. Title II. Series
    W1 KA821P v.7
    [WG 500 A161ca]
    ISBN 3–8055–3910–X

Drug Dosage
    The author and the publisher have exerted every effort to ensure that drug selection and dosage
    set forth in this text are in accord with current recommendations and practice at the time of
    publication. However, in view of ongoing research, changes in government regulations, and the
    constant flow of information relating to drug therapy and drug reactions, the reader is urged to
    check the package insert for each drug for any change in indications and dosage and for added
    warnings and precautions. This is particularly important when the recommended agent is a new
    and/or infrequently employed drug.

Contents

Contents

Foreword

For more than fifteen centuries, the medical world accepted the falla-cies of *Galen, Fabricius,* and *Vasalius* relating to blood flow in man, and it was not until *William Harvey* published his findings on the circulation in 1628 that the true meaning of peripheral vascular diseases evolved.

Since the feet are a prime location for vascular problems, it is essential for us as podiatrists to have a healthy concern for, and deep understanding of, the local circulatory system, especially if a corrective measure, whether medical or surgical, is being contemplated. In fact, few if any of the medical specialties require the detailed analysis of the diagnostic and clinical aspects of peripheral vascular disorders that the field of podiatric medicine and surgery does. Nevertheless, as is also the case in most medical schools in the USA, the curricula of many colleges of podiatry contain inadequate cover-age of this specialty, a lack of which generally continues throughout the postgraduate training period. As a result, the clinician may be poorly pre-pared to cope with the various vascular problems that frequently arise in a podiatric practice. For this reason, it is imperative that we peruse, evaluate, and utilize the information contained in *Circulatory Problems in Podiatry*, written by *David I. Abramson,* MD, FACP.

In his endeavor, Dr. *Abramson* has produced a textbook on vascular disorders solely for the podiatric profession which deals totally with our needs, thus making a distinct contribution to the recognition of our profes-sional growth. His many years of clinical and teaching experience, together with his splendid contributions to the peripheral vascular literature, make him eminently qualified to write such a volume.

The text clearly defines the beneficial and the deleterious effects of many drugs, local applications, and new noninvasive and invasive diagnos-tic techniques. At the same time, detailed history taking, physical examina-tion, and clinical testing are emphasized. Based on scientific and clinical proof, pain of vascular origin located in the lower limbs is discussed in detail, and its differentiation from symptoms which mimic it but are due to nonvascular conditions is presented.

It is my sincere hope that our recent and future graduates, as well as established practitioners of podiatric medicine and surgery, will avail themselves of the excellent, detailed, and comprehensive but still clinical approach to peripheral vascular disorders of the lower limbs found in Dr. *Abramson's* new book.

Philip R. Brachman, DPM
President Emeritus,
Dr. William M. Scholl College of Podiatric Medicine

Preface

As an internist who has spent more than half a century in the medical specialty of vascular disorders of the limbs, I have had the opportunity of maintaining a long and fruitful relationship with practitioners of podiatric medicine and surgery, due, in great part, to the strong and close ties that exist between the two clinical fields. Further reinforcing this interest was my 4-year period spent as a lecturer in peripheral vascular disorders in the Chicago College of Podiatry, under the tutelage of Dr. *Wilfred Danielson,* its president.

From the numerous contacts which have followed, I have developed a general impression that when an abnormality of the arterial, venous, or lymphatic circulation in a lower limb develops in a patient after foot surgery, the podiatrist is not always fully equipped to cope with it. Moreover, in an attempt to prevent vascular complications, there has been a tendency to place too much reliance on the therapeutic effects of reconstructive surgical procedures and to overemphasize their role as a preliminary measure to a podiatric operation. At the same time, the various adverse reactions that may follow such a combined program have not been sufficiently elucidated. Finally, there has been no concerted effort made in the podiatric field to stress the usefulness and advantages of conservative medical therapy in controlling symptoms and signs of vascular insufficiency in the feet.

This monograph, made up of four sections, was developed in the hope that it might help clarify the proper approach to those vascular problems which are found in a conventional clinical practice. It deals with the identification, differential diagnosis, and general principles of therapy of circulatory difficulties affecting the lower extremities, with particular emphasis on the feet. Throughout the volume, the format used in presenting the contents is so oriented as to satisfy almost exclusively the interests and needs of the practitioner of podiatric medicine and surgery.

Section One deals with all aspects of arterial disorders of the lower limbs. The first portion, consisting of four chapters, is devoted, in great part, to the differential diagnosis of symptoms and signs of arterial insufficiency and to these clinical tests which can be performed in the office or at the bedside without the need for expensive instrumentation or technical input. Also included are discussions of noninvasive and invasive laboratory procedures which have become so popular in recent years. In the second portion, made up of six chapters, are presented clinical vascular entities which spontaneously affect the arterial circulation in the lower limbs, with the role of diabetes mellitus in the production of circulatory complications of the feet being especially stressed. Besides descriptions of the various disorders, their differential diagnosis is included, as well as appropriate regimens of therapy presented in general terms and with emphasis placed on prophylaxis rather than on specific dose-related treatment. Such an approach should help the podiatrist better understand the rationale for the therapeutic medical or surgical program instituted for a patient by the physician or surgeon also on the case.

Section Two, consisting of five chapters, deals with the various aspects of venous disorders of the lower limbs and with their complications. The first two chapters are devoted to the clinical and laboratory assessment of the superficial and deep venous circulations and with discussions of the physical signs of venous disorders. The remaining three chapters consist of the presentation of the factors contributing to deep venous thrombosis and their control and a discussion of such clinical entities as phlebothrombosis, iliofemoral and popliteal thrombophlebitis, pulmonary embolism and infarction, and postphlebitic syndrome.

In Section Three, made up of three chapters, the emphasis is on the effects of trauma to various portions of the vascular tree in the lower limbs. Also considered are the untoward systemic and local responses to prolonged bedrest and immobilization of a limb and the iatrogenic vascular complications of podiatric surgery of the feet and ankles, together with steps that must be followed to prevent or minimize their appearance. It is hoped that the latter may possibly help reduce the incidence of malpractice suits having their origin both in nonsurgical and operative procedures. The last chapter in this section deals more specifically with this vexing problem.

Section Four, which consists of one chapter, is devoted to short descriptions of a relatively large number of nonvascular conditions with circulatory components which may be encountered in a medical and surgical podiatric practice.

The reader will soon become aware of the fact that cross-references are extensively interspersed among the contents of this volume, a practice which may prove annoying and cumbersome. However, it does make possible consolidation of the available information on a specific subject, with a minimum of repetition of the same material in different sections of the book.

If this volume makes the podiatrist more acutely aware of the need for determining the exact state of circulation in the feet and legs before initiating any type of therapy, and if he or she becomes more confident and comfortable in dealing with vascular complications should they arise, then its purpose will have been achieved.

I wish to take this means of expressing my profound appreciation to Drs. *Daniel Arenson, Richard A. Bellacosa, Frank M. Passaro, Jack Stern, Gary J. Thomas,* and *Edward Weisman,* all practicing podiatrists who, by their thoughtful suggestions and constructive criticisms, carefully guided my endeavor during its formative stage into pathways useful to members of their profession. I am also most grateful to Dr. *Donald S. Miller* for his generosity in permitting me to utilize photographs from his collection as figures in the book and to Mr. *Charles Hannon* for his assistance in formulating the chapter on medicolegal aspects of podiatry.

David I. Abramson

To Julie, Beth, and John

I Arterial Disorders of the Lower Limbs

1 Symptomatology of Organic and Vasospastic Arterial Disorders in the Lower Limbs

General Considerations

Vascular History

When a routine clinical examination of the arterial tree in the lower limbs reveals an absence or reduction in amplitude of pulsations in the posterior tibial and/or dorsal pedal artery in the foot, frequently there is a tendency to attribute any presenting complaint located in the involved limb or limbs to a lack of local arterial circulation. However, such a reaction may lead to an erroneous diagnosis and the institution of improper, ineffective, costly and, at times, injurious therapy. In order to minimize such a possibility, initially it is essential to obtain a comprehensive and detailed vascular history from the patient, using a fixed and consistent approach, as outlined in table 1/I. Otherwise, pertinent data may inadvertently be omitted.

Aim of Vascular History. Besides dealing with the chief complaint, it is also necessary to probe, through skillful and careful questioning, any valuable leads which may develop during the course of the interview. In this manner, nuggets of information may surface which would otherwise have remained undisclosed. Such findings may greatly assist the interrogator in reaching a proper diagnosis regarding the cause of the patient's difficulties.

Pertinent Points in Vascular History. A number of items listed in table 1/I require some elaboration so as to give basis for the need to question the patient regarding them. For example, it is important to determine whether a cold injury had occurred in the past, since such a state is frequently followed by an increased susceptibility to cold even after exposure to only a moderate reduction in environmental temperature. Information regarding the presence of local orthopedic or neurologic conditions is important, for a number of these may be responsible for symptoms which mimic those produced by arterial occlusive disorders. A history of intravascular clotting suggests predisposition toward subsequent ones of a similar

Table 1/I. Vascular history for the study of arterial circulation in the lower limbs

1   Chief complaints: List

2   Relevant family history: List those conditions which have a relationship to arterial disorders of the lower limbs, such as atherosclerosis in vital organ systems

3   Past history of:
   (a)   Excessive sweating or lack of sweating and dryness of the limbs
   (b)   Changes in hair growth on legs and feet
   (c)   Infrequent need to trim toenails and changes in their appearance
   (d)   Episodes of intravascular clotting
   (e)   Cold injuries (frostbite, trench foot, postfrostbite or post-trench foot syndrome)
   (f)   Trauma to limbs (description of lesions, treatment, outcome)
   (g)   Spontaneous ulcers of legs (cause, treatment, outcome)
   (h)   Spontaneous gangrene of lower limbs (cause, treatment, outcome)
   (i)   Systemic conditions associated with arterial manifestations in the lower limbs (diabetes, hypertension, sickle cell anemia, rheumatoid arthritis, myocardial infarction, atrial fibrillation, congestive heart failure)
   (j)   Episodes of arterial embolization
   (k)   Atherosclerosis in organ systems (heart, brain, kidneys)
   (l)   Atherosclerosis in main arteries elsewhere (carotids and subclavians, thoracic and abdominal aorta)
   (m)   Surgical vascular procedures (sympathectomy, insertion of venous or artificial prosthesis, thromboendarterectomy) and outcome
   (n)   Orthopedic or neurologic conditions affecting the lower limbs
   (o)   Infections in lower limbs, such as cellulitis and lymphangitis and lymphadenitis

4   Habits: Type, duration, and quantity of tobacco smoking, consumption of alcoholic beverages, or drug addiction

5   Occupation: Possibility of injury during daily work activities: routine use of machinery or instruments capable of causing vascular disturbances, such as vibrating tools

6   Present complaints, including:
   (a)   Intermittent claudication: claudication distance in short city blocks, pace of walking, location and description of symptoms, severity of complaint, duration of symptoms after cessation of physical activity, indications of progression of the condition
   (b)   Ischemic neuropathy: positions initiating symptoms, location and description of complaints, severity of symptoms, effect on the well-being of the patient, measures which cause relief of symptoms
   (c)   Ischemic pain in the presence of impending or existing ulcers and gangrene: location, severity, and description of symptoms, conditions which aggravate and relieve them, the effect of the difficulty on the well-being of the patient

nature. Mild trauma to a limb with underlying arterial insufficiency may precipitate ulcers or gangrene in unlikely locations, depending, of course, on the site or sites injured.

Certain systemic conditions may alter the clinical picture of vascular diseases in the lower limbs or even be directly responsible for a reduction in local circulation. For example, the coexistence of diabetes with arteriosclerosis obliterans markedly affects the manifestations, treatment, and prognosis of the primary arterial disorder (p. 112). Hypertension and rheumatoid arthritis are associated with changes in the arterioles of the skin of the lower portion of the legs which lead to ischemic ulcerations (see fig. 2/5a). Atrial fibrillation, congestive heart failure, and myocardial infarction may be followed by the formation and liberation of peripheral arterial emboli, resulting in sudden occlusion of critical arteries of the limbs and elsewhere.

Information regarding previous operative procedures is important for several reasons. If the surgery was performed to increase cutaneous arterial circulation, as through sympathectomy, insertion of a vascular prosthesis, or thromboendarterectomy, data regarding the results of the procedure could be helpful in reaching a conclusion as to the proper therapeutic approach to the current difficulty. Moreover, the previous use of a segment of great saphenous vein in a bypass operation, either in the lower limbs or in the heart, might limit existing options with regard to performing this type of surgery again; the presence of primary varicosities in the lower limbs may also influence the therapeutic operative approach to a local arterial problem.

Detailed questioning regarding the habits of the patient is likewise of value. For example, if he has never smoked, the possibility of his vascular difficulties being due to thromboangiitis obliterans is practically eliminated from the differential diagnosis of the existing condition. Imbibing large quantities of alcoholic liquors may be responsible for the appearance of peripheral neuropathy and neurotrophic ulcers. Repeated intravenous injections of narcotics without aseptic precautions by the drug addict may be followed by numerous ulcerations of the skin of the leg and even gangrene of the foot if some of the material, in high concentration, is inadvertently or intentionally introduced into a peripheral artery of the limb (p. 345). Information regarding the frequency with which the toenails have to be clipped is important, since it gives some insight into the state of nutrition of these structures and hence of the entire foot. However, it is necessary to point out that past trauma to the toenails, such as athletic injuries (particularly in runners and ballet dancers) and previous infections, can also be responsible for their slow growth.

Types of Symptoms. Chronic occlusive arterial disorders are generally responsible for three different gradations of symptoms in the lower limbs, depending solely upon the severity of the vascular impairment and not directly upon the type of underlying causal agent. These are *intermittent claudication, ischemic neuropathy,* and pain associated with serious *trophic disturbances* (*ischemic ulceration* and *gangrene*). All other complaints located in a lower limb with chronic arterial insufficiency can generally be considered to have a nonarterial etiology. It is also important to point out that rarely are even the symptoms associated with a chronic occlusive arterial disorder so typical and specific that such a diagnosis can be made solely on their presence, as elicited by a vascular history. Hence, confirmatory evidence must always be sought through the performance of a selective vascular physical examination (p. 22). In order to facilitate ready identification of the main complaints associated with a chronic occlusive arterial disorder of the lower limbs, their pathogenesis, clinical characteristics, and differential diagnosis are dealt with in the following sections.

Intermittent Claudication

The symptom found in chronic occlusive arterial disorders of the lower limb which most often compels the patient to seek medical advice is pain in the muscles of the lower limbs on walking (intermittent claudication). Since there are a number of conditions, both vascular and nonvascular, which may be either responsible for this complaint or closely mimic it, only through careful questioning of the patient can the actual cause be properly identified. Of importance in this respect is the determination of the factors that initiate, exaggerate, minimize, or eliminate the symptom; its duration after termination of the precipitating agent; and the effect of environmental temperature and humidity on it. The reasons for directing the questions along these lines are explained in the discussion on the pathogenesis of intermittent claudication (p. 7).

Clinical Characteristics of Intermittent Claudication
Definition and Description of Complaint. Intermittent claudication is a symptom complex characterized by pain in a group or groups of exercising muscles in the lower limbs. It has been described in various terms, depending on how well the patient can verbalize his difficulty, as a cramp, a sensation of tightness or compression, a viselike feeling, a sense of paralysis, a

sharp pain, or, in the case of the patient with a high threshold for pain, a dull ache or merely a local sensation of tiredness or fatigue. Occasionally, the discomfort is interpreted as numbness located most commonly in the toes, either alone or in association with pain in the exercising muscles. This type of symptom may result from shunting of cutaneous circulation from the toes into the now widely dilated vessels in the small muscles of the foot, thus further increasing the ischemia of peripheral nerve endings and eliciting neuritic complaints.

Consistently, intermittent claudication is experienced after the patient has walked a certain distance at a specific pace (claudication distance), measured in short city blocks. It is never present on lying down, sitting up, or standing. Nor is it experienced immediately after the patient begins to walk. In most instances, relief from the pain occurs soon after the patient stops walking and stands, attempting to shift the total weight of his body to the uninvolved (or less affected) lower limb. It is not necessary for him to sit down to experience relief from the pain. Generally, if he continues to walk after the symptom appears, it builds up in intensity until he is compelled to stop. Occasionally, however, the symptom levels off, and the patient is then able to walk a long distance, experiencing only moderate discomfort. The explanation for such a response may be that he slows his pace or adopts a shuffling gait. Another possibility is that his vascular tree becomes more efficient on continuing his exercise, analogous to the phenomenon of 'second wind' noted in long-distance runners.

Implications of Location of Complaint. Some gross indication regarding the site of the block in the arterial tree can be derived from the group of muscles in which intermittent claudication is experienced. For example, pain in both buttocks on walking localizes the occlusion to as high as the aortic bifurcation or in the two common iliac arteries (Leriche's syndrome). If the symptom is located in the thigh muscles and does not spread to distal structures despite continued walking, most likely the pathologic obstruction is in the deep femoral artery. On the other hand, if pain is then experienced in the calf muscles as the patient continues to exercise, the block may be in the common femoral artery; or there may be two separate lesions, one in the deep femoral and the other in the distal portion of the superficial femoral or popliteal artery. The order of onset of symptoms may be reversed, with the pain first being experienced in the calf muscles and later in the thigh muscles. Such a situation may also result from a block in the common femoral or the external iliac artery. Intermittent claudication limited to the small muscles of the foot is usually due to complete occlusion of the tibial arteries or of the popliteal artery. However, it is necessary to point out that symptoms in the distal portions of the lower limb can likewise have their origin in obstructive lesions located as high as the common femoral and external iliac arteries or even the aortic bifurcation. When intermittent claudication is experienced simultaneously in the same group of muscles in both lower limbs, it can be inferred that the degree of impairment in the two extremities is about the same.

Pathogenesis of Intermittent Claudication

Pain in exercising muscles of the lower limbs results from insufficient amounts of oxygen being delivered to these active tissues by the blood stream to satisfy their markedly enhanced metabolic needs (15–20 times greater than that required during the resting state). As a consequence of this discrepancy, there is a local formation of abnormal stable products ('P' or pain substances). The exact chemical or physiochemical nature of these materials has not been identified, although in the past, lactic acid, potassium, histamine, and serotonin, among others, have all been implicated. With each muscular contraction, the concentration of such substances is believed to increase, until ultimately there is stimulation or irritation of sensory nerve endings in the tissue spaces in the muscle mass, with the production of pain. It therefore follows that if the patient walks at a fast pace or uphill or carries a heavy valise or groceries on level ground, he will develop pain sooner than when he is walking slowly on a level surface, unencumbered by any packages. For, the onset and severity of the symptoms are directly related to the rate of development and magnitude of the oxygen debt incurred in the exercising muscles.

On termination of the work, there is a rapid return of the metabolic requirements to a resting level, and available blood flow again becomes adequate for basic tissue needs. Hence, there is no further buildup of pain-provoking materials, and the amounts that have accumulated during the period of partial anaerobic work either diffuse into the blood stream or are destroyed locally. With a lowering of the concentration of the 'P' substances, the nerve endings are no longer stimulated and hence the symptoms begin to subside until they are no longer experienced. The duration of the period of recovery in which pain is still present is directly related to two factors: the magnitude of the oxygen debt existing at the termination of the exercise and the efficiency of the systemic and local compensatory cardiovascular mechanisms to cope with it. The length of this period is therefore

grossly a reflection of the degree and severity of the existing vascular difficulty. It generally varies from 2 to 10 min, provided the patient stops walking and rests soon after the onset of pain. Symptoms that persist for hours
after exercise is terminated should make one dubious of the diagnosis of
intermittent claudication. Moreover, those that first appear after physical
effort is terminated and the patient is resting are also not due to vascular
insufficiency.

Clinical Entities Manifesting Intermittent Claudication

Pain in exercising muscles may be found in a variety of different states
and clinical disorders and even in normal persons. In the case of the latter
group, however, the symptom is experienced when the work load is so great
that a normal vascular response to the situation is still not of the magnitude
required to satisfy the resulting rise in oxygen needs, despite a highly efficient local vascular tree and unimpeded blood flow through the large supplying arteries.

Systemic Disorders. A number of these are associated with intermittent
claudication, in the absence of organic changes in the arterial tree of the
lower limbs. For example, the symptom may be present in severe anemia
(including sickle cell crisis) because there are an insufficient number of
oxygen-carrying red blood cells per unit of circulating blood to deliver a
large enough quantity of the gas to the exercising muscles to satisfy their
metabolic needs. In certain types of congenital heart disease, unsaturated
blood passing through active muscles produces a similar lack. Congestive
heart disease is associated with reduced systolic discharge and cardiac output, with the result that, again, adequate amounts of oxygen are not available to the exercising muscles. Local capillary changes and altered tissue
fluid content may also contribute to the deficient oxygen delivery. Patients
suffering from severe hyperthyroidism may experience intermittent claudication, due to the heightened metabolic requirements of all tissues including
voluntary muscles, such a situation being exaggerated during periods of
physical activity. In myxedema, this symptom may likewise be present,
with relief following administration of thyroid medication.

Chronic Occlusive Arterial Disorders. If all of the above diseases can be
eliminated as possible causes for intermittent claudication, then it can be
assumed that the symptom is due to a chronic occlusive disorder obstruct-
ing blood flow through the large arteries supplying the local vascular tree in

the group of involved muscles. Although the pathologic process is generally atherosclerosis (arteriosclerosis obliterans), identical complaints can be initiated by thromboangiitis obliterans (Buerger's disease), postligation of a traumatized artery, and postembolic occlusion. Temporary extrinsic compression of the popliteal artery during walking, as in the popliteal artery entrapment syndrome (p. 369), may also be responsible for the appearance of intermittent claudication; the same applies to disorders in which partial or complete blocks exist in the large proximal arteries supplying the lower limbs, as in the case of coarctation of the aorta and aortoiliac arterial occlusive disease (p. 99).

Differential Diagnosis of Intermittent Claudication
Involvement of Musculoskeletal Structures of Foot and Ankle. Pain with weight-bearing, due to altered dynamics in the ankle joint and the foot (such as forefoot varus or valgus deformity or uncompensated or abnormal subtalar varus or valgus), may mimic intermittent claudication located in the small muscles of the foot. However, it is generally not as severe, and it does not appear only after the patient has walked a set distance, as occurs with intermittent claudication. Moreover, it may persist for a long period after the exercise is terminated, in contrast to the rapid subsidence of symptoms that takes places when the cause is local arterial insufficiency. Of greatest importance as a differential point is the fact that standing, which produces relief in a very short time in the case of intermittent claudication, has no effect on alleviating the symptoms associated with mechanical derangement of the foot. In fact, they generally become more severe as the weight-bearing position is continued. Finally, no signs of arterial insufficiency are noted in the presence of pes planus, arthritis of the ankle joint, callosities, or verrucae, whereas in the case of intermittent claudication due to a local arterial disorder, these are common findings. At the same time, clinical and laboratory abnormalities of the affected musculoskeletal or cutaneous structures are readily identified.

Tendinitis of conjoined origin of intrinsic muscles may also produce pain in the foot on standing or walking, with the symptom developing at the site where the muscles arise from the tuberosity of the os calcis. Although worse on standing, the ache in the heel remains for a while after the patient lies down. Generally, X-ray examination is of little value in the diagnosis of the condition. Of importance is the finding that the arterial circulation to the leg and foot is always normal. Also to be considered in this category are *bursitis* and *fasciitis.*

In the presence of an *abnormal subtalar-midtarsal joint complex,* the feet are comfortable upon first arising in the morning but may then become painful as soon as the patient stands or walks, to become less intense after the exercise is continued. However, later, following more physical activity during the day, the feet again become painful. The explanation for such a sequence of events may be that at night the muscles that guard an abnormal talonavicular joint are relaxed and so with assumption of the upright position in the morning, the unprotected joint becomes weight-bearing, producing local pain. With continued standing or walking, the muscles again go into spasm, splinting and restricting joint movement and, as a result, the pain lessens temporarily. With further physical effort, the protective mechanism is no longer able to operate, and symptoms return. Again, no signs of local impairment of arterial circulation is noted in the disorder. Hence, the typical sequence of events and the absence of vascular involvement should offer no difficulty differentiating the pain due to an abnormal subtalar-midtarsal joint complex from intermittent claudication.

In the case of *Morton's neuralgia,* the typical finding is pain in the toes on standing or walking, which is sharp, shooting, crippling, burning, or cramp-like in type. Frequently the symptoms subside when the shoe is removed. The complaint originates in the region of the third or fourth metatarsophalangeal joint, at times extending up the leg as far as the knee. An important clinical sign is the finding of a crepitant mass which is generally palpated in the vicinity of the web between the third and fourth toes at the point where the web joins the foot proper. To determine its presence, the toes are dorsally extended, and the mass between the metatarsal heads is pinched, eliciting typical symptoms, as described above. Because of the characteristic history, the positive Mulder's sign, and the absence of vascular abnormalities, there should be no difficulty differentiating the pain of Morton's neuralgia from vascular intermittent claudication.

Involvement of Musculoskeletal Structures of Leg. A number of conditions affecting the different tissues of the leg are associated with symptoms which may be mistaken for intermittent claudication in the calf muscles. One of these, *tennis leg,* generally develops acutely shortly after some type of trauma to the calf, as while playing tennis or running. The injury consists of partial tearing of the medial gastrocnemius muscle belly at or near the musculotendinous junction. The condition is usually ushered in by the appearance of severe lancinating pain in the posteromedial segment of the calf, midway between the knee and ankle, on taking a step. A characteristic clinical finding is a defect palpated in the medial muscle belly of the gastrocnemius at or above the musculotendinous junction. Ecchymosis over the medial aspect of the calf and extending distally along the course of the Achilles tendon to the ankle may be observed several days later, associated with slight edema. The typical clinical pattern and the absence of signs of local arterial insufficiency should be very helpful in differentiating the symptoms of tennis leg from vascular intermittent claudication.

The pain of *shin splints,* a condition causing symptoms in the antero-lateral mid-third of the tibialis anterior muscle, may mimic intermittent claudication. The clinical entity is generally noted after violent athletic exertion, particularly in the untrained individual. It results from either tearing of the tibialis anterior muscle away from the bone or a hemorrhage, tear, or strain of the muscle itself. The mechanism responsible for the pathologic changes is the development of considerable tension in the gastrocnemius muscle which, in turn, places undue stress on the tibialis anterior muscle. For, the two are opposing muscles, one pulling the front part of the foot down and the other pulling it up. If runners do not initially perform stretching exercises to counteract existing tight muscles, the added tension on the tibialis anterior muscle when they run very fast or very long on a hard surface may damage this structure and produce the described abnormalities. The clinical picture consists of pain and discomfort in the leg, associated with induration and swelling of the pretibial muscles, the complaints generally being controlled by rest, strapping, elevation, and cold packs. No signs of local arterial insufficiency are present, and hence there should be no difficulty differentiating shin splints from intermittent claudication. However, it should be mentioned that in severe cases, overuse of the muscles of the leg has resulted in the anterior tibial compartment syndrome (p. 313).

Intermittent Limping. This is a nonvascular syndrome, produced by a number of unrelated conditions, that may mimic intermittent claudication of the calf muscles. Its clinical pattern consists of the development of a cramp-like pain or a sense of exhaustion in one or both legs, brought on after the patient has walked several blocks, which requires him to come to a complete halt. One of the etiologic agents is a shortened Achilles tendon or triceps surae muscle, producing an inability to dorsiflex the foot and an imbalance of the metatarsal heads. Another responsible factor is wearing high heels or the existence of some type of congenital abnormality having the same structural effect. Pain in an arthritic ankle joint may result in disuse of the limb for fear of eliciting symptoms, which will eventually result in extreme contraction of the gastrocnemius and its tendon and the appearance of intermittent limping. The presence of a painful plantar wart, causing the patient to assume a protective habitus, may also produce the problem. The typical clinical findings common to the different conditions and the good therapeutic results from nonvascular procedures all support the view that the symptoms are not due to impairment of local circulation, signs of which are never noted in the presence of intermittent limping.

Among other nonvascular conditions responsible for pain in the calf is a group of *muscle enzyme deficiency disorders,* such as muscle phosphorylase deficiency (McArdle's syndrome), muscle phosphofructokinase deficiency, and muscle glucosidase deficiency. In all of these disorders, painful cramps are produced in active muscles with physical effort, associated with local weakness, easy fatigability, and stiffness. The diagnosis of *McArdle's syndrome* can be made be determining the absence of a rise in venous blood lactate levels after ischemic exercise of the affected muscles. Signs of arterial insufficiency are not present in muscle enzyme deficiency disorders.

Another deficiency condition associated with pain in the muscles of the leg is severe *vitamin B_1 deficiency.* At the beginning, local weakness is experienced only when the patient walks a long distance. However, with development of a greater state of deficiency, difficulty in walking becomes more and more marked, until even a distance of 100 feet may have a profound effect. Generally such abnormalities as burning of the soles and numbness of the dorsum of the feet and, at times, foot drop are also present. The dramatic therapeutic response to hyperalimentation may help identify the condition, together with the absence of signs of impairment of local circulation.

Involvement of Nervous Structures in Lower Back. Several neurologic conditions affecting large nerve trunks in the lumbar region which innervate structures in the lower limbs are associated with pain in the buttocks and thighs and hence may be mistaken for classic intermittent claudication located approximately in the same sites. One of these is a *herniated lumbar disk,* which may cause symptoms first in the buttocks and then radiation of the pain down the posterior aspect of the thigh and leg to the ankle (in the sciatic nerve distribution). Of diagnostic importance is the fact that the complaints become worse on change of posture, as from the horizontal to the upright position, and on bending, lifting, coughing, or straining, and not particularly on walking, as is the case with intermittent claudication. Also, signs of pressure and irritation of nerve trunks are present, such as decreased sensation to cotton wool and pin prick, reduced vibration sense perception, decreased or absent ankle and knee jerks, spasm of the muscles of the lower back, positive Lasegue's and crossed Lasegue's signs, and weakness in extension of the great toe, among others. At the same time, there are no findings indicative of a reduced local arterial circulation.

A clinical neurologic entity associated with symptoms that closely resemble vascular intermittent claudication is neurospinal compression (*intermittent ischemia of the cauda equina* or *pseudoclaudication syndrome*), causing *neurogenic intermittent claudication.* The condition results from some type of abnormality of the lumbar spine, generally a herniated nucleus pulposus or a vertebral spine bony alteration. The actual mechanism responsible for the clinical picture has not been determined, but a number of possibilities have been proposed, among which is compression of nerve roots in the cauda equina during exercise, producing ischemic neuropathy. It has been suggested that such a response occurs due either to protrusion of the involved disk, to pressure induced by marked hypertrophic ridging in the intervertebral canal, or to congenital narrowing of this structure. Another explanation offered is that during physical exercise involving the lower limbs, there is a relative neural ischemia of the spinal cord.

The history and clinical findings in neurogenic intermittent claudication consist of the following: On walking a distance, the patient experiences pain in the buttocks and, at times, in lower segments of the limbs, which is relieved by rest, thus mimicking the typical characteristics of intermittent claudication. However, the distance the patient covers before experiencing the symptom may become smaller and smaller with each subsequent attempt. Furthermore, the complaint is described as a sensation of numbness, tingling, weakness, or incoordination, resembling a neuritic type of symptom rather than one localized to a muscle mass, as occurs in true intermittent claudication. Of great importance is the fact that the pain experienced with walking also develops in the hip or thigh on straightening the back while in bed or on prolonged standing. Moreover, the symptoms initiated by walking are generally relieved by sitting or lying down and not by standing, and total subsidence of pain occurs only after 20 or 30 min have elapsed.

Besides the symptoms described above, neurogenic intermittent claudication may be associated with some of the signs of a herniated disk, such as absent or reduced ankle jerks, at least during exercise, and elevated cerebrospinal fluid protein. However, the usual manifestations of a herniated disk, including a positive coughing or sneezing effect and a positive leg-raising maneuver, are not elicited. Because of the lack of clear-cut findings, at times it may be necessary to perform a myelogram to demonstrate a partial or complete block in the lumbar region. The most important differential point is the fact that in neurogenic intermittent claudication, the arterial circulation in the involved lower limb is normal.

Ischemic Neuropathy

A small percentage of patients suffering from a chronic occlusive arterial disorder of the lower limbs, previously manifested solely by long-standing intermittent claudication, may now also begin to experience a new type of symptom – rest pain in the feet. This complaint, termed ischemic neuropathy, generally becomes so severe as to overshadow any other of the difficulties associated with local impairment of arterial circulation. It is an ominous sign, indicating that there has been a rapid advancement of the occlusive process in the vascular bed without a corresponding development of an effective compensatory collateral circulation.

Clinical Characteristics of Ischemic Neuropathy
The complaints of ischemic neuropathy reflect a state of ischemia in which nervous elements in the feet are stimulated, with the result that the patient experiences paresthesias, formication, burning, prickling, tingling, coldness, or numbness in the toes, associated with severe lancinating sensations which travel down the limb. At the beginning they appear within 15 min after the patient lies down in bed in preparation for sleep. Unable to fall asleep under such circumstances, he soon learns that relief can be obtained by sitting up in bed, with his lower limbs dangling over the edge, or by getting out of bed and walking around the room for several minutes. However, recurrence of symptoms takes places shortly after he returns to the horizontal position in bed. He finds that the only practical solution to achieving a longer period of comfort and hence an opportunity to fall asleep is to sit in a reclining chair with his feet on the floor. Since this position is now maintained all night long and for a good part of the day, dependency edema will inevitably develop and increase in amount until there is significant mechanical obstruction of the cutaneous microcirculation and exaggeration of the already existing severe ischemia. Under such conditions, some slight trauma to the limb is enough to initiate an ischemic ulceration or gangrene, with practically no possibility of subsequent healing of the lesion.

Patients suffering from ischemic neuropathy always manifest signs of a marked impairment of circulation to the involved limbs, including absent arterial pulsations, zero oscillometric readings, poor or no hair and nail growth, nutritional changes in the skin, low skin temperature, and abnormal skin color changes in the toes (cyanosis or pallor). Besides such vascular abnormalities, there may be signs of involvement of peripheral nerves, consisting of reduced or absent vibratory sense perception in the toes.

Pathogenesis of Ischemic Neuropathy

The reason the patient first experiences the severe symptoms only on lying in bed is that in this position, the beneficial hydrostatic mechanism existing on standing or sitting, which helps drive blood into the diseased and partially obliterated arteries of the lower limbs, is lost. At the same time, systemic systolic blood pressure falls 10–15 mm Hg. As a consequence of both alterations, the head of pressure in the stenotic arteries in the lower limb falls and perfusion through the tissues becomes even less efficient. Such a situation exaggerates an already existing severe degree of ischemia. This is particularly true in the case of peripheral nerve endings, which are very responsive to lack of oxygen and react by becoming irritated, stimulated, or in the presence of extreme anoxia, nonconductive.

Clinical Entities Manifesting Ischemic Neuropathy

As already indicated, ischemic neuropathy is a terminal manifestation of a state of severe arterial insufficiency of the lower limb, the most common cause being arteriosclerosis obliterans. When diabetes mellitus coexists, difficulty may be encountered in differentiating the neuritic symptoms of ischemic neuropathy from those produced by peripheral neuropathy (p. 121). Ischemic neuropathy is much less often observed in thromboangiitis obliterans than in arteriosclerosis obliterans.

Differential Diagnosis of Ischemic Neuropathy

Peripheral Neuropathy. The symptoms associated with this state, whether caused by diabetes mellitus, serum sickness, chronic alcoholism, or drugs, may resemble those experienced by the patient with a chronic occlusive arterial disorder suffering from ischemic neuropathy. However, the involvement is generally more extensive, affecting the upper, as well as the lower, limbs. Also, the pain may be present continuously during the day and is not precipitated solely by assuming a horizontal position in bed, as in the case of ischemic neuropathy. Nor is uncomplicated peripheral neuropathy associated with intermittent claudication, a relationship which always exists in the case of ischemic neuropathy. Moreover, the signs of a marked local reduction in circulation, noted in the latter state, are absent in peripheral neuropathy. At the same time, neurologic abnormalities in the lower limbs may be extensive and severe, including calf tenderness, hyperesthesia of the entire limb, loss of vibratory sense perception in the foot, reduced or absent ankle and patellar reflexes, depression of nerve conduction velocity, and diffuse peripheral nerve damage as identified by electromyographic studies. In the advanced case, atrophy of local groups of muscles and foot drop may develop. In contrast, ischemic neuropathy is associated with only minor abnormal neurologic signs.

Trauma to, or Pressure on, Peripheral Nerves. Irritation or partial destruction of sensory components of peripheral nerves to the lower limbs may cause very severe rest pain which resembles ischemic neuropathy, as, for example, in the case of major causalgia and post-traumatic vasomotor disturbances (pp. 326, 329). The development of a neuroma at the site of trauma or of an operative procedure may also initiate symptoms which mimic those found in this state (p. 190).

Pressure on nerve trunks in their course to the limb can be produced by arthritis of the spine, bursitis, neurofibromatosis, neoplasms within the lower segment of the spinal canal, tumors of the cauda equina, and herniated nucleus pulpus in the lumbar region. Constriction or compression of the lateral femoral cutaneous nerve where it enters the fascia lata after having passed beneath the lateral portion of the inguinal ligament may cause uncomfortable paresthesias along its cutaneous distribution on the outer aspect of the thigh (neuralgia or meralgia paresthetica). In all of the above conditions, the arterial circulation in the lower limbs is normal, and hence there should be no difficulty differentiating them from ischemic neuropathy.

Restless Legs Syndrome ('Jitter Legs'). This difficulty is characterized by unpleasant, distressing paresthesias and formications located either in the calf, lower portion of the leg, or occasionally in the thigh, the distinctive feature being that they are experienced at rest, generally while lying in bed [1, 2]. Frequently they are severe enough to interfere with proper rest. Associated complaints are a sensation of coldness in the feet; muscular weakness and fatigue in the lower limbs; and a sense of aching, restlessness, numbness, burning, and a drawing, pulling sensation. The condition is found in all age groups, although mostly in the fifth to seventh decades, men and women being equally represented. Besides the difficulties in the legs, as a group, individuals suffering from the restless legs syndrome are tense, depressed, and compulsive, often also complaining of symptoms which may be of a functional nature, including tension headaches, indigestion, and extreme tiredness to the point of total exhaustion.

In most instances there is bilateral and symmetric discomfort in the legs in the restless legs syndrome. Although the symptoms are primarily experienced at night, they may also be present during the day when the patient is not actively occupied, as while reading or watching television. Difficulty in falling asleep is a very common symptom; however, some individuals do not complain of this but instead are awakened within a few hours by the distress in their legs. In many cases, some relief is experienced by either making voluntary twitching movements with the lower limbs, by getting out of bed and moving around, or by waving the lower limbs several times while sitting on the edge of the bed.

The cause of restless legs syndrome is not known, although a large number of conditions and states have been implicated, including diabetes mellitus, cholesterol microemboli, vitamin deficiencies, carcinoma, iron-deficiency anemia, chronic venous insufficiency, uremic neuropathy, and pregnancy, and following gastrectomy, among others. The possibility has also been raised that it is a disease of peripheral nerves, although nerve conduction velocity and electromyographic studies have always been found to be normal. Another view, which has been proposed by a number of investigators [1, 2], is that the restless legs syndrome has a psychogenic origin. In one series of cases, it was found in 5% of healthy people [1]; and in another, more than 90% of the patients suffering from it had associated diagnoses of a functional nature [2]. Nevertheless, as a general rule, a psychogenic basis for the symptoms should be entertained only after all possible organic causes have been eliminated in the differential diagnosis.

The characteristic discomfort at rest, the relief afforded by movements of the lower limbs, the localization of the symptoms to the legs, and the absence of signs of local arterial insufficiency should readily differentiate restless legs syndrome from arterial insufficiency of the lower limbs. Nor should there be any difficulty in separating the condition from nocturnal leg cramps (p. 287). The symptoms of peripheral neuropathy may simulate those of restless legs syndrome, but relief with movement does not occur in this state; moreover, there are always definite signs of nerve involvement, which are not noted in the restless legs syndrome. The complaints associated with tension fibrositis may resemble those of restless legs syndrome, such as aching in the back of the calves and thighs, but this is increased with activity and relieved by rest.

Since there is no known etiology in restless legs syndrome, no specific treatment is available. A number of medications have been suggested in the control of the symptoms, including hypnotics, sedatives, muscle relaxants, histamine liberators, vasodilators, dextran, vitamins, oxycodone hydrochloride (Percodan), iron preparations, quinine, diazepam (Valium), aspirin compound, and codeine. Unfortunately, none of these has consistently produced relief of symptoms. Of the group, analgesics and tranquilizers have proved to be the most effective, although they have certain disadvantages when given over a protracted period.

Musculoskeletal Disorders. The rest pain of ischemic neuropathy must also be differentiated from that found in a number of musculoskeletal disorders involving the structures of the lower limbs. Among these are myositis and fibrositis and disorders of the bone, including Paget's disease (p. 375), gout, osteoid osteoma, periostitis, decalcification following hyperparathyroidism, chronic osteomyelitis, and multiple myeloma and other tumors of bone. In most instances, the differential diagnosis can be made by roentgenographic and blood chemistry examinations. Another important point in the case of all these conditions is the absence of signs of local arterial insufficiency.

Pain of Chronic Ischemic Ulceration or Ischemic Gangrene

The second type of rest pain observed in severe chronic occlusive arterial disorders is that associated with the appearance of nutritional lesions, such as ischemic ulcerations and gangrene, generally of the foot and particularly of its distal segment.

Clinical Characteristics of Pain of Chronic Ischemic Ulceration or Ischemic Gangrene

The pain associated with impending or existing ischemic ulceration and ischemic gangrene is frequently very intense and unremitting, originating in the vicinity of the lesion. At times it may also be intermittent and lancinating in type. Although present at rest, it becomes much worse on walking. The latter type of response is due to the stretching of inflamed tissues and to shunting of blood from the cutaneous circulation in the affected site into dilated vessels in the neighboring muscles, thus further exaggerating the ischemia of nerve endings in the tissues at the periphery of the lesion. Elevation of the involved limb above heart level also increases the severity of the symptoms, since in this position, hydrostatic pressure is working against the movement of blood through stenosed arteries in the limb. Lying down in bed, in preparation for sleep, has a similar effect. This is due, in part, to the loss of the beneficial hydrostatic mechanism and, in part, to the drop in blood pressure occurring under such circumstances; both factors contribute to further reduction in perfusion of already ischemic tissue, including the peripheral nerve endings. Moreover, when the patient is in bed, the number of impulses from his body and of stimuli from his environment bombarding his sensorium are significantly reduced, thus permitting him to concentrate his attention fully on his difficulty which, as a result, becomes exaggerated in his mind.

Besides the state of local circulation, the severity of the symptom may be significantly influenced by a variety of unrelated factors. For example, an individual with a high threshold for pain may minimize the difficulty, whereas one with a low threshold may react so markedly to it that he becomes a narcotic addict in an attempt to control his symptoms. Or he may try to coerce his physician (on occasion, successfully) into initiating steps for a major amputation at a time when the physical findings do not warrant such a heroic approach. If the underlying occlusive process is associated with peripheral neuropathy, as may be the case in the patient with both arteriosclerosis obliterans and diabetes, the pain of an ulcer or gangrene may be minimal or even absent, provided the changes in the peripheral nerves are extensive. On the other hand, the clinical pattern may be exaggerated if functional sensory pathways still exist. As a general rule, an ischemic ulcer in a patient with thromboangiitis obliterans produces much more intense pain than does an identical lesion in the individual suffering from arteriosclerosis obliterans.

The pain of impending or existing ischemic ulceration or gangrene is easily differentiated from intermittent claudication, which in practically all patients has preceded the appearance of nutritional disturbances by several years. Although the pain associated with an ischemic ulcer becomes worse on walking, it is also present at rest, in contrast to intermittent claudication which is experienced only with physical effort. Moreover, in the latter state, the complaint is localized to the exercising muscles and not to a site of impending or existing ulceration or gangrene.

In case the ulceration or gangrene has not as yet become clinically apparent, there may be some difficulty in making the diagnosis, since at times there may be few localizing signs in the site from which the pain is arising. Usually, however, the preulcerative or pregangrenous area manifests localizing signs, such as abnormal skin color changes (intense cyanosis, not altered by digital pressure or elevation of the limb, or pallor), a significant reduction in cutaneous temperature as compared with that of surrounding tissues, and local swelling. With loss of continuity of the surface layers of the skin, there is no longer any doubt as to the cause of the pain. Associated with such abnormalities, there are always signs of a markedly impaired cutaneous blood flow in the involved limb, particularly the foot, equal to the degree of severity noted in the case of ischemic neuropathy (p. 15).

Pathogenesis of Pain of Chronic Ischemic Ulceration or Gangrene

The pain associated with an ischemic ulcer originates in the surrounding viable inflammatory tissue. In the case of gangrene, irritation or partial destruction of small sensory nerve endings located in the transition zone between living and necrotic structures is responsible for initiation of the symptoms. The more extensive the area of destruction, the larger the transition zone and the greater the number of nervous elements affected by the local ischemia; as a consequence, the more marked the pain.

Clinical Entities Manifesting Pain of Chronic Ischemic Ulceration or Gangrene

Pain due to ischemic ulceration or gangrene is present most frequently in individuals suffering from both arteriosclerosis obliterans and diabetes. With good local care of the feet and abstinence from smoking, the patient with arteriosclerosis obliterans should only infrequently demonstrate ulcers and gangrene and, hence, pain on this basis. In the case of thromboangiitis obliterans, the incidence of such lesions is high if smoking is continued, and the associated pain is usually quite severe. Generally with abstinence from smoking, nutritional disturbances no longer develop.

Differential Diagnosis of Pain of Chronic Ischemic Ulceration or Gangrene

The differentiation of pain of ischemic ulceration or ischemic gangrene from that associated with ulcers and gangrene having other etiologies (p. 45) will depend primarily on the history and physical examination. In the presence of ischemic ulcers and gangrene, a history of intermittent claudication is almost always present, this symptom having existed for many years before the appearance of the nutritional disturbance. Moreover, physical examination invariably reveals the existence of a markedly impaired arterial circulation in the involved lower limb. In contrast, in the case of ulcers or gangrene of nonvascular or of venous origin, a history of intermittent claudication is not elicited and the arterial circulation in the foot is normal. At the same time, there are symptoms and signs present implicating other etiologic agents. (For a discussion of the pain associated with spasm of small arteries, see p. 37; for a discussion of pain associated with sudden embolic occlusion of normal or diseased critical arteries, see p. 81.)

References

1   Ekbom, K.A.: Restless legs syndrome. Neurology, Minneap. *10:* 868 (1960).
2   Young, J.R.; Humphries, A.W.; Wolfe, V.G. de: Restless leg syndrome. Geriatrics *24:* 167 (1969).

2 Clinical Assessment of the Nutritional Circulation in the Lower Limbs

At present there is, unfortunately, a definite trend toward the utilization of and dependency upon noninvasive vascular laboratories in order to determine the state of the arterial circulation in the lower limbs. Such a practice is associated with many disadvantages and, most importantly, is not necessary or generally warranted. For, in approximately 95% of patients, the proper assessment of the local circulation can be achieved through a detailed vascular history (p. 1) and a selective physical examination, together with a few simple clinical tests requiring no costly equipment or technical knowledge. In fact, the entire procedure can be carried out in the office. As an added dividend, such an exercise leads to the development of greater skills in physical diagnosis, thus making perception of vascular signs in the lower limbs more acute and accurate.

Again, as in the case of a vascular history, in each instance it is necessary to follow painstakingly a comprehensive outline, as listed in table 2/I, in order to carry out an effective physical examination. Two different types of arterial beds in the lower limbs must be studied separately: the nutritional circulation, particularly to the skin, made up of small arteries, arterioles, capillaries, and venules, which directly supplies the tissues with nutrients and helps remove products of metabolism; and the large arteries and their main branches, which together constitute the distributional system. Whereas in the normal individual, the former is wholly dependent upon the state of the larger vessels feeding it, in the case of patients suffering from a chronic occlusive arterial disorder, this type of relationship no longer exists. Under such circumstances, the blood supply to the tissues may be adequate even in the face of an almost complete or complete occlusion of the main arteries and their major branches. This situation is possible because generally an extensive collateral arterial circulation develops simultaneously with a slow, progressive, obstruction of the distributional system (fig. 2/1). The stimulus for the growth of such a compensatory vascular network is the usually present persistent state of chronic mild or moderate ischemia of distal tissues.

Table 2/I. Vascular examination for the study of the arterial circulation in the lower limbs

---

1 Inspection: for the study of the nutritional circulation
   (a) General appearance of the skin
   (b) Skin color in horizontal, elevated, and dependent positions (normal pink color, rubor, cyanosis, pallor)
   (c) Hyperhidrosis; normal sweating pattern; anhydrosis
   (d) Nail changes (deformity, increased thickness, ridging, brittleness, deposition of pigment)
   (e) Hair growth on legs, feet, toes (normal, reduced, absent)
   (f) Presence of dermatophytosis between toes and elsewhere on feet
   (g) Signs of local inflammation (rubor, swelling)
   (h) Presence of minor nutritional changes of skin and subcutaneous tissue (parchment appearance of skin, calcinosis, scar tissue, loss of normal wrinkling over small joints of toes)
   (i) Presence of major nutritional changes of skin and subcutaneous tissue (ulceration; superficial and deep gangrene, 'wet' or 'dry')

2 Palpation: for the study of the nutritional circulation and the distributional system
   (a) Skin temperature (differences in various toes and between the feet, presence or absence of normal skin temperature gradient, abrupt changes in skin temperature)
   (b) Determination of pulsations in abdominal aorta and its main branches and in common femoral, popliteal, posterior tibial, and dorsal pedal arteries; examination for aberrant vessels
   (c) Palpation of arteries, scars, and masses for thrills
   (d) Determination of texture and consistency of skin (persistence of dimpling of skin after removal of digital pressure)

3 Auscultation: for the study of the distributional system
   (a) Examination for presence of bruits over the abdominal aorta and its main branches and the femoral and popliteal arteries (intensity, duration, location)
   (b) Examination of all local scars and masses for bruits

4 Clinical testing: for the study of the nutritional circulation and the distributional system
   (a) Oscillometry performed at 3 levels on the lower limbs
   (b) Venous filling time and return of color
   (c) Reactive hyperemia test
   (d) Subpapillary venous plexus filling time
   (e) Plantar pallor test

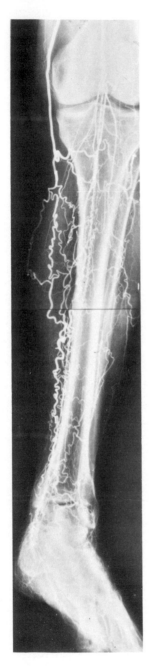

Fig. 2/1. Arteriographic demonstration of extensive development of collateral circulation in the leg and foot of a patient with arteriosclerosis obliterans in response to a slow, progressive, obstruction of the main arterial tree. Complete occlusion of popliteal, anterior tibial, and posterior tibial arteries is present, as indicated by nonvisualization.

It is clear, therefore, that only by the study of the two different types of circulations can a realistic evaluation of the local circulation be achieved. This chapter is devoted to a discussion of the clinical means for collecting information on the state of the nutritional circulation in the lower limbs, and in chapter 3 is found a description of clinical measures useful in evaluating the rate of blood flow through the main arteries and their branches. Chapter 4 deals with the laboratory study of both the nutritional and the distributional vascular systems.

General Considerations of the Nutritional Circulation

For the most part, direct means of studying the nutritional circulation of the skin are not clinically available. Hence, information regarding the state of this vascular bed can only be derived through an indirect approach, utilizing mainly inspection and palpation of the skin and subcutaneous tissue and several simple clinical tests.

In order to collect definitive and consistent data with most of the procedures, it is essential to maintain controlled conditions in the examining room, including a physiologic environmental temperature (72–75 °F; 21–24 °C) and elimination of drafts. The patient should be placed on the examination table in a relaxed and comfortable position, with his lower limbs exposed to the air for about 30 min before collection of data is begun, in order to allow acclimatization to occur. It is also essential to have good illumination, preferably from a natural source.

Postural Skin Color Changes

Physiologic and Pathologic Bases for Skin Color Changes
The color of the skin is a reflection of the rate of blood flow through the two uppermost layers of superficial venules, which together are termed the subpapillary venous plexus, and, to a lesser extent, through the cutaneous capillary bed. The tint of the skins is dependent upon the relationship of the quantity of oxyhemoglobin to that of reduced hemoglobin in the blood circulating through these vascular beds. The greater the concentration of oxyhemoglobin, the redder the skin; the greater the concentration of

reduced hemoglobin, the bluer the skin. Complete cessation of cutaneous blood flow results in pallor or a cadaveric appearance as the subpapillary venous plexuses and cutaneous capillaries are emptied of blood. The more rapid the rate of blood flow through the microcirculation, the less the opportunity afforded for removal of oxygen from each unit of blood as it passes through the tissues; hence, the greater the amount of oxyhemoglobin in the venous blood, thus resulting in rubor (a more intense shade of red) of the skin. Conversely, the slower the rate of movement of blood through the microcirculation, the greater the removal of oxygen, thereby raising the amount of reduced hemoglobin in venous blood, a situation responsible for the appearance of cyanosis of the skin.

Normal Variations in Skin Color with Changes in Limb Position. In order to evaluate abnormal cutaneous color alterations with different positions of the lower limbs, it is necessary first to describe the normal responses to such a procedure. In the horizontal position, the skin has a pink color. When the limb is elevated and maintained in this position for a relatively long period (supported by the hands of the examiner), the hue diminishes somewhat in intensity. Even repeated dorsiflexion of the foot while elevated does not elicit any actual pallor, although this step may further reduce the intensity of the pink color. When the extremity is then placed and maintained in dependency, the color deepens to a normal degree, but signs of cyanosis do not appear even after a prolonged period in this position.

Abnormal Variations in Skin Color with Changes in Limb Position. The limb suffering from an organic impairment of arterial circulation may demonstrate a variety of color changes with alterations in position, depending upon the degree of insufficiency. In the presence of a mild reduction of blood flow and with the limb in the horizontal position, the skin of the leg and foot generally manifests a normal pink color. Following maintenance of the limb in the elevated position, there may be a slight but discernible decrease in the intensity of the pink color, bordering on pallor, as arterial inflow through stenosed arteries is further reduced by opposing hydrostatic forces. Repeated dorsiflexion of the foot while elevated may exaggerate the pallor somewhat. When the limb is then placed in dependency, facilitating arterial inflow, the skin transiently becomes slightly red, due to reactive hyperemia. With maintenance of this position for any period of time, the rubor is replaced by slight cyanosis.

In the limb with a moderate degree of local arterial insufficiency, a normal pink skin color may also be present in the horizontal position. However, with persistent elevation, this is replaced by a definite pallor, particularly on the plantar surface of the foot (positive plantar pallor test). If such a change does not develop with prolonged elevation, the patient should be asked to dorsiflex his foot repeatedly, since this maneuver will frequently bring out the color change. When the limb is now placed in dependency, the pallor may remain for 45–60 s or longer and then it is replaced by an irregular and patchy red discoloration, rather than the normal uniform pink color appearing within 10 s (time of return of color). Maintaining the abnormal limb in dependency will often elicit an initial rubor, almost immediately replaced by cyanosis which deepens as the extremity remains in dependency.

In the case of the limb suffering from a severe degree of organic arterial impairment, pallor is generally present even in the horizontal position, particularly in the toes, due to the fact that even under such circumstances, there is insufficient arterial inflow to fill the subpapillary venous plexuses with blood. On elevation, this response rapidly becomes exaggerated, giving the limb a cadaveric appearance. When placed in dependency, the pallor persists initially and is then followed in sequence by transient rubor and then intense cyanosis as the low or absent tone in the cutaneous venules and capillaries permits immediate pooling of poorly oxygenated blood in them.

Precautions in Interpretation of Results. Certain conditions may result in the collection of misleading information. For example, in the patient who suffers solely from primary varicosities, cyanosis may be noted in the dependent position because of venous stasis. Other states which may demonstrate abnormal color changes in the feet in the presence of normal local arterial circulation are the cyanotic type of congenital heart disease, congestive heart failure, a pneumonic process interfering with oxygenation of the blood, blood dyscrasias, carbon monoxide poisoning, and shock.

Persistent vasospasm (p. 36) may also be responsible for varying degrees of cyanosis in all three positions, in the absence of local organic arterial insufficiency. However, the differentiation can readily be made by utilizing any one of the clinical means for removal of vasomotor tone (p. 69), such a step causing disappearance of the cyanosis if it is due to vasospasm and having little effect on the abnormal color changes produced by chronic organic arterial disorders.

Changes in Cutaneous Temperature

Physiologic Basis for Cutaneous Temperature Changes

As in the case of skin color, cutaneous temperature is a reflection of local cutaneous arterial inflow. Under resting conditions, it is the resultant of the total heat brought to the skin by the circulating blood and of the part lost to the environment through radiation, convection, and vaporization. With ambient temperature maintained at a constant physiologic level, the skin temperature now becomes a qualitative index of the rate of cutaneous circulation.

Technique of Procedure

A relatively gross determination of cutaneous temperature can best be obtained using the back of the hand applied to the plantar surface of the toes, the dorsum of the foot, and the leg. For accurate results, as required in the procedure for determining whether vasospasm exists, the use of some type of skin thermometer is required (p. 69). It is necessary to compare identical areas on the two limbs, since in this manner, small differences (as little as 1–2 °F; 0.55–1.1 °C) can be identified between corresponding toes. Such information has more significance than the general impression that a foot is cold.

Interpretation of Results

After exposure to physiologic conditions for about 30 min, the normal foot demonstrates a rise in skin temperature if previously exposed to a low outside temperature or a fall in temperature if the weather is warm. In the individual who has minimal sympathetic activity, the limb may become quite hot.

If the foot remains cool after prolonged exposure to a normal room environment, the possibility of raised vasomotor tone (vasospasm) must be considered, the low skin temperature being contributed to, in part, by evaporation of sweat (produced in greater than normal amounts in the presence of high sympathetic tone), and, in part, by the reduced local blood flow. Since the patient suffering from organic arterial disease will also have low skin temperatures in the feet initially, it may be necessary to perform one of the tests for removal of vasomotor tone (p. 36) to make the differentiation. In the case of vasospasm, such an approach will cause a rapid rise in skin temperature to a normal level, whereas in the presence of permanent arterial occlusive disease, there will be only a slight increase following the procedure.

It is important to call attention to the fact that decreases in arterial inflow through main channels may exist without any corresponding reduction in cutaneous temperature, probably the result of the development of a very efficient cutaneous circulation in the affected limb in response to a chronic state of local ischemia. Hence, a normal skin temperature does not necessarily rule out the presence of an occlusive process in the large arteries of a lower limb.

Nutritional State of Skin and Subcutaneous Tissue

Old or Recent Trophic Changes

Valuable information regarding the cutaneous and subcutaneous tissue circulations can be derived from inspection and palpation of the limbs. For example, healed, depressed scars on the toes or loss of digits (fig. 2/2a) should make one suspicious of the presence of local arterial impairment, provided, of course, that trauma, venous or lymph stasis, and burns can be ruled out as etiologic agents. At the same time, one must eliminate from consideration a number of nonvascular systemic disorders which demonstrate significant trophic changes in the skin as one of the facets of their clinical pattern (pp. 45, 46).

Also to be studied are the texture and consistency of the skin and subcutaneous tissue. As a general rule, firmness and normal elasticity of these structures can be attributed to adequate local circulation and good nutrition. On the other hand, areas of softness, persistent dimpling of the skin after application of digital pressure (in the absence of edema), or flabbiness may indicate a reduction in local blood flow. The loss of wrinkling over the small joints of the foot and a decrease in the normal range of motion may be due to abnormal attachment of the skin to the subcutaneous tissue (again if swelling is not present), as occurs in scleroderma, or to ankylosis resulting from irreversible changes in these structures (fig. 2/2b).

State of Toenails

Changes Resulting from Arterial Disorders. Of significance in regard to the efficiency of the cutaneous nutritional circulation is the state of the toenails. In the presence of a local organic arterial disorder, these structures generally demonstrate slow growth, deformity, brittleness, vertical and horizontal ridging, deposition of calcium or pigment, and an increase in thickness of the nail substance. In vasospastic conditions, the most frequent abnormality is thinning of the proximal nail folds, with gradual merging into a widened cuticle (pterygium).

Changes Resulting from Nonvascular Conditions. It is necessary to keep in mind that a number of nonvascular disorders, including trauma, may also be associated with alterations in toenail structure. A common offender is a fungus infection (onychomycosis), in which the nail may be painful, loose, and brittle, with a piled-up irregular appearance of the free edge. Initially there is scaling of the nail under the overhanging cuticle, and in time the whole nail plate may become involved, with yellow or dark brown or small chalky-white spots appearing. In onychomycosis due to Monilia, the disease begins under the lateral nail fold, and pus may be expressed from beneath this structure. When the condition is present in conjunction with local arterial insufficiency, difficulty may be encountered in determining the role played by each disorder. Another nonvascular condition which may alter toenail structure is hypothyroidism in which horizontal grooves and ridging commonly develop, with the nails becoming white and fragile, associated with separation of the nail plate. Psoriatic arthritis may be responsible for marked distortion of the nails, splinter hemorrhages, and yellow discoloration. Local trauma may result in an irregular, thickened structure or the development of claw nails, also caused by neglect. Pigmentation of the nails may be found following administration of certain drugs and chemicals and in the presence of some systemic disorders, such as Addison's disease.

State of Hair Growth

The quantity of hair growing on a lower limb may also be affected by impairment of local arterial circulation. In the presence of a severe degree of involvement, hair growth may stop entirely; with mild to moderate reductions, however, growth may be normal. It is necessary to point out that in some races or ethnic groups, like the North American Black and some Asiatic groups, including the Chinese, absence of hair growth on the toes, feet proper, and even legs may be a normal phenomenon. What has the greatest significance is the presence of adequate hair growth on one foot and its absence on the other. Finally, it must also be kept in mind that in the

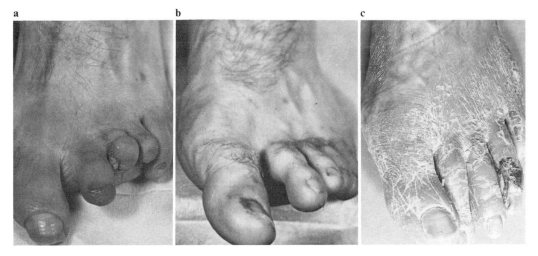

Fig. 2/2. Manifestations of nutritional alterations in the foot. **a** Loss of portions of digits in a diabetic, with complete healing of operative sites. **b** Ankylosis of the toes following frostbite and disuse. **c** Dryness and scaliness of the foot and superficial gangrene, due to a marked compromise of arterial circulation to the sweat glands, oil glands, and skin in a patient with arteriosclerosis obliterans.

case of sudden occlusion of a critical artery by an embolus (p. 81), hair growth on the toes may still appear normal despite the acute absence of adequate local blood flow.

State of Sweat and Sebaceous Glands

Since sweat and sebaceous glands of the skin derive their basic components from the blood, the quantity of their secretions is also a reflection of local blood flow. It follows, therefore, that the limb with a seriously impaired local blood flow can be expected to demonstrate reduced or even absent sweating (anhidrosis), resulting in extreme dryness and scaliness of the limb, especially the foot (fig. 2/2c). Conversely, any improvement in local circulation manifests itself in the disappearance of the latter signs and the return of normal sweating patterns.

It is necessary to point out, however, that anhidrosis may also be caused by a number of nonvascular conditions or states, such as atrophy of the skin affecting the sweat glands; permanent elimination of the sympathetic nervous system control over the sweat glands, as by lumbar sympathectomy; and complete destruction of peripheral nerves (including post-ganglionic efferent sympathetic fibers), as in peripheral neuropathy.

Excessive sweating (hyperhidrosis) is frequently present when increased sympathetic activity exists. It is generally found in the limb manifesting signs of vasospasm (p. 36). There are also a number of physiologic and nonvascular states in which hyperhidrosis may be present. For example, profuse sweating is elicited in normal people on exposure of the body to heat and high humidity and after severe exercise, when there is need for body heat dissipation through evaporation of perspiration. Such a response is also noted when the body temperature rises, as during a fever. Feet which function abnormally with ambulation and, as a result, are subjected to undue stress often demonstrate hyperhidrosis due to a pathomechanical fault. Anxiety, fear, or joy may also be associated with excessive sweating, as is an anxiety state or neurocirculatory asthenia. Finally, certain types of hyperhidrosis are familial or congenital.

Clinical Testing of State of Nutritional Circulation

Reactive Hyperemia Test. Among the simple clinical procedures which can readily be performed in the office or at the bedside and which give pertinent information regarding the cutaneous circulation is the reactive hyperemia test. It is based on the principle that a short period of artificially produced total anoxia of a limb will be followed by a marked increase in local blood flow immediately after reestablishment of circulation (state of reactive hyperemia). This response represents an attempt on the part of the body to repay the oxygen debt incurred during the period of cessation of local blood flow. The vascular change probably occurs in the terminal arterioles and capillaries as the result of the action of slowly diffusible substances accumulated in the extravascular fluid during the period of arterial arrest.

The reactive hyperemia test is performed as follows: An ordinary pneumatic blood pressure cuff is wrapped snugly around the thigh above the knee, the limb is elevated for several minutes to facilitate venous drainage of the subpapillary venous plexuses, and an arterial occlusion pressure is rapidly allowed to enter the system. Then the limb is placed on the examining table and the pressure is maintained for 3 min, at the end of which time it is suddenly released by disconnecting the blood pressure manometer from the system. The color changes in the skin are then studied. In the limb with a normal circulation, a bright red flush appears at the level just below the cuff almost immediately after removal of the arterial occlusion pressure, the change progressing rapidly and uniformly down the limb until it envelops the toes in a matter of 10–15 s. The response remains for 10–40 s and then recedes in the same order that it spread over the limb, the entire color change being completed within 2 min.

In the presence of organic arterial disease or intense vasospasm, the resulting flush may have a cyanotic hue instead of rubor and its advancement is delayed, the color change spreading slowly downward in a patchy manner. As long as 2–3 min may elapse before the toes manifest the change, some of the digits changing color later than others. The recession of color is also slowed. In the presence of complete occlusion of a large artery but with the existence of an efficient collateral circulation, there is a delayed onset of the flush, followed by the development of full color. The appearance of a diffuse faint color suggests narrowing of the finer vessels, whereas marked mottling may indicate very severe impairment of the local blood supply. Vasospasm may manifest itself in the form of a prompt appearance of the flush which then disappears quickly. It is noteworthy to mention that the reactive hyperemia test only gives information regarding the state of the cutaneous circulation and hence cannot be utilized in the study of muscle blood flow.

Subpapillary Venous Plexus Filling Time. This test is useful in determining the state of tone of the cutaneous microcirculation (primarily the superficial venules). It consists of applying firm digital pressure to the skin for several seconds and then studying the color changes which follow sudden removal of the finger. Normally the procedure causes local transient pallor of the skin, resulting from displacement of blood from the compressed venules into the surrounding and deeper tissues, followed by return to normal color within a second or two. A delay of 4–5 s may be observed in the presence of paralysis of the subpapillary venous plexuses (the two uppermost layers of venules), associated with either vasospasm or structural changes in the large vessels supplying the microcirculation. If the abnormal response is present even after removal of vasomotor tone, then it is due to organic arterial disease or to local low or absent tone in the microcirculation.

Besides giving considerable information regarding the turgor of the skin, the subpapillary venous plexus filling time also helps differentiate between living and nonliving tissues. For example, application of digital pressure to an apparently cyanotic area with no appearance of transient pallor indicates that an irreversible change has occurred and that gangrene will ultimately develop in the involved site.

Vasospasm

Vasospasm may cause a marked reduction in nutritional circulation to the skin of the lower limbs and, hence, may be responsible for the appearance of a clinical pattern which closely resembles that resulting from a severe degree of organic arterial occlusive disease. However, since the vascular responses to vasospasm are transient and generally entirely reversible, whereas those due to organic occlusive disease are not, the prognosis is completely different for the two types of conditions. For this reason, it is essential to make an early differentiation between them.

Physiologic Basis for Normal Vasomotor Tone

To understand the pathogenesis of vasospasm in the lower limbs, it is necessary first to review the mechanisms responsible for maintaining normal vasomotor tone, at least in the cutaneous vessels.

Role of Vasomotor Center. Under physiologic conditions, the arterioles in the skin, particularly of the digits, are maintained in a partial state of contraction, due to intermittent discharge of vasoconstrictor impulses originating in the vasomotor center in the medulla and reaching the peripheral vessels via the sympathetic nervous system (fig. 2/3). The nervous impulses terminate in neuroeffector organs (alpha-receptor fibers) located in the vicinity of the circular muscle fibers of the blood vessel wall. At this site, in response to the electrical effect, a chemical neurotransmitter, norepinephrine, is liberated. This hormone accumulates in the cleft of the neuroeffector organ until the proper concentration is reached; at this point, stimulation of the circular muscle fibers occurs, with a resulting reduction in lumen size of the blood vessel and a similar change in local blood flow. Such a mechanism provides a peripheral resistance to the movement of blood into the cutaneous capillaries, venules, and veins from the arterial tree.

Role of Higher Centers in the Brain. The vasomotor center, in turn, is markedly under the control of higher centers, such as the temperature-regulating center in the hypothalamus and numerous sites in the cerebral cortex. As a consequence, various emotions (including embarrassment, fear, and anxiety) and mechanisms which maintain a constant body temperature in the face of significant variations in environmental temperatures and in heat production and dissipation influence the rate of vasoconstrictor impulse formation in the vasomotor center. Because of responses to such

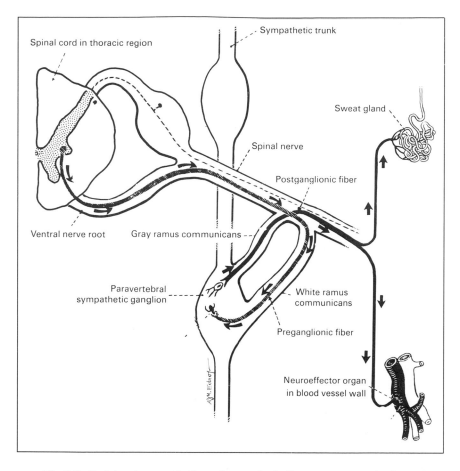

Fig. 2/3. Peripheral sympathetic pathways, including gray communicating ramus, paravertebral sympathetic ganglia, white communicating ramus, and postganglionic fibers innervating blood vessels and sweat glands. Reproduced from ref. [2] with permission.

influences, normally there are variations in the state of vasomotor tone of the cutaneous vessels and hence in the rate of movement of blood flow through the microcirculation in the skin, particularly of the digits.

Normal Variations in Vasomotor Tone. People ordinarily manifest varying degrees of vasomotor tone. There are those with low tone, demonstrating warm, dry, well-colored hands and feet, and there are those with a high, but still normal, degree of tone, as reflected in cool or even cold, perspired, limbs, with slight cyanosis of the toes. The great majority of normal individuals, however, demonstrate fairly warm, fairly dry, pink hands and feet when exposed to a physiologic environment and signs of increased vasomotor tone in a cool or cold environment.

Pathogenesis of Vasospasm

Responsible Mechanism. When, for whatever reason, the rate of vaso-constrictor impulse formation in the vasomotor center in the medulla is persistently increased, there follows a quickly rising norepinephrine concen-tration at the neuroeffector organs in the microcirculation, triggered by the flood of impulses reaching the latter. The accumulation of the large quantity of the hormone causes a much greater than normal constriction of the cir-cular muscle fibers in the walls of the cutaneous arterioles, particularly in the digits, a resulting decrease in lumen size, and a corresponding reduction in local cutaneous blood flow. A state of vasospasm now exists.

Clinical Changes Produced by Vasospasm. The alteration in cutaneous circulation found in vasospasm manifests itself in the form of a fall in cutaneous temperature of the lower limbs, especially the toes; cyanosis or pallor, depending upon the degree of interference with arterial inflow; and increased reactivity of cutaneous vessels to vasoconstrictor impulses or stimuli. With persistent severe vasospasm, edema of the foot may develop (fig. 16/5a and p. 330). Because the sweat glands are simultaneously stimu-lated by sympathetic nervous impulses, excessive sweating (hyperhidrosis) accompanies vasospasm.

Differentiation of Vasospasm. The symptoms and signs of vasospasm can be distinguished from those of acute or chronic organic arterial disor-ders by temporarily removing vasomotor control over the peripheral ves-sels, as by blocking the lumbar paravertebral sympathetic ganglia, spinal or caudal block, or peripheral nerve block (posterior tibial nerve block at the ankle), using a local anesthetic. Reflex or indirect vasodilatation, produced by body warming (p. 200), can also be used for this purpose. If vasospasm is responsible for the clinical picture, temporary destruction of the continuity of the sympathetic pathway produces complete disappearance of the abnor-mal findings, with replacement by rubor, increased cutaneous temperature, and dryness of the skin. On the other hand, in the presence of organic arterial occlusive disease, only slight changes will be noted following removal of vasomotor tone.

Conditions and Situations Favorable to the Appearance of Vasospasm. In the susceptible individual, many types of stimuli and situations may initiate vasospasm. Among these are exposure to cold, emotional excitation, physical inactivity, contemplation and dread of a surgical procedure, and the trauma, both mental and physical, associated with the actual operation itself (postoperative vasospasm). Generally, there is a greater tendency for females, especially young women, to manifest signs of vasospasm than for males to do so. It is necessary to point out that even people who have no predilection toward vasospasm may demonstrate it, provided the initiating stimulus is forceful enough. For example, a blow to a normal exposed artery during an operative procedure may cause the vessel to go into such marked contraction that there is complete obliteration of the lumen (p. 38).

Clinical Disorders or States Manifesting Signs of Vasospasm
The functional or vasospastic arterial disorders are characterized by a reduction in cutaneous blood flow, particularly to the toes, which exists either intermittently or spasmodically or more or less continuously, as a result of a state of exaggerated control of peripheral vessels by the vasomotor center.

Raynaud's Disease. This is the most common of the vasospastic disorders seen in clinical practice. It is characterized by color changes in the digits, primarily the fingers and, much less often, the toes, precipitated by exposure of the limbs or the body to cold or by emotional excitation. Of prime importance in arriving at a proper diagnosis is the fact that no etiologic agent is identifiable, even after at least 3 years of clinical and laboratory observation. The condition affects mostly young women between the ages of 10 and 25 years and, only rarely, men [1].

The episodes of color changes are limited to the digits, with no extension onto the hand or foot proper. The clinical picture results from spasm of the digital arteries, brought on by the precipitating stimulus. This temporary response almost totally or totally prevents movement of blood into the affected digits. As a result, the subpapillary venous plexus is emptied of blood, since venous drainage is not involved, and the digit becomes pale or cadaveric. If there is intermittent release of digital artery spasm, cyanosis will replace the pallor or it may precede it. When the spasm is released, due to removal of the precipitating stimulus, the digit is flooded with blood, causing the skin to assume an intense red color. This change is a manifestation of reactive hyperemia, a rapid means of repaying the oxygen debt incurred during the period of ischemia, the response representing a state of vasodilatation of the digital artery and its branches. With subsidence of the reaction, the skin of the digit returns to a normal pink color. The triple color change (pallor, followed by cyanosis, and then rubor) is the typical response. However, other equally diagnostic combinations are pallor and then rubor, cyanosis and then rubor, and pallor and then cyanosis, but no rubor. During the periods when pallor and cyanosis are present, the involved digits feel numb due to the state of ischemia of peripheral nerve endings. There may also be a sense of fullness and swelling locally. With return of circulation, the patient experiences severe paresthesias, as sensory nerve conduction is reestablished, and then disappearance of symptoms. In a small percentage of patients with Raynaud's disease, very painful superficial ulcerations will develop on the fingertips and rarely on the toes.

The prognosis of Raynaud's disease is good, provided the precipitating stimuli can be eliminated. In this regard, the condition must be differentiated from Raynaud's syndrome, which is associated with a great variety of unrelated conditions, some of which have a very grave outlook. Since the clinical manifestations are the same in Raynaud's disease and Raynaud's syndrome, the differentiation is based on eliciting an etiologic agent in the case of the latter. Some of the conditions in which Raynaud's syndrome is one facet of the clinical picture are: the organic arterial occlusive disorders (arteriosclerosis obliterans, thromboangiitis obliterans); the connective tissue disorders (progressive systemic sclerosis or scleroderma, polyarteritis nodosa, systemic lupus erythematosus, dermatomyositis, rheumatoid arthritis); the neurovascular compression syndromes of the shoulder girdle causing changes solely in the fingers (cervical rib, scalenus anticus, hyperabduction, costoclavicular, and scapulocostal syndromes); postcold injuries (following common frostbite, trench foot, immersion foot); use of high-frequency vibratory tools (pneumatic hammer, pneumatic drill, chain saw), and cryoglobulinemia and cold agglutinins.

Acrocyanosis. This interesting and relatively rare functional disorder is characterized by a persistent uniform cyanotic rubor of the skin of the extremities, associated with a reduced cutaneous temperature. Although noted in both a warm and cold environment, the color changes are much more intense in the cold. Besides the cyanosis, there may be swelling and stiffness of the toes and localized tender areas. Ulceration or gangrene is never noted. The condition is found more often in young women than in men, its only bothersome clinical feature being the unesthetic appearance of the involved limbs. The cause of acrocyanosis is not known, although it has been suggested that the clinical manifestations result from persistent spasm of cutaneous arterioles, associated with capillary and venular dilatation and paralysis.

Livedo Reticularis. This is another unusual vasospastic disorder affecting the lower limbs. In contrast to acrocyanosis (see above), the cyanosis takes the form of a mottled, blotchy pattern instead of being uniform. Symptoms are not present, although the patient, frequently a young woman, is affected psychologically by the unsightly appearance of the skin of her lower limbs.

On occasion there may be recurrent ulcerations on the back of the legs which become indolent and unresponsive to treatment. Initially the lesion is a tender nodule in the skin or a circumscribed bluish or purplish area on which a blister may develop. Despite such findings, all the clinical signs indicate the presence of a normal circulation through the main arteries of the lower limbs.

The characteristic hemodynamic abnormality in livedo reticularis is a marked and widespread vasospastic involvement of the arterioles of the skin of the limbs, producing a moderate degree of ischemia, followed by atonic dilatation of the capillaries and venules supplied by these vessels and stasis of local circulation. The latter change is responsible for the cyanotic mottling with normal skin color intervening. In the presence of ulceration, permanent changes may be found in the cutaneous circulation in the form of an arteritis or arteriolitis. Removal of vasomotor tone, as by lumbar sympathectomy, has no effect on the color changes and hence is not indicated in livedo reticularis.

Other Conditions or States Manifesting Vasospasm. Such post-traumatic painful vascular disorders as major causalgia and post-traumatic vasomotor disorders (pp. 327, 330) always demonstrate varying degrees of vasospasm, some of which may be due to disuse of the limb, a commonly associated finding in these conditions. Vasospasm also plays a significant role in the clinical picture of common frostbite (p. 319) and the post-frostbite and post-trench foot syndromes.

As mentioned above, in different conditions in which the lower limb remains immobile, whether due to fear of eliciting pain or because of the application of a mechanical device to prevent movement, such as a cast, vasospasm may become quite marked, due to disuse alone. The latter factor may also play a role in the appearance of vasospasm in the postoperative limb, although other conditions, such as fear, apprehension, and trauma to tissues incurred during the surgical procedure, may also contribute to this state. Naturally, under such circumstances, it is always necessary to make certain that the coldness, cyanosis, pallor, or local pain is produced by vasospasm and not by associated organic arterial disease or to injury of arteries locally sustained during the operation. Such a distinction can be readily made by removing vasomotor tone by one of the procedures available for this purpose (p. 36). (For a discussion of the clinical manifestations of acute spasm of main arteries, see p. 308.)

Ischemic Ulceration and Ischemic Gangrene

Two of the most serious nutritional disturbances found in the presence of a compromised cutaneous circulation are ischemic ulceration and ischemic gangrene of the lower limbs.

Pathogenesis
Although ischemic ulceration and ischemic gangrene differ in physical characteristics (p. 42), the underlying causative factor is the same in both, namely a marked impairment of local arterial inflow. When the circulation falls to a level incompatible with its ability to satisfy the metabolic needs of resting tissues, then even minimal trauma or a minor infection may be sufficient to initiate a lesion. Or, in the case of gangrene, the process may even develop apparently spontaneously, as when the systolic blood pressure and, hence, perfusion pressure, drops precipitously, particularly in a stenosed vessel. In general, the arterial impairment is of a more marked degree in the presence of gangrene than in the case of ischemic ulceration. Since any reduction in arterial circulation to a lower limb is ordinarily most severe in the distal segment, it is understandable why the toes and heel are common sites for either type of lesion (fig. 2/4). However, an ulceration or, less frequently, gangrene may also develop elsewhere on the limb if the skin locally is extensively devitalized by trauma. Rarely is spontaneous gangrene found on the leg, except possibly when there is a severe localized arteritis or arteriolitis of the cutaneous circulation (p. 44).

Aside from the gradually increasing state of anoxia produced by the inevitable advancement of the atherosclerotic process, several other factors

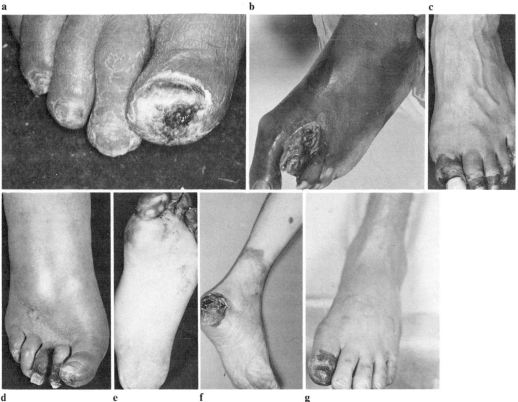

Fig. 2/4. Examples of severe ischemic changes in the feet. **a, b** Ulcerations in the toes due to arteriosclerosis obliterans and diabetes. **c–e** Gangrene of the toes in patients with arteriosclerosis obliterans. **f** Gangrene of the heel with ischemic necrosis of the foot and lower part of the leg in a patient with arteriosclerosis obliterans in whom the femoral artery was acutely occluded by a rapidly growing thrombus. **g** Gangrene of a toe in a patient with thromboangiitis obliterans who continued to smoke.

may initiate gangrene, even in a limb suffering from only a mild or moderate degree of arterial impairment. Two such very important agents are the local application of heat (see fig. 8/1e and p. 197) and prolonged exposure of the limb to a moderately cold environment (see fig. 8/1f and p. 138). Moreover, it is necessary to point out that if a limb with occlusive arterial disease is placed in forced extension or in a cast, as in the management of a podiatric condition, this may also precipitate ischemic gangrene (see fig. 17/1b and p. 338). The possibility of such untoward complications emphasizes the fact that in the presence of an impaired blood supply to a lower limb, vigilance must be exercised at all times in order to prevent gangrene.

Clinical Manifestations

General Considerations. As already indicated (p. 18), the formation of an ischemic ulceration or ischemic gangrene of the foot is associated with varying degrees of pain. The severity of the symptom is influenced by the etiologic agent, the extent and depth of the lesion, and the patient's threshold for pain. The appearance of the ulcer or gangrene depends upon whether superimposed infection and inflammation exist; also important are the precipitating factor and the underlying pathologic process. Naturally, in the case of the diabetic with severe peripheral neuropathy, an ischemic lesion may be associated with little or no pain (p. 121).

Description of Ischemic Ulceration. Second in frequency only to venous stasis ulcers (p. 296), the ischemic ulceration of the lower limbs can be described as an epithelial defect with a base composed of necrotic material, secretion, and pus (fig. 2/4a, b), generally surrounded by viable or poorly viable skin which demonstrates signs of inflammation (rubor, swelling, slight increase in cutaneous temperature, and tenderness to pressure). However, in the presence of a severely compromised local circulation, the inflammatory reaction may only be minimal since blood flow is required for its development. If healing begins to occur, the various abnormal manifestations become less obvious and the necrotic tissue is replaced by granulation tissue which covers the base and wall of the lesion. Eventually the granulation tissue reaches the level of the surrounding skin, at which time it is epithelialized by the inward growth of skin from the edges of the lesion.

Description of Ischemic Gangrene. Generally the gangrenous process manifests its presence by the appearance of cyanosis of the skin in the involved site which, although originally reversible, soon develops irreversible signs as the necrotic process progresses. Then the local tissues become distended with fluid and almost fluctuant, particularly if the gangrene is in the distal segment of a toe. Such a change is followed by absorption of the fluid, with the superficial tissues becoming dry and shrivelled (fig. 2/4c–e, g). This stage of mummification is termed 'dry' gangrene. As the process advances, the deeper structures, including bone, are similarly affected, until eventually a clear-cut line of demarcation or separation may develop between viable and necrotic tissue (fig. 2/4c, d). Little or no local odor is present.

If the area of necrosis becomes secondarily infected, however, the course of events is different. Signs of inflammation develop at the periphery of the lesion and these may extend for some distance into the surrounding viable skin. Lymphangitis may also be noted. The dry appearance of the lesion is lost as the necrotic tissue is broken down by bacterial action, with the production of purulent material. The process is now considered to be 'wet' gangrene.

There is some question as to whether the clinical designations 'dry' gangrene and 'wet' gangrene should be utilized. Actually, even in the case of mummification of tissues, debridement generally reveals that the deeper structures are moist and soft as destruction takes place in them. However, the differentiating point is that in 'wet' gangrene, superimposed infection plays a significant role, whereas in 'dry' gangrene, this factor is minimal. In most instances, when diabetes is present, alone or in conjunction with arteriosclerosis obliterans, 'wet' gangrene is the predominant feature, whereas when arteriosclerosis obliterans is the only underlying cause for the lesion, generally 'dry' gangrene is present.

Clinical Entities or States Associated with Ischemic Ulceration or Ischemic Gangrene
Chronic Occlusive Arterial Disorders. Arteriosclerosis obliterans is the most common cause of ischemic ulceration and gangrene of the lower limbs (fig. 2/4c–e and p. 104). When diabetes mellitus coexists with arteriosclerosis obliterans, the incidence of ischemic ulceration (fig. 2/4a, b) and ischemic gangrene significantly rises, due to the vulnerability to infection and the poor healing response contributed by this disorder (p. 118). The frequent presence of peripheral neuropathy in diabetes also increases the seriousness of ischemic ulceration in this condition because the usual painless character of the lesion and its frequent location on the plantar surface of the foot work against early recognition of the lesion, at a time when appropriate treatment might have prevented extensive destruction of local structures.

Thromboangiitis obliterans, a chronic inflammatory arterial disease (p. 104), is also associated with the appearance of ischemic ulceration or gangrene on the toes and elsewhere on the foot, similar to those seen with arteriosclerosis obliterans (fig. 2/4g). Of interest is the finding that severe pain in the vicinity of the lesion is much more frequent than in arteriosclerosis obliterans.

Acute Occlusive Arterial Disorders. Sudden obliteration of a critical peripheral artery by a large embolus (p. 81) or by a rapidly forming thrombus (p. 90 and fig. 2/4f) may be followed by gangrene of the foot and even lower segment of leg if the available arterial collateral circulation is unable to supply adequate nutrition to the affected tissues to maintain viability. Following occlusion of the microcirculation to the skin of the toes by atherothrombotic or cholesterol emboli (p. 83), small areas of superficial gangrene or ulceration will almost invariably develop on the tips and distal segments of the digits (see fig. 5/4 and p. 84). (For development of ischemic gangrene following trauma to main arteries, see p. 308.)

Arteritis and Arteriolitis. Involvement of the small cutaneous arteries and the arterioles by an inflammatory obliterative process may be responsible for the development of ischemic ulcerations and necrotic patches on both the foot and the leg. For example, in some of the connective tissue disorders, including progressive systemic sclerosis (scleroderma), systemic lupus erythematosus, polyarteritis nodosa, and rheumatoid arthritis (pp. 372, 373, 375), a vasculitis of cutaneous vessels may be responsible for the development of ischemic ulcerations of the lower segment of the leg (pretibial area) and of the toes and of ischemic gangrene of the toes. The ulcers are characteristically small, multiple, painful, and indolent. The pathologic thickening of the walls of the arterioles in the subcutaneous fat, generally found in connective tissue disorders, may contribute to the formation of ulcerations, since such a change interferes with the ability of the skin to withstand minor trauma and to heal ischemic lesions. The formation of the gangrenous plaques on the toes in these conditions is usually due to thrombosis of small terminal arteries and arterioles by the vasculitis. The appearance of ischemic lesions is related to periods of exacerbation of the underlying disorder, as well as to repetitive minor trauma to the limb.

An unusual form of ischemic ulceration of the leg is the *hypertensive ischemic ulcer,* which is generally found in the female patient suffering from severe hypertension, with a significantly elevated diastolic pressure. The lesion, which is usually present on the anterolateral aspect of the leg above the external malleolus (fig. 2/5a), begins either as a pigmented spot of varying size or as a reddish patch which soon becomes cyanotic. As a result of slight trauma to the area or even spontaneously, a superficial ischemic necrotic eschar develops in the original site, which on surgical removal leaves an ulcer with a grayish base [3, 4]. The lesion is almost always very painful and resistant to therapy. Changes in the main arterial tree are not present, but histologic studies of the involved tissues reveal subendothelial hyalinosis and stenosis of arterioles similar to the vascular changes found in various organs of the body in severe arterial hypertension. The pathologic alterations evidently cause thrombosis of the affected vessels, the end result being localized infarction of the skin. (For a discussion of ischemic lesions produced by compression of the cutaneous microcirculation by external forces, see p. 338.)

Differential Diagnosis of Ischemic Ulceration

A large number of unrelated conditions are associated with ulcerations of the lower limbs, most of which are nonvascular. Hence, there should be no difficulty differentiating such lesions from those due to arterial ischemia, since the local arterial circulation is intact, whereas the ischemic lesion resulting from large artery disease is invariably associated with obvious signs and symptoms of a markedly compromised cutaneous and muscle blood flow in the foot and leg. At the same time, other etiologic factors can generally be identified in the case of nonvascular ulcerations.

Venous Stasis Ulceration. This type of lesion is due to the presence of chronic venous hypertension and can readily be differentiated from ischemic ulceration by: its location, mainly on the medial aspect of the leg over the internal malleolus; the history of either primary varicosities or of an old occlusion of a main collecting vein; and in the latter case, of other signs of chronic venous hypertension associated with postphlebitic syndrome (p. 287). At the same time, signs of arterial insufficiency are absent. The clinical manifestations of the venous stasis ulceration are presented on pages 296–302.

Neurotrophic (Neuropathic) Ulcers. These lesions are primarily noted in patients with peripheral neuropathy, due particularly to diabetes mellitus (p. 122 and fig. 7/1c–e), as well as to other etiologic agents, such as chronic alcoholism, certain drugs, and exposure to toxic chemicals. Other etiologic factors are anterior poliomyelitis, syringomyelia, disseminated sclerosis, spinal cord injury, tabes dorsalis, and leprosy. Characteristically, despite extensive destruction of skin, subcutaneous tissue, and even bone, the lesion is painless. Its clinical manifestations are described on page 124. Generally there is a superimposed low-grade bacterial infection which contributes to further destruction of local structures.

Systemic Disorders. A number of unrelated conditions may be associated with ulcerations, primarily of the leg. Among these are congestive heart failure with marked edema of the legs and feet, ulcerative colitis during periods of exacerbation of the disease, and hematologic disorders, such as pernicious anemia, sickle cell anemia (fig. 2/5b), chronic hemolytic anemia, cryoglobulinemia, and the dysproteinemias.

Ulcerations Secondary to Infection. Pyogenic infections may be responsible for the development of ulcerations of the lower limbs, especially pseudomonas organisms, frequently associated with immunologic deficiency. The type of lesion resulting from such etiologic agents is usually characterized by the formation of purulent exudate from which the causative organism can be cultured.

Pyoderma gangrenosum (Meleney bacterial ulceration) [3], which is generally found on the dorsum of the foot or in the pretibial area, is an unusual bacterial lesion due to the synergistic action of gram-positive streptococci and gram-negative bacilli (synergistic gangrene). Quite often the ulcerations are associated with debilitating diseases, such as ulcerative colitis.

The lesion first manifests itself as an erythematous papule, less than 0.5 cm in diameter, which becomes edematous and pustular and then develops into an ulcerative lesion within 48 h. The center becomes necrotic, the base appearing red and granular. A blue halo surrounds the lesion, and beyond it the skin is erythematous. There is rapid progression of the ulcer until it becomes quite large. Therapy consists of large doses of appropriate oral and parenteral antibacterial drugs, combined with local management and possibly the local and parenteral administration of corticotropins.

Currently ulcerations due to *Treponema pallidum* and the tubercle bacillus are rare. They occur over the pretibial area, generally are painless, and produce a moderate amount of serous exudate. In the case of the syphilitic lesion, darkfield illumination of smears taken from the ulcer bed usually reveals the classic spiral organism. In most instances the tuberculous ulcer is a small punched-out lesion with a hemorrhagic central area and an elevated edge.

Differential Diagnosis of Ischemic Gangrene

A number of other factors besides local impairment of arterial circulation may be responsible for the development of gangrene of the lower limbs.

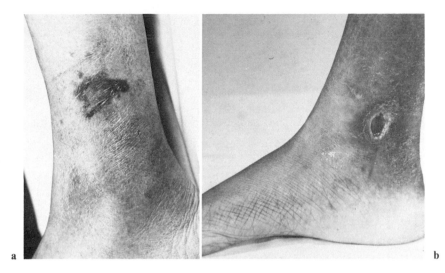

a   b

Fig. 2/5. Ulcerations of the leg. **a** Hypertensive ischemic ulcer. **b** Sickle cell anemia ulcer.

Drug Gangrene. Certain medications which can be given intravenously or intramuscularly with impunity will cause gangrene of the foot and leg if inadvertently or purposely (as by an addict) injected intra-arterially in the lower limb. Drugs which have elicited such a response are amphetamine sulfate (Benzedrine), amobarbital (Amytal), secobarbital, pentobarbital (Nembutal), merperidine hydrochloride (Demerol), chlorpromazine hydrochloride (Thorazine), promazine hydrochloride (Sparine), ether, hydroxyzine hydrochloride (Atarax), sodium thiopental (Pentothal Sodium), and propoxyphene hydrochloride (Darvon). When delivered to the tissues in high concentrations, these medications produce extensive necrosis of distal structures, the response occurring within minutes after completion of the intra-arterial injection. The basis for the rapid production of gangrene is unclear, although it has been suggested that a chemical inflammatory reaction is elicited in the capillary bed, the arterioles, and the small arteries, followed by rapid thrombosis, acute ischemia, and death of tissues. When the medications are given intravenously, there is thorough mixing and dilution of the material by the venous blood before it reaches the microcirculation. However, there are several drugs which, if even given intravenously, may cause necrosis of tissues, for example, continuous intravenous administration of norepinephrine (Levophed).

Such vasoconstrictor medications as ergotamine tartrate may produce gangrene of digits when given orally or by suppository (Cafergot) over a protracted period of time, generally in the management of migraine headaches. First, the pulses in the main arteries of the limbs disappear, followed by the onset of intermittent claudication, and then cyanotic mottling develops on the skin of the leg and foot, as well as elsewhere. If the medication is continued, the color changes become irreversible and gangrene forms. The basis for such changes is severe vascular spasm which eventually leads to widespread thrombosis of small arteries and of the microcirculation, followed by intense ischemia and necrosis of the skin and subcutaneous tissue. Discontinuation of the medication before this stage is reached will generally cause reversal of the pathologic process.

Gangrene Produced by Infectious Processes. Certain infectious diseases, such as meningococcic, staphylococcic, or streptococcic bacteremia, cholera, typhus fever, typhoid fever, pneumonia, and trichinosis, may be associated with thrombosis of digital arteries in the toes, resulting in gangrene of distal tissues (see fig. 5/5a). The etiologic agent may be exotoxins elaborated by the bacterial organisms which cause damage to the endothelium of the blood vessels and subsequently the development of thrombus occluding the artery. (For the production of gangrene by mechanical obstruction or compression of the vascular tree, see p. 338; for venous gangrene, see p. 261 and fig. 14/3b; for gangrene produced by congenital bands, see p. 369 and fig. 19/1c.)

References

1   Abramson, D.I.; Shumacker, H.B., Jr.: Raynaud's disease in men. Am. Heart J. *33:* 500 (1947).
2   Abramson, D.I.: Peripheral arterial vascular disorders; in Zimmerman, Levine, Physiologic principles of surgery; 2nd ed. (Saunders, Philadelphia 1964).
3   Meleney, F.L.: Clinical aspects and treatment of surgical infections (Saunders, Philadelphia 1949).
4   Martorell, F.: Hypertensive ulcer of the leg. J. cardiovasc. Surg. *19:* 599 (1978).

3 Clinical Assessment of the Arterial Distributional System in the Lower Limbs

In contrast to the study of the nutritional circulation (p. 22), the large proximal arteries supplying the vessels of the lower limbs and those located in these sites lend themselves readily to direct identification and examination. Hence, it is possible to obtain an accurate assessment of their state of patency by several simple clinical measurements. The following sections are devoted to this approach.

Palpation of Peripheral Arterial Pulses

Technique of Procedure

One of the most important steps in the study of the main arteries of the lower limbs is palpation of these vessels in order to determine the amplitude and force of pulsations in them. Every artery that lends itself to such an examination should be checked even though the abnormal vascular changes may appear to be limited to a single limb. Moreover, it is necessary to compare a vessel with the corresponding one on the opposite side. Only experience can determine what is a normal pulsation for any single artery.

Among the important steps in the study of arterial pulsations is the assumption of a comfortable position during the vascular survey, for, otherwise, the strain on the muscles of the body resulting from utilizing an improper stance may dull the perceptive senses of the examiner and lead to misleading interpretations of the results. Another cause for drawing improper conclusions is that when firm digital pressure is applied to the skin overlying an artery, the pulse in the fingers of the observer may become prominent to him or her and thus be mistaken for the one in the artery of the patient. The differentiation can readily be made by having the examiner count the beats aloud, while an assistant checks the rate and rhythm against a different pulse in the patient, preferably the corresponding one on the opposite side. Finally, the pressure applied to the skin should be varied, depending upon the known depth of the vessel. This step is especially important in the presence of weak pulsations, which may be obliterated and not perceived by the observer's fingers if strong persistent force is utilized in the examination.

For the lower limbs, it is necessary to palpate the following arteries: abdominal aorta and the external iliac, common femoral, popliteal, posterior tibial, and dorsal pedal. In the abdomen, the aorta can be palpated in the midline approximately at the level of the umbilicus; the external iliac artery is felt by applying deep palpation over the lower lateral aspect of the anterior abdominal wall. The remaining vessels, found in the lower extremity, the deep femoral, superficial femoral, anterior tibial (with the possible exception of its most distal segment), and peroneal arteries generally do not lend themselves to this type of examination because of their inaccessible location in deep tissues and so have to be studied by other means (p. 72).

Examination of Specific Vessels in the Lower Extremity. The *femoral artery* can be readily palpated in the groin below Poupart's ligament (fig. 3/1a), demonstrating the strongest pulsations of all the peripheral arteries. Because the *popliteal artery* is commonly found deeply placed in the fatty tissues within the diamond of the popliteal space, it is generally palpated with difficulty, unless the patient is turned on his abdomen and the leg being examined crossed over the back of the other to relax the tissues in the popliteal space (fig. 3/1b). Then the digits of the observer's other hand are placed over the examining fingers and used to apply sufficient pressure to make the pulsations in the vessel felt by the palpating digits. If, instead, the latter were performing the dual function of exerting force to compress the tissues and of determining whether pulsations were present, their perceptive sense would have been dulled.

In the foot, the *dorsal pedal artery,* a continuation of the anterior tibial artery, is usually felt in its course over the dorsum (fig. 3/2a), its position with respect to the bony landmarks being quite variable. In most instances, however, it lies somewhat medial to the midline. In each instance, the entire dorsal surface of the foot should be examined before concluding that the vessel is absent. The *posterior tibial artery* is generally palpated behind and beneath the medial malleolus (fig. 3/2b). To determine whether it is present, the examiner must stand on the same side of the patient as the vessel he is studying. To be in a position to palpate the vessels on both sides, it is therefore necessary for the bed or examination table to be so placed as to allow the observer to move to either side of it. In the case of the right posterior tibial artery, with the observer on the right side, the fingers of his

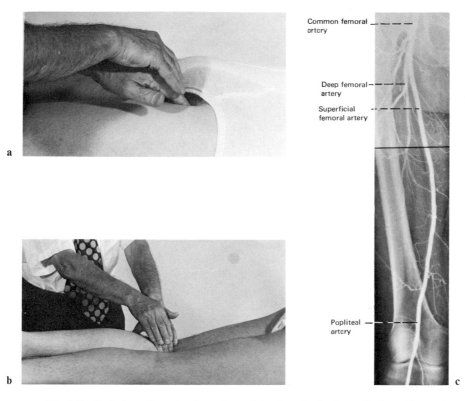

Fig. 3/1. Technique for palpation of arterial pulses in the lower limbs. **a** Femoral artery. **b** Popliteal artery. **c** Arteriographic representation of the location of the vessels. Modified from ref. [1]; reproduced with permission.

left hand are cupped over the medial malleolus so that the fingertips slide off to enter the groove below. At the same time, the foot is dorsiflexed and plantar flexed with the examiner's right hand. The latter maneuver places the vessel on stretch and then relaxes it, thus increasing the possibility of palpating it. Generally, firm pressure is necessary to feel the artery. In the case of the left posterior tibial artery, the left side of the patient and the right hand of the examiner are utilized, with the left hand being in position to dorsiflex and plantar flex the foot.

Search for Aberrant Arteries. Examination of the pulses should always include a step to seek aberrant or anomalous arteries, since their presence when pulsations are absent in main arteries of the limb markedly enhances the prognosis. For example, following slow occlusion of the popliteal artery, the lateral and medial genicular arteries may become prominent in their course over the knee. In some instances, in the absence of the posterior tibial artery at the ankle, a vessel may be palpated on the superior aspect of the lateral malleolus (fig. 3/2c), which is an enlarged perforating branch of the peroneal artery (lateral tarsal artery).

Interpretation of Results

Reductions in amplitude of pulsations or even their absence does not always have the same connotation. For example, the dorsal pedal artery is not present on one or both feet in from 6 to 18% of normal people [4]. When this vessel cannot be palpated, it is advisable to examine more proximally over the anterior surface of the ankle joint for the anterior tibial artery, of which it is a continuation. The posterior tibial artery is normally absent in only about 0.2% of cases. However, in some individuals, pulsations are not felt because of abnormal changes in overlying nonvascular tissues, such as pitting edema, induration and brawniness of the skin, and fatty pads located in the vicinity of the ankle (table 3/I). At times, also, the posterior tibial artery may be present but impalpable behind a prominent medial malleolus found in individuals with severely pronated feet demonstrating calcaneal eversion. Similarly, the popliteal artery may not be felt because of anatomic alterations in the popliteal space. Under such circumstances, pulsations in the dorsal pedal and posterior tibial arteries in the foot confirm the presence of a patent popliteal artery.

Also of importance to point out is that reduction in, or complete absence of, pulsations in an artery does not necessarily denote permanent organic local changes in the walls. For example, vasospasm (p. 36), which is reversible, can produce either effect, as do changes in nonvascular tissues overlying the arteries, including hypertrophy of voluntary muscles locally (table 3/I). Moreover, calcium deposits in the media of medium-sized blood vessels, as in Mönckeberg's sclerosis (p. 109), has a damping effect on pulsations in the involved artery, at the same time that this condition causes no interference with the movement of blood through the lumen of the vessel. Syndromes involving the large arteries in the abdomen and chest, such as coarctation of the aorta, dissecting aortic aneurysm, and slow occlusion of the aortic bifurcation (table 3/I), are responsible for absent pulses in the tibial arteries of the feet, without pathologic changes necessarily being found in the latter. Extrinsic pressure on the abdominal aorta or its main branches, as by tumors or other solid structures, will have a similar effect.

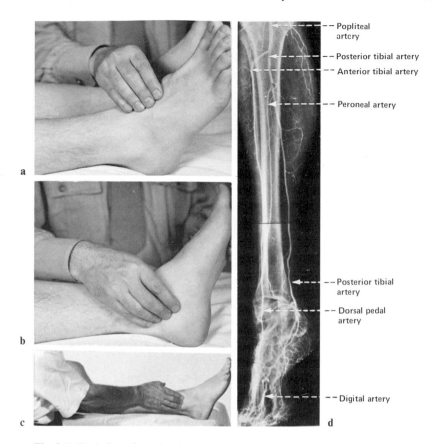

Fig. 3/2. Technique for palpation of arterial pulses in the feet. **a** Dorsal pedal artery. **b** Posterior tibial artery. **c** Penetrating branch of the peroneal artery (lateral tarsal branch). **d** Arteriographic representation of the location of the arteries in the leg and foot. Reproduced from ref. [2] with permission.

Finally, there are distant influences exerted by certain systemic conditions (table 3/I) which alter the amplitude of arterial pulsations in the lower limbs. Among the disorders which have such an effect, unrelated to any local changes in the vessels, are arterial hypertension and aortic insufficiency, which increase peripheral pulsations due to a widened pulse pressure, and aortic stenosis, shock, atrial fibrillation, constrictive pericarditis, pericardial effusion with tamponade, myocarditis, the terminal stage of congestive heart failure, and tachycardia, all of which depress or cause disappearance of the pulses, generally as a result of reduction in systolic output.

Table 3/I. Factors or states affecting amplitude of arterial pulsations in the lower limbs[1]

I Systemic conditions influencing peripheral pulses
   A Those decreasing amplitude of pulsations
      (1) Congestive heart failure
      (2) Rapid atrial fibrillation
      (3) Numerous premature contractions
      (4) Paroxysmal tachycardia
      (5) Aortic stenosis
      (6) Shock
      (7) Myocarditis
   B Those increasing amplitude of pulsations
      (1) Hyperthyroidism
      (2) Hypertension
      (3) Aortic insufficiency
      (4) Marked anemia
      (5) Fever
      (6) Physical exertion
      (7) Erythromelalgia

II Lesions in or extrinsic pressure on proximal segments of main arterial tree
    Those decreasing amplitude of pulsations
      (1) Coarctation of the aorta
      (2) Leriche's syndrome
      (3) Dissecting aneurysm of the aorta
      (4) Tumors in abdominal cavity compressing arteries

III Local nonvascular changes
   A Those decreasing amplitude of pulsations
      (1) Normal increases in thickness of skin overlying arteries
      (2) Hypertrophy of muscles overlying arteries
      (3) Presence of local fatty pads
      (4) Lipedema
      (5) Induration and brawniness of the skin overlying the artery
      (6) Pitting and nonpitting edema
      (7) General obesity
   B Those increasing amplitude of pulsations
      (1) Local inflammation (acute cellulitis, erysipelas)

IV Local vascular changes
   A Those increasing amplitude of pulsations by removal of normal or
     exaggerated vasomotor tone (vasospasm)
      (1) Lumbar sympathectomy
      (2) Early stage of frostbite
      (3) Early stage of major causalgia and post-traumatic vasomotor disorders
      (4) Paget's disease of bone

Table 3/I (continued)

B	Those decreasing amplitude of pulsations or producing absence of pulsations
	(1) Vasospasm (resulting from exposure to cold, Raynaud's disease, acrocyanosis, livedo reticularis, later stages of frostbite, causalgia, post-traumatic vasomotor disorders, disuse atrophy)
	(2) Chronic occlusive arterial disorders affecting large arteries (arteriosclerosis obliterans, thromboangiitis obliterans)
	(3) Acute occlusion of large arteries (arterial embolism, rapid arterial thrombosis)
	(4) Organic occlusion of small arteries (diabetes, hypertension, rheumatoid arthritis and other connective tissue disorders)
	(5) Proximal congenital or acquired arteriovenous fistula
	(6) Mönckeberg's sclerosis
	(7) Trauma to large arteries (contusion, laceration, thrombosis)

[1] Since oscillometry is dependent upon the amplitude of the arterial pulsations, the readings obtained with this instrument are influenced in a similar manner by the various factors or states listed here.

Bounding peripheral pulsations may follow removal of normal or abnormal vasomotor tone, as by lumbar paravertebral sympathetic blocks or sympathectomy, provided extensive organic occlusive disease is not present locally.

Auscultation of Peripheral Arteries and Scars

Examination by auscultation of arteries supplying, or located in, the lower limbs is an essential routine step in determining the state of blood flow through them. By so doing, sites of partial occlusion (stenosis) can readily be recognized.

Pathogenesis of Bruits

When normal movement of blood is interfered with because of the presence of a segmental partial obstruction in a large artery, locally turbulent nonlaminar flow is produced. This type of disturbance is responsible for the development of high-frequency vibratory energy appreciated by the ear, through the use of a stethoscope, as a bruit or murmur. Such a sound is heard only when there is a pressure drop, and hence a pressure gradient, across the partially occluded portion of the artery. The resulting disturbance varies both with the degree of stenosis and the rate of movement of blood through the narrowed portion of the vessel. It is therefore clear that complete obstruction, and hence total cessation of blood flow locally, eliminates bruits at or below the point of occlusion. Similarly, over a main artery with normal lumen size throughout, no high-frequency vibrations will be set up by the unimpeded flow of blood and so again no bruits will be heard.

With varying degrees of block, the intensity and duration of the bruit will be altered. For example, under resting conditions, a slight stenosis in a main artery introduces no significant impedance to blood flow and therefore only a negligible pressure drop across the involved segment; as a consequence, no sound produced by the movement of the blood is heard under such circumstances. However, if the patient is now exercised, resulting in an augmentation of circulation through the stenotic segment of the artery, a sound may become audible. With a greater degree of partial occlusion, the blood stream must accelerate in its passage through the involved portion and hence acoustic vibrations will be heard even when the patient is resting. Under such conditions, the bruit exhibits a crescendo in intensity during the early part of systole and a decrescendo during the latter part. The more extreme the stenosis, the louder and harsher does the sound become. At the same time, its duration is lengthened, so that with a severe degree of partial occlusion, the bruit may extend into early diastole. From such findings, it can also be assumed that an inadequate collateral circulation exists distally, with most of the blood flow having to pass through the highly stenotic main vessel. On the other hand, if an adequate secondary system exists, a significant portion of the local circulation will be diverted along this pathway, with much less passing through the involved channel. As a consequence, the bruit produced by the stenosis in the latter vessel becomes definitely reduced in intensity.

Location of Bruits

Over the anterior abdominal wall, bruits can be heard at a point corresponding to the location of the aortic bifurcation (centrally between lower rib margin and the umbilicus) and, laterally, over the common and external iliac arteries. In the lower limb, they may be audible in the groin over the common femoral artery and, less frequently, in the popliteal space over the popliteal artery. In examining for bruits, the diaphragm or the bell of the stethoscope should be placed in contact with the skin overlying the vessel under study, using the least amount of compression to make the abnormal sound audible to the ear.

Interpretation of Results

Certain precautions must be taken in interpreting the auscultatory findings. First it must be kept in mind that bruits may be transmitted in a distal direction from the site of narrowing, provided the vessel below is patent. Hence, it does not necessarily follow that the presence of a murmur over an artery always indicates that the stenosis is located immediately beneath the site being examined. Also, it is necessary to point out that bruits over vessels are not produced solely by narrowing, for an arterial aneurysm and an acquired arteriovenous fistula (pp. 309, 310) are both associated with the same type of acoustic phenomenon. If the lumen of the vessel under examination is distorted by too much pressure applied to the overlying skin by the bell or diaphragm of the stethoscope, iatrogenic bruits will be elicited. It is likewise important to remember that the less interposed nonvascular damping tissue present over the vessel, the better the conductance of the sound and hence the more likely its intensity to reach audible levels. Finally, it must be pointed out that the presence of a bruit over an artery cannot always be interpreted as indicative of clinically significant stenosis or of other abnormal states [3, 5].

Examination of Scars

Auscultation should also be routinely used in the examination of old or recent scars in the vicinity of arteries, to determine whether the original trauma had at the same time caused vascular injury, with the production of a false arterial aneurysm (recognized by the presence of a systolic bruit) or an arteriovenous fistula (identified by a continuous murmur with systolic accentuation). Examination of injured soft tissue masses should also be performed in order to determine whether bruits exist, especially if the trauma was caused by a high-velocity missile.

*Evaluation of Data Derived from Combined Auscultation and
Palpation of Arteries*

Valuable conclusions can be reached by comparing the results obtained by auscultation with the data collected from palpation of peripheral pulses. For example, the presence of a bruit heard over the external iliac artery in the lower portion of the abdomen, when associated with a reduced pulsation in the femoral artery in the groin, probably indicates a stenosis of the former vessel. If the absence of bruits over the lower part of the abdomen is associated with no pulsations in the femoral artery in the groin, this may mean either that the external iliac artery is completely occluded or that it is wide open but that the common femoral artery is blocked. Of course, such information is available only if the abdominal wall is relatively thin. Otherwise, absence of bruits may merely mean poor or no conduction of the sound through a thick layer of subcutaneous fat.

Oscillometry

General Considerations

Oscillometry is another approach which gives pertinent information regarding the state of circulation through the main arteries in the lower limbs. *Unfortunately, it has not received the clinical applicability that it rightfully deserves.* In fact, it has been practically discarded by the podiatric profession and without good reason, as will be demonstrated below. The instrument is relatively inexpensive as judged by the cost of other diagnostic procedures and it is simple to operate, requiring no specialized technical expertise. Hence, it should be routinely used in office and hospital practice.

The apparatus consists of a sensitive aneroid capsule capable of recording small volume changes which are magnified and noted on an arbitrary degree scale of the instrument. A number of oscillometers are available commercially, being manufactured by the Boulitte Co., the UMA Inc., the P. Propper Manufacturing Co., Inc., and the W.M. Welch Scientific Co., among others.

Physiologic Basis for Procedure

The principle upon which the clinical use of the method is based is the fact that with each cardiac systole, there is a sudden thrust of blood into the peripheral arteries, this momentarily causing an increase in the volume of the limb. The oscillometer is capable of recording such a change, the magnitude of the response being a reflection of the amount of blood transiently filling the main arteries. It follows that if the lumens of the vessels in the limb are pathologically reduced in size, the readings obtained by oscillometry will be correspondingly decreased. No movement of blood into an artery completely occluded by clot or atherosclerotic plaques will result in a zero oscillometric reading. It is necessary to point out that the instrument is not sensitive enough to be influenced by the pulsatile alterations occurring in collateral arterial beds because of the small-calibered vessels generally making up such compensatory systems. Thus, the information that is obtained is a qualitative and indirect index of the rate of blood flow only through main arteries.

Technique of Procedure

Steps in Collection of Readings. A modified pneumatic cuff is carefully and snugly wrapped around each of three levels on the lower limb: the thigh above the knee, the maximal circumference of the calf, and the leg above the ankle. Air pressure is introduced into the system to a level approximately above the systolic blood pressure, using a blood pressure bulb, and then lowered in steps of 10 mm Hg by means of an escape valve. Following each drop, the pneumatic cuff is connected to the recording aneroid capsule and the range of movement of the recording needle is noted. The important reading is the one indicating the greatest excursion of the needle, the height of pressure in the pneumatic cuff at which this occurs appearing to have little clinical significance. In fact, the pressure in the system merely acts as a coupling agent for transmission of the limb volume changes to the recording aneroid.

Determination of a Reference Point. Since oscillometric readings are affected by the magnitude of pulse pressure of the blood, systemic disorders, as well as local vascular pathologic changes, can influence them. For example, hypertension and aortic insufficiency are associated with high oscillometric readings, whereas aortic stenosis, tachycardia, shock state, and atrial fibrillation have the opposite effect. For this reason, it is necessary to obtain a reference reading from an arm above the elbow, provided that there are no abnormalities of the circulation in the upper limbs. The figure thus obtained can be considered to reflect purely systemic changes; hence, those from the thigh and upper portion of the leg should be the same if the blood flow in them is normal. If, instead, the figures from the lower limbs are significantly less, then it can be assumed that the difference is due to local pathology in the main arteries traversing these segments of limb or in the large vessels supplying them.

Range of Readings. The normal figures have a wide range: 5–15 arbitrary units or higher for the thigh above the knee and for the leg at the level of the calf, and 3–8 units or higher for the leg above the ankle. The figures for corresponding sites on both lower limbs should normally be approximately the same.

Steps for Collection of Significant Data. Certain precautions must be taken in order to obtain accurate and reproducible results. Room temperature should be physiologic (70–75 °F; 21–24 °C). The patient should be relaxed and in a supine position on the examining table, and the same type machine and, if possible, the same instrument should be used on the patient at all times. If such measures are taken, it is possible to determine whether there has been progression of the occlusive process in the intervals between routine examinations by observing whether the readings are becoming smaller at specific sites or remaining stationary.

Pertinent Information Derived from the Procedure

Oscillometry is a very valuable diagnostic tool in regard to a number of aspects of occlusive arterial disorders. First, it helps determine whether an obstruction of a main channel exists and, if present, grossly the site of the difficulty, thus enlarging upon the information derived from palpation of pulses alone. For example, if normal pulsations are present in the femoral artery in the groin and no bruits are heard over this vessel, it can be assumed that an oscillometric reading of zero obtained from the thigh above the knee indicates that the superficial femoral artery is completely obstructed as it passes through the adductor canal. Such reasoning is based on the fact that the oscillometric reading obtained from the thigh just above the knee reflects almost completely the pulsatile blood flow through the superficial femoral artery, for the hemodynamic changes in the numerous small branches of the deep femoral artery located at this level do not materially influence the results. Further convincing evidence on this point can be collected by obtaining an oscillometric reading as high up on the thigh as possible, so that the pneumatic cuff now encompasses the common femoral and the upper segments of the superficial and deep femoral arteries. A fairly normal reading from this level would support the impression that when a zero reading is obtained from the segment of thigh immediately above the knee, the block is limited to the distal segment of the superficial femoral artery.

A normal reading at the level of the thigh above the knee, combined with a zero figure for the calf level, indicates that the popliteal artery is completely occluded, with or without obstruction of the origin of the tibial vessels. If a normal reading is obtained from the level of the calf and a zero figure from the leg above the ankle, the assumption is that the anterior and posterior tibial arteries are completely occluded at some site or sites in their course down the leg.

Precautions in Interpretation of Results

Certain conditions may result in the collection of misleading data and others contraindicate the use of oscillometry. For example, the presence of edema of the thigh and leg may damp the readings, causing lower than normal figures to be recorded (table 3/I). Under such circumstances, it is necessary to apply the cuff in the usual fashion and raise the pressure in it to above the systolic level, maintaining it for several minutes. This will drive the fluid out of the segment of limb being compressed, thus loosening the cuff. The latter is then reapplied snugly, thus allowing for the collection of accurate oscillometric readings. In the presence of induration and brawniness of the skin of the leg, however, no maneuver is available to counteract the damping effect of such changes in skin consistency. Allowing the room temperature to fall below a physiologic level will initiate a degree of vasospasm and hence result in lower than normal readings. Fever will have the opposite effect (table 3/I). If phlebothrombosis (p. 257) is suspected as being present in the venous plexus of the calf, it is inadvisable to attempt an oscillometric reading at this level because of the possibility of dislodging a clot by the compression of the tissues by the cuff. A similar precaution should be taken when foreign bodies, like shell fragments (shrapnel), are embedded in the tissues ordinarily subjected to oscillometry.

Evaluation of Procedure

In summary, it can be stated that oscillometry is a simple and inexpensive noninvasive procedure which generally supplies pertinent information regarding the presence or absence of chronic or acute occlusive arterial disorders affecting the main arteries of the lower limbs. Moreover, it is very useful in grossly localizing the site of obstruction and, through repeated testing at intervals, information is gained as to whether progression of the obliterative process is occurring. However, it is of no value in determining whether collateral circulation is developing in response to the resulting ischemia, and it is not useful in arriving at a proper conclusion regarding the prognosis of a limb. Also, it is necessary to repeat that a diminution in readings can be caused by vasospasm, as well as by organic arterial diseases (table 3/I). However, the differentiation can readily be made by removing vasomotor tone through one of the clinical measures available for such a purpose; this immediately produces a rise in oscillometric readings to a normal level if the original low figures were due to vasospasm, while eliciting only a slight increase in the presence of permanent changes in the vessel wall. Finally, oscillometry does not help in making an exact diagnosis of a specific disorder, but it does act as an adjunctive procedure in determining whether or not a partial or complete obstruction to blood flow exists in the main arteries of the lower limbs, thus substantiating and enlarging upon the information derived from palpation of peripheral pulses. With it, a readily reproducible record is available, which is expressed quantitatively, in contrast to the purely qualitative and subjective appraisal that results from palpation of an artery. Moreover, the procedure is of value in ascertaining mild degrees of impairment of arterial inflow, not reflected in sufficient reduction in amplitude of pulsations to be obvious by palpation of the vessels. In many respects, the information derived from oscillometry is similar to that obtained by the Doppler ultrasonic flowmeter (p. 65).

Other Clinical Tests of Arterial Patency

Venous Filling Time

Information regarding the state of the main arteries can also be derived from a study of the rate of filling of the superficial veins on the dorsum of the foot after the limb has been elevated for several minutes to drain blood out of the venous tree and then placed in dependency. Normally the superficial veins fill with blood and become visible within 10 s (venous filling time). Delays beyond this period are due to interference with movement of blood primarily through the arterial tree and hence into the venous system. The coexistence of varicosities negates the value of the test since, under such circumstances, the superficial veins will immediately fill with blood on assumption of the dependent position because of regurgitant flow from incompetent proximal vessels.

Return of Color Time

The rate of return of color to the skin of the foot on placing the previously elevated lower limb in dependency is a reflection of the rapidity of blood flow through the main arteries, as well as an indicator of the state of cutaneous microcirculation (p. 26). In the normal limb, the pink color, which was maintained in the elevated position, persists or deepens as the foot remains in dependency. In the case of the patient with arterial insufficiency, who previously demonstrated pallor of the foot in the elevated position, there may be a delay beyond the normal limit of 10 s to as much as 45–60 s or more before the color reappears (return of color time). Moreover, the change is not uniform, but instead the return of the pink color takes the form of an irregular and patchy discoloration. It can be assumed that the greater the delay in return of color to the foot, the more marked the atherosclerotic process in the main arterial tree. As in the case of the venous filling time (p. 62), the test is of no diagnostic value if primary varicosities coexist.

References

1   Abramson, D.I.: Vascular disorders of the extremities (Harper & Row, Hagerstown 1974).
2   Abramson, D.I.; Miller, D.S.: Vascular problems in musculoskeletal disorders of the limbs (Springer, Berlin 1981).
3   Ratschow, M.: Importance of phonoangiography for the evaluation of arterial stenosis. Angiology *13:* 290 (1962).
4   Silverman, J.J.: Incidence of palpable dorsalis pedis and posterior tibial pulsations in soldiers: an analysis of over 1,000 infantry soldiers. Am. Heart J. *32:* 82 (1946).
5   Stead, E.A., Jr.; Greenfield, J.C., Jr.: Pressures and pulses. Physiol. Physns *2:* 1 (1964).

4 Laboratory Assessment of the Arterial Circulation in the Lower Limbs

In recent years a large number of noninvasive and invasive laboratory procedures have been developed for the purpose of assessing the arterial circulation in the lower limbs. Some are carried out with no discomfort to the patient, whereas others may be associated with serious untoward responses and complications. All are costly, thus significantly adding to already spiralling medical expenses. Moreover, in every instance, they require either the use of outpatient laboratory facilities or a hospital environment. Several have important but limited application, whereas others are time-consuming and frequently unnecessary. However, because of the popularity that some of these diagnostic procedures enjoy, it is deemed necessary to devote this chapter to a discussion of the common methods, the principles on which they operate, the importance of the information derived from their application, and any untoward responses and complications that might follow their use.

Noninvasive Vascular Diagnostic Laboratory Procedures

Role of the Noninvasive Vascular Diagnostic Laboratory
Currently noninvasive vascular diagnostic laboratories are available in most general hospitals and even in private facilities. More and more reliance is being placed upon them, their prevalence and popularity being a reflection of the insecurity from which both podiatrists and physicians appear to suffer in regard to their ability to make a correct clinical diagnosis of arterial insufficiency in the lower limbs of their patients or conclusively to rule out such a possibility. It is realized, of course, that the increase in incidence of malpractice suits also plays a role in this respect.

The data derived from a session in a noninvasive diagnostic laboratory, for the most part, confirm and document the results already collected by a careful clinical vascular examination of the lower limbs. In addition, at times, pertinent information may be obtained which is helpful in arriving at a more comprehensive assessment of the state of local arterial circulation.

However, the common practice of having the patient routinely visit a noninvasive laboratory at 3- or 4-month intervals, in order to determine whether any progression of the occlusive arterial process is occurring, has no firm basis of support and should be discarded. Adequate data of this sort can readily be collected by clinical means alone.

Another point which must be considered is that noninvasive vascular testing has great potential for the collection of improper data by laboratory technicians who are not always as meticulous and skilled as the procedures require. It is necessary to point out that such an approach does not fall into the category of routine laboratory measures, as for example, obtaining an electrocardiogram, which from the technical point of view is practically foolproof. Interpretation of the results by the physician is based on the assumption that the records are valid and correctly collected, which may not necessarily always be true. The current rapid expansion in noninvasive laboratories has produced the need for a large number of well-trained operators, but at the moment such a demand cannot be satisfactorily met. As a consequence, the quality of the data originating from some of the facilities, particularly the privately run ones, has deteriorated and this may lead to loss of trust in all of them.

In conclusion, it can unequivocally be stated that a noninvasive vascular diagnostic laboratory should not at any time supplant the need for a thorough history and selective physical examination (see chapters 1–3). While the results collected by such a facility are generally accurate, the laboratory is not an essential ingredient in the diagnostic armamentarium [1]. Moreover, dependence upon data obtained in this manner, rather than on the basis of patient evaluation, may contribute to a reduction in diagnostic skills and acumen of the neophyte in the field.

Doppler Ultrasonic Flowmeter

The Doppler ultrasonic flowmeter is by far the most commonly utilized instrument in most noninvasive vascular laboratories. In fact, in some facilities it is the sole approach to the measurement of flow velocity in major arteries in the lower limbs. One of its advantages is that the desired information can be obtained at the bedside without the need to use an expensive recording system.

Basis for Test. The principle on which the method is derived is the Doppler phenomenon, namely that sound reflected from a moving object undergoes a shift in frequency which is proportional to the velocity of the object. The instruments available commercially all consist of a probe containing two piezoelectric crystals (transducers). One of these is driven by an electronic oscillation and projects a 2- to 10-MHz ultrasonic beam (at a frequency in the range of 9 MHz) which is directed transcutaneously through the overlying tissues to the artery under study. The moving cells in the blood cause the ultrasonic beam to be back-scattered and reflected back to the other crystal in the probe, but at a different frequency. By appropriate filtering, a third signal is produced, equal to the difference between the entry and the projected frequencies. This is then converted to an audible signal which is heard through a loudspeaker or headphones, and the response is recorded visually on a chart. The instrument is thus able to identify changes in velocity of flow pattern, the rate of blood flow being proportional to the difference between the two frequencies. With additional electronic circuitry, it is possible also to determine the direction of blood flow (directional Doppler flow velocity meter).

Technique. The test consists of placing the Doppler probe on the skin directly over the location of an artery and studying the character of the sound. In order to facilitate conduction of the signals, a water-soluble gel is placed between the probe and the skin. In some instances, besides the collection of data under resting conditions, other sets of readings are obtained after a period of exercise on the treadmill or following 5 min of arterial occlusion in the limb under examination, in order to study the effect of physical stress on the local vascular tree.

Application of Method to the Study of Local Arterial Circulation. Examination of a normal artery with the Doppler ultrasonic flowmeter reveals the presence of a multiphasic sound, consisting of a high-pitched hissing sound heard during systole and one or two short, medium-pitched sounds, during diastole. All sounds become higher-pitched if there is an increase in blood velocity.

As the probe is passed over the skin overlying a stenosed artery, the intensity of the sound tends to become greater, the increase in pitch being due to the accelerated velocity of the blood passing through the narrowed segment of vessel. In the case of a total occlusion, the sound, which has been increasing in intensity as the obstruction is approached, disappears at the level of the lesion and beyond it. In areas where flow is dependent solely on movement of blood through collateral arteries, the probe generally detects a sound which has a blunted and dull quality, as compared with the sharp, clear-cut sound heard over a normal vessel. It is necessary to point out, however, that the ultrasonic flowmeter gives no pertinent information regarding the volume of blood passing through the artery under study per unit of time.

Application of Method to the Study of Blood Pressure in Feet. The ultrasonic flowmeter can also be used in determining the height of systolic blood pressure in distal vessels, such as the posterior tibial and dorsal pedal arteries in the ankle and foot. The data are collected in the following manner: A blood pressure cuff is wrapped around the middle or upper part of the leg and the probe, being used as a stethoscope, is positioned either over the usual site for the posterior tibial artery, just distal to the internal malleolus, or over the dorsal pedal artery on the dorsum of the foot. Then the pressure in the blood pressure cuff is raised to above systolic level and dropped in a stepwise fashion until a sound is heard over the vessel. The level at which this first occurs is read off the blood pressure manometer, being considered to be the systolic pressure in the vessel. In normal individuals, resting ankle blood pressure is approximately the same as that in the brachial artery in the arm. In the case of a partial block in the artery feeding the vessel under study or in the vessel itself, the local blood pressure will fall significantly, the degree of change depending upon the severity of the occlusion. Hence, an 'ischemic index' can be derived through the ratio of the brachial arterial pressure to the tibial arterial pressure.

In the presence of equivocal results, the patient is instructed to walk on a treadmill for a specific period of time, and then the data obtained immediately after termination of exercise are compared with the control readings collected before the physical work was begun. Another set of figures is collected 10–25 min in the postexercise period. In patients with either no or minor atheromatous changes, physical exertion in general produces an increase in ankle blood pressure, a reflection of the rise in systemic blood pressure elicited by the work. In the presence of a significant degree of stenosis of the artery under study or of complete occlusion of the vessel supplying it, exercise causes an immediate moderate reduction in ankle blood pressure and a return to the control level in 5 min. Such a response, however, is noted only when there is a highly developed collateral circulation and adequate outflow. If there is a less efficient secondary circulation, as well as involvement of the external iliac or common femoral artery, ankle blood pressure may fall to zero after exercise, to return to the control level within 7–15 min. Further progression of the atherosclerotic process, associated with poor development of a collateral circulation, also causes a fall in ankle blood pressure to zero following exercise, but with the readings returning to the resting level only after a delay of 15–22 min.

Summary and Evaluation. The Doppler ultrasonic flowmeter is helpful in determining whether an occlusive arterial disorder exists in the lower limbs and in detecting the sites of partial or complete obstruction. In these regards, the instrument appears to elicit practically the same type of information derived from the use of the much less complicated and less costly oscillometer (p. 58). It is also useful in obtaining the height of systolic blood pressure at the level of the ankle, information of great importance in determining the proper therapeutic course to follow when an uncontrolled ulcer or gangrene exists on the toes or foot proper (p. 182) [3]. However, there is a possibility for error when using the method in the study of a lower limb of a diabetic suffering from peripheral neuropathy. Under such conditions, vascular calcification or increased arterial stiffness is frequently found in the arterial tree of the foot, a change which may result in falsely elevated readings. Hence, eliciting a high ankle blood pressure in such a case does not necessarily exclude the possibility of an obstructive lesion in the main arteries.

It is necessary to point out that the Doppler ultrasonic flowmeter cannot replace contrast angiography (p. 73) for the collection of pertinent technical information preliminary to a reconstructive vascular procedure. Moreover, because the instrument is extremely sensitive, an audible signal is not always equivalent to a palpable arterial pulse; nor does it represent an amplified bruit (p. 55).

Three major limitations have been found with regard to the application of the Doppler ultrasonic flowmeter to clinical practice [2]. First, the ultrasonic beam is unable to penetrate atherosclerotic plaques reliably and, second, the scans are time-consuming to perform. Finally, the images include motion artifacts because the systems are not real time. For the latter reason, a real-time echo system has been proposed [2].

Skin Temperature Changes following Removal of Vasomotor Tone
Aims. Since a reduction in local cutaneous blood flow results from excessive vasomotor tone (vasospasm) (p. 36), and since the latter process is reversible and hence amenable to management, it becomes of paramount

importance to ascertain at an early stage to what extent this state is responsible for the presence of an abnormal clinical picture suggestive of arterial insufficiency. Such information becomes available by temporarily removing vasomotor tone (as outlined below) and determining the resulting rise in cutaneous temperature. The assumption is made that the observed change in skin temperature is a reflection of the augmentation in cutaneous blood flow that follows passive dilatation of skin vessels on removal of normal or exaggerated vasomotor tone.

Technique. The limb under study is exposed to a constant, physiologic environmental temperature for at least 30 min, with drafts eliminated. Then control skin temperature readings are collected from the toes, the dorsum of the foot, and several levels on the leg, using either a thermistor, some type of electromotive thermocouple, or, if neither is available, a modified mercury thermometer with a flat, widened recording surface. When the figures become constant, vasomotor tone is inhibited by means of one of several clinical procedures. Among these are procaine blocking of the lumbar paravertebral sympathetic ganglia; reflex or indirect vasodilatation (p. 200); block of sympathetic nerves by spinal or caudal anesthesia, and anesthetization of the posterior tibial nerve, in its location behind and below the medial malleolus, with a 1% procaine solution.

Within 15 min after a successful block of vasoconstrictor impulses, the skin temperature readings in the feet of normal persons begin to rise from a level around 25 °C (77 °F) to at least 30 °C (86 °F) and generally to between 31.1 and 35 °C (between 88 and 95 °F). In the patient with excessive sympathetic activity, there will be a maximum rise to approximately the same level as that observed in the normal person. The only difference between the two types of responses is that the magnitude of the increase will be much greater because of the considerably lower pretest reading of about 20 °C (68 °F) generally found in the individual manifesting vasospasm. If the existing impaired circulation is due solely to an organic occlusive arterial disorder, removal of vasomotor tone generally results in a rise to only 26.7 or 27.8 °C (to 80 or 82 °F) but not higher, since the permanent structural obstruction in the involved vessels prevents a normal arterial inflow even after removal of vasomotor tone.

Evaluation of Procedure. Although the method of temporarily blocking sympathetic vasoconstrictor impulses and studying the skin temperature rise is very helpful in differentiating a primarily organic arterial disorder from a vasospastic entity, it is of no use in assessing the state of the circulation in the underlying muscle. The reason is that removal of vasomotor tone has little if any effect on blood flow in this tissue.

Graphic Representation of Pulse Waves

The study of the contour and amplitude of the recorded pulse wave is helpful in determining the state of local circulation in various segments of the lower limb, including the toes. To collect the data, a number of instruments are commercially available. These consist of a simplified strain-gauge plethysmograph, an impedance plethysmograph, a recording oscillometer, and a pneumatic cuff connected to a transducing system, among others. The strain-gauge plethysmograph and the impedance plethysmograph (rheograph) have had the widest clinical application in the study of the pulse wave.

Method for Collection of Data. The strain-gauge plethysmograph consists of a sealed strand of silicone (or of a piece of latex tubing) filled with mercury or electrically conductive alloy of gallium and indium. The instrument provides a simple and reliable method for sensing and recording transient percentage changes in limb or toe volume, as reflected in alterations in circumference of the part under study occurring during a cardiac cycle. The data are collected by encircling a segment of limb with the strand of silicone or latex tubing. As the instrument is stretched by an increase in limb volume, the electric pathway through the enclosed conductive material becomes lengthened and thinner, thus causing a rise in electric resistance of the gauge. By formula, the percentage increase in electric resistance is found to be proportional to that of limb volume at the level being examined. The variable resistance of the conductive column in the tubing is arranged to form one side of a Wheatstone bridge, the latter being coupled to an alternating-current bridge circuit to permit vacuum-tube amplification of the resistance change. The resulting response is charted on a recorder in the form of a pulse wave.

The *impedance rheograph* utilizes a different principle from that described for the strain-gauge plethysmograph (see above). Since the method is based on alterations in peripheral resistance of the various contents of the limb, including blood, a better name for the apparatus is impedance rheograph rather than impedance plethysmograph, which implies that changes in limb volume are being measured. The technique consists of the application of 4 limb electrodes, by means of which a high-frequency, low-current signal is passed through the tissues locally. Variations in the volume of blood in the limb cause corresponding changes in electric impedance, thus producing an analog signal which is directly related to the volume of the segment of extremity at the moment the tracing is recorded. As in the case of the strain-gauge plethysmograph, the impedance rheograph is able to detect or analyze simple waveforms at the bedside.

Analysis of Various Types of Pulse Waves. A recorded arterial pulse wave obtained from a normal lower limb consists of the following components: a rapidly rising upstroke (anacrotic limb), with a sharply rounded peak occurring early in cardiac systole, and a downstroke (catacrotic limb), which is concave upward and contains a dicrotic notch.

In the presence of chronic occlusive arterial diseases, certain changes occur in the contour and amplitude of the pulse wave. In the early stage, the anacrotic limb ascends more slowly than normally and demonstrates a reduction in amplitude, with a rounding of the peak. The catacrotic limb manifests a slow descent and a shallow dicrotic notch. With progression of the obstructive process, further rounding of the peak occurs, even to the point of becoming saw-toothed or umbrella-shaped. At the same time, there is slow development of the entire curve. Severe stenosis of the artery results in the loss of the dicrotic notch, and far-advanced disease may cause complete absence of the pulse wave. It is necessary to mention that in the presence of a short segmental occlusion, good collateral flow, and absence of disease in distal small arteries, the pulse wave curve may be normal in all respects. When an inadequate secondary circulation exists, the first portion of the curve becomes flattened.

At times it may be necessary to place a load on the local vascular tree to bring out abnormalities in the pulse wave not present under resting conditions. This may be accomplished by applying an arterial occlusion pressure, using a pneumatic cuff, to a proximal segment of limb for 3–8 min and then releasing it and immediately recording a pulse wave. In both normal individuals and in patients with a chronic occlusive arterial disorder, initially there is disappearance of the dicrotic notch. However, this reappears in a very short time in the normal person (1–8 s), whereas in the individual with local arterial insufficiency, there is a significant delay (9–300 s), with the magnitude of the control peak not being reached until 2–3 min after release of the arterial occlusion pressure.

In the presence of a vasospastic disorder or of vasospasm associated with other difficulties, the pulse wave record may demonstrate large slow deflections which are probably due to rhythmic alterations in vasomotor activity. The existence of an active reflex initiated by deep inspiration may also be noted, the change probably being caused by vasoconstriction of small arteries and arterioles. Following a period of arterial occlusion, in contrast to the response observed in patients with chronic occlusive disease (see above), the pulse record approaches that of the normal individual obtained under similar circumstances.

Invasive Vascular Diagnostic Laboratory Procedures

Contrast Angiography

Radiographic visualization of the arterial tree in the lower limbs by means of the intra-arterial injection of radiopaque contrast material is an invasive technique which provides detailed anatomic information of the larger arteries. Since it is not infrequently associated with untoward responses and, at times, even serious complications (p. 74), it has no role either as solely a diagnostic procedure or as a means of determining whether progression of the occlusive process is occurring in the main arteries of the lower limbs, information on both points being readily collected using clinical means. (For indications for angiography, see p. 73.)

Technique. Since angiography of the lower limbs is routinely performed either by the radiologist or by the vascular surgeon in a hospital setting, no attempt will be made to describe the method except in a general way, only stressing principles involved.

Most of the currently available contrast media, if properly administered, are quite safe and produce very few side reactions. Among those commonly used are different concentrations of Hypaque-M, Hypaque Sodium, Renografin-76 and -60, and Angio-Conray. All are iodine compounds which have a low toxicity and are readily excreted by the kidneys. The basis for their application in arteriography is that they absorb the X-ray beam to a greater or lesser degree than do the surrounding tissues, with the result that the arterial tree is visualized on the exposed film following their intra-arterial injection. Since the intensity of opacification will depend upon the concentration of the contrast media in the blood, as a general rule, the injection is made as close to the area under study as possible. In the unanesthetized patient, the administration of the radiopaque medium usually elicits unpleasant symptoms, such as a hot, burning sensation that travels down the limb into the foot. At times, the response may be so severe that he will not give permission for a second trial, even if the need is essential for a proper therapeutic approach, unless promised that a general anesthetic will be given beforehand. The cause of the symptoms is not entirely clear, although it may be related to transient ischemia of tissues, this despite the fact that contrast media have been found to have a vasodilating effect when studied on laboratory animals.

Angiography for the abdominal arteries and the arterial tree in the lower limbs consists of: *translumbar aortography,* a blind procedure in which the contrast medium is directly injected into the abdominal aorta at the level of the lumbar region of the spine, and *arteriography,* in which the femoral arteries in the groin are entered. There are several other routes which are used only occasionally. *Pedal angiography,* which is helpful in visualizing the tibial arteries at the ankle and the digital vessels (fig. 4/1), requires some modification of the technique used in conventional arteriography. One approach involves passage of a small catheter introduced into the common femoral artery into the distal segment of the popliteal artery and delivering the bolus from this point. Another consists of performing femoral arteriography under sodium thiopental (Pentothal Sodium) anesthesia. Preliminary production of reactive hyperemia by the application of an arterial occlusion pressure for 5 min and the initial intra-arterial injection of tolazoline hydrochloride (Priscoline) will also help visualize the arterial tree in the feet.

Role of Angiography as a Diagnostic Procedure. Radiographic visualization of the arterial tree in the lower limbs (see fig. 3/1c, 3/2d, chapter 3) is very useful and even essential in a number of different situations. For example, it is helpful in determining whether main arteries have been injured as a result of trauma or following a surgical procedure (p. 306). It is also valuable in making the diagnosis of congenital arteriovenous fistula (p. 363) and in initiating the proper surgical therapeutic regimen. The procedure has its greatest clinical application as a preliminary measure to reconstructive vascular surgery in patients with arteriosclerosis obliterans who have satisfied the clinical criteria for such an approach (p. 153) and must now be studied to ascertain whether an operation is technically feasible. It likewise plays a role during the operative procedure in identifying technical surgical errors which can then be corrected at once, thus minimizing the possibility of subsequent thrombosis of the prosthesis. In summary, con-

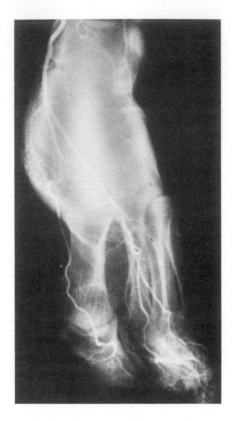

Fig. 4/1. Arteriographic demonstration of the posterior tibial artery at the ankle and the digital vessels.

trast angiography should be reserved only for those situations in which the required information cannot be collected by safer clinical and noninvasive measures.

Precautions in Interpretation of Angiograms. It is important to point out that since conventional angiography involves visualization of a two-dimensional image, the procedure may not always record a true picture of the degree of occlusion in a vessel. Another precaution to consider in the evaluation of an angiogram is that spasm of the artery produced by inser-tion of the needle may cause changes in lumen size which mimic filling defects of organic stenoses, thus requiring radiographic expertise for differentiation. It is also important to consider that angiography supplies only anatomic information regarding the vascular tree and that it does not necessarily yield quantitative data of the actual state of the circulation, such as the distribution of perfusion of blood to the tissues. For example, the presence of a visualized segment of posterior tibial artery at the level of the ankle, filled with radiopaque material by way of an extensive collateral circulation, does not indicate that under physiologic conditions, such a vessel plays an important role in conveying nutrient to the tissues. For its effectiveness in this regard is significantly impaired by the fact that the blood reaching it has passed through the circuitous, tortuous, and extensive secondary vascular tree and in the process its head of pressure has been markedly reduced due to the high resistance encountered. Hence, on entering the visualized segment of patent posterior tibial artery, its ability to perfuse the distal microcirculation is also diminished.

Complications from Contrast Angiography. About 5–10% of the patients on whom angiography is performed develop some type of complication from the technique. A relatively frequent occurrence is extravasation of radiopaque medium at the site of administration, with infiltration of adventitial or periarterial tissues. Moist applications and external heat should be used to encourage rapid resorption of the material, for otherwise an inflammatory reaction will develop, followed by induration and fibrosis. Hematomas at the site of injection are treated in a similar fashion. A much more serious complication is local destruction of the arterial wall which may be followed by thrombosis of the vessel, requiring immediate reconstructive surgery if the artery is a critical one. Local dissection of the vessel wall may be caused by partial extrusion of the needle from the arterial lumen, a result which has no serious consequences since the local blood pressure compresses the intima and media against the adventitia.

The needle puncture itself may produce trauma to the artery or the force of injection may cause marked distention of the vessel. At times either mechanism may be responsible for spasm of the artery, identified by the complaint of severe local pain and the appearance of blanching, followed by the development of scattered violaceous plaques on the skin below the point of injection and subcutaneous hemorrhages. Associated neurologic findings may consist of motor paralysis, loss of deep reflexes, and anesthesia of the foot. In most instances, this clinical picture clears up in a week or 10 days, although prolonged spasm may lead to arterial thrombosis and even superficial gangrene.

Among other complications is infection resulting in the formation of a local abscess at the puncture site; if left untreated, it may result in arterial thrombosis. Finally, there are some systemic complications of arteriography, such as acute renal failure if a large quantity of contrast medium (more than 150 ml) has been injected. It is therefore imperative to diurese patients routinely following arteriography so as to remove the radiopaque material as rapidly as possible. Allergic responses or anaphylactoid reactions to the contrast material have also been reported, and for this reason, an intravenous test quantity should precede the administration of the total dose. Moreover, medications should always be available in the arteriographic room to combat such a possibility. (For the various precautionary measures necessary to control or minimize some of the complications of angiography, see p. 358.)

Electromagnetic Blood Flowmeter

Technique. The electromagnetic blood flowmeter has a very limited use as a diagnostic tool, since it is only applicable to the measurement of blood flow through exposed, unopened arteries or vascular prosthesis during the time when the patient is still on the operating table. The principle of the method is based on Faraday's law that the movement of an electric conductor through a magnetic field induces a voltage across the conductor proportional to the number of magnetic lines of force cut per unit of time. The technique consists of establishing a magnetic field across the artery or an inserted vascular prosthesis, and with the blood passing through the vessel or tube acting as a conductor, a voltage is generated which is proportional to the strength of the magnetic field, the diameter of the vessel, and the mean velocity of the blood stream. The induced voltage can be picked up from electrodes in contact with the outer surface of the exposed blood vessel or graft wall.

Application to Study of Blood Flow. The electromagnetic blood flowmeter is of value mainly in determining whether a newly inserted arterial prosthesis is functioning at the time of operation. Through its use, technical difficulties can be identified and immediately remedied, thus increasing the possibility that the graft will remain patent. The instrument is also useful in the study of the efficiency of the vascular bed after the insertion of a prosthesis. This is accomplished by proximally injecting 10–30 mg of papaverine intra-arterially and determining the percentage increase from the basal flow elicited by the drug [4]. The magnitude of this figure is a reflection of the rate of distal 'runoff' and inflow capacity and of the functional state of the prosthesis.

Radioactive Tracer Technique

The use of radioactive tracers gives information regarding the physiologic state of the arterial tree, in contrast to angiography which visualizes its anatomic architecture. The procedure also assesses the efficiency of the collateral circulation developed in response to impairment in blood flow through main arterial channels, thus providing an objective, reliable test of blood perfusion through local tissues.

Technique. A number of radioactive tracers are available for the study of the peripheral circulation. Some are particulate in nature, and since the particles are larger in diameter than the lumen of a capillary, they are trapped in the first capillary bed they encounter, being distributed in proportion to the perfusion present in this site. Among the particulate tracers are ^{131}I-MAAA or ^{99m}Tc-MAA, ^{99m}Tc-albumin microspheres, and ^{113m}In-albumin microspheres. All of these materials temporarily cause obstruction of the local microcirculation, but they are quickly reduced to smaller particles which now readily pass through the capillary bed to be excreted from the body. The nonparticulate tracers include ^{99m}Tc-labeled serum albumin, ^{99m}Tc-labeled red blood cells, and ^{113m}In-labeled transferrin.

The method involves the intra-arterial injection of the radioactive tracer, followed by scintillation scanning of the vascular bed under study. The procedure is performed at rest and then when stress is placed on the vascular tree, as during reactive hyperemia elicited by a short period of total ischemia or after a bout of physical exercise.

Application to the Study of Blood Flow. The use of particulate radioactive tracers is especially helpful in the study of small artery disease, since the procedure visualizes the relative perfusion of capillary beds, information not available with arteriography.

Radioisotope Disappearance Rate

Technique. Radioisotopes have also been used for diagnostic purposes in patients with impaired circulation by locally depositing them under the skin or into a muscle mass of the lower limbs and determining the rate of removal of the material through external counting. Radioactive gases, such as ^{133}zenon and ^{85}krypton, have replaced the freely diffusible isotopes originally used. The radioactive material is injected into the site under study and the amount of radioactivity centered over the area is measured with a scintillation probe and registered on a ratemeter connected to a linear recorder. The disappearance rate of the radioactivity from the injection site is measured in terms of half-life.

Application to the Study of Blood Flow. For the most part, the method is helpful in determining whether the reduction in blood flow is present either in the skin or in the muscle. Its usefulness as a routine clinical diagnostic approach is limited.

References

1   Baker, W.H.; String, S.T.; Hayes, A.C.; Turner, D.: Diagnosis of peripheral occlusive disease: comparison of clinical evaluation and non-invasive laboratory. Archs Surg., Chicago *113:* 1308 (1978).
2   Hashway, T.; Raines, J.: Real-time ultrasonic imaging of the peripheral arteries: technique, normal anatomy, and pathology. Cardiovasc. Des. Bull., Tex. Heart Inst. *7:* 257 (1980).
3   Lennihan, R., Jr.; Mackereth, M.: Ankle pressure in arterial occlusive disease involving the legs. Surg. Clins N. Am. *53:* 657 (1973).
4   Welsh, P.; Repetto, R.: Intraoperative blood measurements following revascularization of the lower extremities with chronic arterial occlusive disease. Cardiovasc. Surg. *19:* 515 (1978).

5 Spontaneous Acute Occlusive Arterial Disorders: Arterial Embolism and Arterial Thrombosis

Sudden occlusion of a critical artery to or in the lower limbs, whether due to an organized clot arising elsewhere in the vascular tree or to a local rapidly forming thrombus, can be considered to be one of the few real emergencies in the field of peripheral vascular disorders. Consequently, its early recognition is imperative so that a proper therapeutic program can be instituted immediately. Otherwise, if the obstruction remains untreated, loss of viability of distal structures can usually be expected, especially if the cause is an embolus. In the presence of a thrombus, generally the prognosis is much less serious, provided the etiologic agent responsible for the production of the lesion is a chronic occlusive arterial disorder, such as arteriosclerosis obliterans or thromboangiitis obliterans. For, under such circumstances, frequently a collateral arterial system already exists and is functionally capable of supplying the tissues with blood, although not as efficiently as the now obstructed main channel. Such a secondary circulation develops in response to a persistent, progressive state of low-grade ischemia in the involved structures, produced by the underlying local arterial impairment.

Arterial Embolism

In arterial embolism, particulate matter of varying size becomes liberated from its site of origin in the cardiovascular system, to enter the systemic blood stream and cause total obstruction of a peripheral artery above a point at which the diameter of the involved vessel is smaller than that of the embolus. In the case of a critical artery, total cessation of blood flow through it produces a typical clinical pattern of acute ischemia of distal structures (p. 81).

Sites of Embolic Origin

Heart. This organ is the source of peripheral arterial emboli in about 80% of cases. Common sites of origin of such agents are diseased mitral and aortic semilunar valves, the cause for the development of excrescences or thrombi being either rheumatic heart disease or atherosclerosis. Infected emboli may form in the presence of bacterial endocarditis superimposed upon the involved cusps. Another etiologic agent in the production of emboli is some type of abnormality of the left atrium, such as atrial fibrillation or a widely dilated chamber with normal sinus rhythm. In both instances, conditions are conducive to the growth of clots in the auricle of the left atrium. In at least half the cases in which emboli arise in the heart, myocardial infarction is the cause, the pathologic process extending to the endocardium and being responsible for the development of mural thrombi on the involved site. Other less common locations are the cavity of a left ventricular aneurysm and left atrial myomas. The insertion of artificial valve replacements may also be a source of peripheral arterial emboli, as a result of the deposition of aggregates of platelets and fibrin on the surface of the prosthesis which then separate and enter the blood stream.

Vascular Tree. The cavity of a thoracic or abdominal aortic aneurysm or a similar lesion in a main artery in a lower limb may also be the source of peripheral arterial emboli, as well as thrombosed vessels and ulcerated surfaces of the abdominal aorta. Rarely, thrombi originating in a deep venous plexus in the calf (phlebothrombosis) will pass into the main venous system and through a patent foramen ovale in the heart into the peripheral arterial system (paradoxical emboli).

Sites of Embolic Occlusion

Emboli generally occlude arteries at a bifurcation or, less often, where a vessel suddenly becomes appreciably narrower in diameter. In the case of the abdominal aorta, the most common site for lodgment of a clot is at its bifurcation (fig. 5/1). This also applies to the arteries supplying the lower limbs, the common femoral above the origin of the deep femoral artery being most often occluded (fig. 5/2a, c). The other vessels supplying or located in the lower limbs are affected in the following order of reducing frequency: popliteal, common iliac (fig. 5/2b), external iliac, superficial femoral, posterior tibial, and, finally, anterior tibial arteries [6].

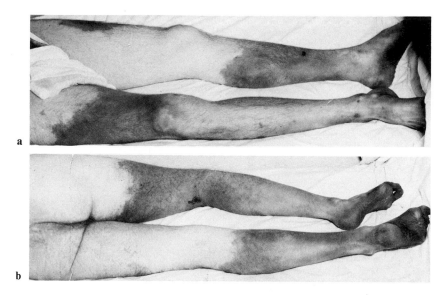

Fig. 5/1. Untreated saddle embolus at bifurcation of aorta causing gangrene of both lower limbs. **a** Anterior view. **b** Posterior view. Reproduced from ref. [1] with permission.

Clinical Manifestations of Embolic Occlusion of Critical Arteries to or in the Lower Limbs

Symptoms. Usually total occlusion of such vessels as the abdominal aorta, common femoral, superficial femoral, or popliteal artery by an embolus elicits an abrupt and dramatic onset of acute ischemic pain in the foot, particularly the toes, associated with a 'dead' feeling and paresthesias in the digits. In the case of obstruction of the popliteal artery, there may be an associated ache in the calf, approximately at the level of the bifurcation of the vessel. With persistence of the state of acute anoxia, the symptoms become more intense until the peripheral nerves become nonfunctioning, as manifested by disappearance of the severe pain and replacement by numbness, especially of the foot.

Vascular Signs. The objective changes in the involved limb are characteristic of the existence of a severe degree of ischemia. The most marked abnormality is a waxy pallor of the foot, with the height of the color change in the remainder of the limb grossly corresponding to the level of arterial

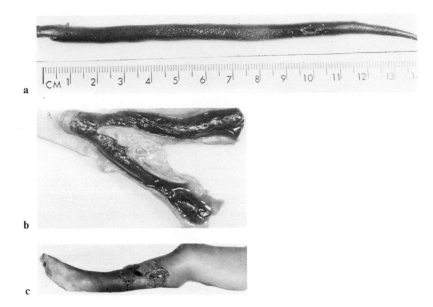

Fig. 5/2. a Embolus removed from left femoral artery. **b** Embolus at the bifurcation of the left common iliac artery with propagation into the external and internal iliac arteries. **c** Gangrene of a leg and foot following occlusion of the common femoral artery by an embolus. **a, b** Reproduced from ref. [1] with permission.

occlusion. The alteration in skin color is due to absence of blood in the superficial venules (subpapillary venous plexuses) resulting from interference with or absence of arterial inflow and from a superimposed vasospasm of cutaneous microcirculation which almost invariably accompanies organic occlusion of a main artery. Interspersed small islands of cyanosis are frequently noted, resulting from trapping of blood in some of the small cutaneous vessels. Because of the absence or significant reduction of arterial inflow, venous outflow is likewise minimal, as reflected in collapsed cutaneous veins. For the same reason, the circumferences of the involved limb are smaller than those of the opposite normal limb. Cutaneous temperature is markedly decreased, dropping to a level only somewhat higher than environmental temperature, particularly in the foot and toes. In the upper part of the limb, coldness of the skin gradually becomes less obvious. Palpation of the skin frequently identifies a zone of demarcation between normal and decreased cutaneous temperature which grossly reflects the level at which the occlusion exists in the artery. In the segments of limb below the block, no arterial pulsations are present, the same being true for oscillometric readings. Above the point of obstruction, pulsations are generally present but reduced in amplitude because of the superimposed vasospasm which affects the large arteries in the extremity, as well as the cutaneous microcirculation. At times, however, the proximal pulsations may be greater than those at the same level in the opposite normal limb, for reasons that are not entirely clear.

Besides clinically determining the level at which there is a significant demarcation in cutaneous temperature and skin color and the level at which pulses can no longer be palpated, further pertinent information can be obtained with the oscillometer (p. 58) and the Doppler ultrasonic flowmeter (p. 65), both of which are helpful in locating the site of occlusion. Arteriography is rarely required for the latter purpose; furthermore, it has the disadvantage that the delay incurred in performing the procedure may result in progressive limb ischemia to the point of placing the viability of distal tissues in jeopardy.

Neurologic Signs. As the state of anoxia deepens, objective signs of sensory and motor deficits become more marked, due to the untoward effects on peripheral nerves of such a situation. A relatively early finding is a stocking-glove type of hypesthesia or anesthesia which bears no relationship to normal anatomic nerve distribution to the skin. An area of hyperesthesia may be noted above the upper level of reduced sensation. The location of the latter finding may help in identifying the site of the occlusion in the main artery.

Impairment in motor function is associated with a further increase in the severity of the existing ischemia. It takes the form of difficulty or inability to move the toes and varying degrees of foot drop. The presence of such findings indicates that the prognosis with regard to limb viability is much poorer than if there are only sensory deficits. (For differential diagnosis of large artery embolism, see p. 91.)

Clinical Manifestations of Embolic Occlusion of the Microcirculation
Atherothrombotic or cholesterol embolization elicits a clinical pattern which is different from that produced by embolic occlusion of a main arterial channel. In this state there is liberation of minute emboli into the systemic circulation, causing obstruction of arterioles and capillaries, generally in the skin of the toes and in the voluntary muscle of the leg.

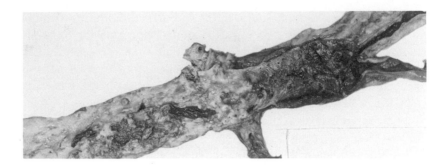

Fig. 5/3. Saddle thrombus at bifurcation of aorta, associated with marked atheromatous changes in proximal portion of vessel and demonstrating ulceration, a common site for the liberation of microemboli. Reproduced from ref. [1] with permission.

Etiologic Factors. The particulate matter responsible for embolism to the microcirculation has its origin in fragmented atheromatous plaques or debris from ulcerated sites in the infrarenal or terminal portion of the abdominal aorta (fig. 5/3). It consists of a variable combination of lipoid material, cholesterol crystals, adherent red blood cells, and fibrin aggregates. The condition is usually found in older men suffering from generalized atherosclerosis.

Local Clinical Picture. Following occlusion of portions of the microcirculation in the skin of the foot, the patient generally complains of very severe ischemic pain in the tips of the toes, associated with reversible or irreversible cyanosis or dusky discoloration of entire digits ('blue toe' syndrome). Later the condition progresses to superficial ulceration or necrosis of the tips of the toes (fig. 5/4), which is ringed by a dark halo formed by hemorrhage into the subcutaneous tissue. Mottling of the skin of the leg and, to a lesser extent, of the thigh, buttock, and lower portion of the trunk is a commonly associated finding. The change, which resembles livedo reticularis (p. 39), is caused by an inflammatory reaction to the cholesterol crystals deposited in the microcirculation of the skin as microemboli. The mesh-like red-to-blue pattern is not affected by elevation of the lower limbs or by digital compression, although its appearance varies from week to week. Occlusion of arterioles and capillaries in the muscles of the leg and elsewhere manifests itself in the form of myalgias and muscle tenderness,

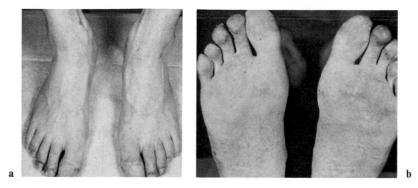

a   b

Fig. 5/4. Atherosclerotic or cholesterol emboli producing blue-toe syndrome in several toes of both feet. **a** Dorsal surface. **b** Ventral surface, with the superficial necrosis clearly demonstrated. Reproduced from ref. [2] with permission.

associated with the development of elevated, hard, tender nodules on the limb, covered by reddish-blue skin. The changes represent areas of necrosis of muscle. Microscopic examination of a biopsied tender nodule by polarized light reveals clefts of cholesterol crystals, presented as multiple lance-shaped parallel or criss-crossing voids [3].

In the mild form, the symptoms in the legs may resemble those of the restless legs syndrome (p. 16). In fact, microemboli have been implicated as one of the causative agents in the development of this condition.

Despite extensive signs of a severe degree of local acute ischemia of skin and muscle, there are no findings to indicate any impairment of circulation through the main arterial channels in the involved limbs. Arterial pulsations are present in the feet and oscillometric and Doppler ultrasonic flowmeter readings are normal for the thigh and leg. Aside from the changes noted in the affected areas of skin and muscle, no nutritional abnormalities are present elsewhere on the limb. If arteriography is performed in an attempt to determine the cause of the difficulty, no stenosis or occlusions are found. Aortography will almost invariably reveal ulceration of atherosclerotic plaques in the abdominal aorta.

Systemic Responses to Microemboli. Aside from the changes in the lower limbs, microemboli may produce acute renal insufficiency from release of crystals into the renal arteries, as during surgery on the abdominal aorta or following aortography. Chronic renal insufficiency may also occur in response to repeated liberation of microemboli into the renal vascular tree. Entrance of the particulate material into the gastrointestinal system may cause such difficulties as hemorrhage, vomiting, and abdominal pain. If only the pancreas or the spleen is involved in the process, the patient generally remains asymptomatic.

General Principles of Therapy for Large Artery and Microcirculation Embolism

Prophylactic Measures for Large Artery Embolism. The first approach to the management of arterial embolism is its prevention in people who are potential candidates for liberation of clots into the systemic blood stream. As already mentioned, patients with myocardial infarction may develop mural thrombi that can become separated from their site of origin and cause obliteration of peripheral arteries. For this reason, such individuals should be placed on anticoagulation therapy at the onset of the acute episode to inhibit the growth of thrombi. In the presence of atrial fibrillation, attempts should be made to reestablish normal sinus rhythm, although there is some risk associated with such a step in the case of the longstanding type, since liberation of thrombi in the auricle of the left atrium may follow. Furthermore, rarely is such a regimen successful if the condition has been present for a long time. Surgical means of dealing with mitral stenosis may be useful in controlling the development of clots in the heart, although the substitution of an artificial valve may, by itself, introduce another source for the formation of emboli – on the surface of the prosthesis.

In the active treatment of large artery embolism, the goal is rapid restoration of blood flow through the involved vessel, before permanent loss of viability of distal tissues occurs. Such a therapeutic program first requires an intravenous injection of heparin to prevent a thrombus from developing at the site of the embolic occlusion and propagating both proximally and distally in the artery. To protect the limb from injury, it is covered with several layers of cotton padding to form a loosely fitting boot. The head of the bed is raised about 20 cm (8 in) so as to increase local arterial inflow. Large doses of narcotics are generally necessary to control the pain originating in the foot. At the same time, preparations are being made for surgical intervention, which involves the insertion of a Fogarty balloon catheter [5] above the site of obstruction, in order to remove the embolus and any accompanying thrombus that may already have formed. Immediately following a successful attempt to remove the embolus, the clinical picture improves dramatically although pulses may not return for several days. Nevertheless, nonpulsatile movement of blood into the limb is occurring, the damping of pulsations probably being due to the superimposed vasospasm almost invariably present with embolic occlusion of large arteries.

Whether heparin should be given postoperatively is still a moot question, although most of the available evidence supports the view that it should, despite the possibility of initiating bleeding in the operative site. Since frequently the cause of the embolic phenomenon cannot be eliminated, it is advisable under such circumstances to initiate a long-range oral anticoagulant program with warfarin sodium (Coumadin) while the patient is still in the hospital and then to continue it on an outpatient basis, terminating heparin administration at the time of discharge. This regimen should be continued indefinitely or until the underlying causative cardiovascular condition is appropriately treated. Otherwise, it is almost inevitable that subsequent episodes of peripheral embolic episodes will occur, perhaps to such critical organs as the brain and kidneys. The outpatient program must be carefully medically supervised at all times to prevent bleeding episodes or loss of protection from intravascular clotting because of inadequate anticoagulant administration. To maintain an appropriate therapeutic state, it is essential to have prothrombin times taken at least every other week and the dosage of Coumadin altered accordingly if necessary. (For further discussion of outpatient oral anticoagulant therapy, see p. 282.)

Treatment of Embolic Occlusion of the Microcirculation. In obstruction of the microcirculation in the skin and muscles of the lower limb, early therapy, for the most part, is symptomatic. It involves the use of narcotics to control the pain associated with the ischemic lesions on the toes, protection of the feet from injury, and debridement of the separated necrotic tissue. A 2% nitroglycerine ointment (Nitrol ointment) should be applied to the base of the involved toes 3 times a day, in an effort to increase blood flow into the digits by its vasodilating effect on the digital arteries. There is a real question as to whether heparin and Coumadin should be given, since these drugs prevent organization of a fibrin layer over the ulcerated lesions in the aorta and iliac arteries from which the microemboli generally arise and hence may be responsible for recurrence of the condition. Instead it is necessary in the near future to identify the exact location of the source of the emboli, using angiography (fig. 5/3), and then to carry out appropriate surgical correction, in the form of endarterectomy, insertion of a bifurcation graft to replace an area of atherosclerotic ulceration in the abdominal aorta or, in the presence of an aneurysm of this vessel or its main branches, excision of the lesion and reestablishment of circulation [4].

Prognosis

Untreated Embolic Occlusion of a Major Artery. Whether the distal tissues will remain viable under such conditions depends upon the size and previous role of the obstructed vessel in supplying blood to the limb, the degree and duration of superimposed vasospasm, and the effectiveness and efficiency of an existing collateral circulation, if any (fig. 5/1).

Treated Embolic Occlusion of a Major Artery. Following an embolectomy, the prognosis with regard to maintenance of viability of the involved limb depends upon the skill and celerity of the surgeon in performing the procedure, including removal of clots from distal branches, and the duration and severity of the superimposed vasospasm in the postoperative period. Of significance with regard to longevity is the seriousness of the cardiovascular disease responsible for the development of the peripheral embolus.

Atherothrombotic and Cholesterol Embolic Occlusion of the Microcirculation. Under these circumstances, the prognosis with regard to viability of the involved limb is good, since blood flow through the main arteries to the foot is normal. Careful aseptic treatment of the lesions on the toes will generally result in complete healing, with little or no loss of toe tissue. However, if the source of the microemboli is not eliminated, repeated showers of particulate matter can be expected, these eventually producing enough obstruction of the cutaneous microcirculation to cause extensive lesions in the skin of the toes and elsewhere.

Spontaneous Arterial Thrombosis

In spontaneous arterial thrombosis, changes take place in the intima of an artery which are responsible for the growth of a thrombus locally, this process ultimately producing complete occlusion of the lumen of the involved vessel.

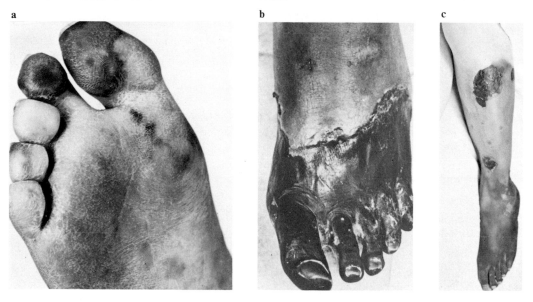

Fig. 5/5. Arterial thrombosis produced by different etiologic agents. **a** Gangrene of first and second toes due to thrombosis of small arteries in the foot, associated with trichinosis. **b** Gangrene of foot following thrombosis of a popliteal arterial aneurysm and of the artery itself in a patient with arteriosclerosis obliterans. Clear line of demarcation noted. **c** Gangrene of foot and leg produced by thrombosis of the left femoral artery following prolonged vomiting and diarrhea in a patient susceptible to intravascular clotting. Reproduced from ref. [1] with permission.

Etiologic Agents

Spontaneous thrombosis of large or small arteries may occur as a result of a number of unrelated mechanisms. Some of the etiologic agents are inflammatory in nature, such as thromboangiitis obliterans (p. 104) and the connective tissue disorders (p. 370); others are infectious (meningitis, trichinosis [fig. 5/5a], staphylococcic or streptococcic bacteremia, typhoid fever, and pneumonia); while most are degenerative (arteriosclerosis obliterans [fig. 5/5b] and cystic adventitial disease). A number of systemic disorders, such as congestive heart failure, cardiac arrhythmias, and the nephrotic syndrome, are also associated with episodes of spontaneous arterial thrombosis. Certain abnormal states, including prolonged immobilization of a limb and severe dehydration (fig. 5/5c), likewise predispose to this condition, as does the administration of drugs which affect the coagulation mechanism, including oral contraceptives [7].

Pathogenesis

Underlying the development of a spontaneous arterial thrombosis is a slowing of blood flow and a loss of the axial stream in laminar flow pattern of the movement of the blood. Contributing to such a state are hemorrhage into an atherosclerotic plaque rapidly enlarging it, arterial dissection causing projection of the inner layers of the wall into the lumen of the vessel, and growth of a clot originating in the cavity of an aneurysm into the lumen of the artery from which the lesion arises, occluding it.

When thrombi obstruct terminal vessels, such as digital arteries, gangrene of a portion or of an entire toe is a good possibility. This is due to the fact that no other vascular channels are available under such circumstances for supplying the digit with blood, even if the remainder of the arterial tree in the limb remains open. This type of response has been noted in various types of infectious diseases (p. 89). Under such conditions, the thrombotic episode may be initiated by exotoxins, elaborated by bacterial organisms, which produce damage to the endothelium of the blood vessels. Such a change, together with the slowing of the blood stream and deposition of fibrin, may be responsible for the development and growth of a thrombus that eventually obliterates the lumen of the involved artery.

Clinical Manifestations

The clinical picture associated with a spontaneous arterial thrombosis is greatly influenced by both the rate at which the lesion develops and the efficiency of the existing collateral circulation at the time when the process is completed.

Sudden obliteration of a large, previously *normal,* artery by a rapidly forming thrombus produces a severe degree of acute ischemia of distal tissues, the clinical manifestations resembling those elicited by sudden obliteration of a normal vessel by an embolus (p. 81). For, under both conditions, there is no existing effective collateral circulation to take over the function of supplying the tissues with blood.

If rapid, complete obliteration of a previously *diseased* and stenotic artery occurs – as for example by development of a hemorrhage in a small atheroma, markedly distending it and filling the entire lumen of the vessel – the clinical picture is much less severe. This is due to the existence of an already developed secondary circulation, formed in response to a persistent chronic, low-grade state of tissue ischemia due to the underlying arterial disorder. After a short period of vascular readjustment, this secondary circulation assumes the function of delivering generally adequate amounts of blood to the distal tissues, although not as efficiently as the critical, now occluded, artery. As a consequence, the signs of acute ischemia rapidly diminish in severity and almost complete clinical recovery usually occurs. If the collateral vessels are poory developed and incapable of maintaining an adequate blood supply to the tissues, then the manifestations of acute ischemia become much more marked, resembling those of a rapidly developing thrombus in, or an embolus to, a normal artery.

If the thrombus in a critical artery develops very slowly, as is the case in most of the patients with arteriosclerosis obliterans, sufficient time is available for the growth of a compensatory collateral circulation, generally adequate for supplying the tissues with the necessary quantity of nutrition. As a result, total thrombosis of large arteries may occur without significant changes in symptoms, except possibly some decline in claudication distance. If the patient is leading a sedentary existence, as many elderly individuals with arteriosclerosis obliterans do, this deterioration may not even become apparent to him. The only objective findings of such an occurrence are generally disappearance of pulses in vessels previously manifesting reduced ones and oscillometric readings changing from low to zero levels. Significant alterations in nutritional circulation are usually not noted.

Differential Diagnosis of Large Artery Thrombosis

Arterial Embolism. The clinical entity which most closely resembles spontaneous arterial thrombosis is large artery embolism (p. 81). Since the treatment of both conditions is quite different, it is of paramount importance to make the differentiation between the two conditions early in their inception. Arterial embolism is invariably associated with some type of cardiovascular disorder capable of discharging particulate material into the systemic circulation, a situation which does not necessarily exist in the case of arterial thrombosis. Moreover, in the great majority of patients, a history of intermittent claudication or of objective signs of arterial insufficiency in the lower limbs cannot be elicited, whereas in most people with arterial thrombosis due to a chronic occlusive arterial disorder, such findings invariably antedate the onset of the acute episode by months or years. Another differential point opposed to the diagnosis of arterial embolism is the finding of significant arterial disease in the contralateral unaffected limb, an observation definitely supporting arterial thrombosis as the etiologic cause for the current difficulty. In the case of the younger patient with arterial embolism, the circulation elsewhere is normal. As a general rule, the degree of anoxia initially observed in the limb with an occluded main artery can be expected to be more marked in arterial embolism than in sudden obliteration of a previously diseased artery by a thrombus. For example, there is a waxy pallor of the skin of the foot in arterial embolism, whereas in the presence of arterial thrombosis, the color is less cadaveric and more cyanotic in hue. A possibility which must always be considered in the case of the elderly patient is that arteriosclerosis obliterans and a precursor for arterial embolism may coexist, thus making the cause for an episode of acute ischemia of a limb difficult to identify correctly.

Vasospasm. Spontaneous arterial thrombosis, as well as arterial embolism, must be distinguished from vasospasm following trauma to a large artery or to the tissues in the vicinity of the vessel, since such an abnormal response produces a marked reduction in arterial circulation to the limb (p. 308). Besides the history of injury to the limb, another important differential point is that in the vasospastic state, there is frequently a proximal border of pallid or mottled cyanotic skin which is irregular and not as sharply delineated as in organic arterial occlusion. If the vasospasm is neurogenic in origin, then a lumbar paravertebral sympathetic block will be followed by almost immediate improvement in the clinical picture, whereas in the case of arterial thrombosis or embolism, the changes produced by such a procedure are minimal. In myogenic vasospasm, this diagnostic procedure is of no value, since the clinical picture is not altered by it. (For discussion of neurogenic and myogenic vasospasm, see p. 308.)

General Principles of Therapy

In the early stage of spontaneous arterial thrombosis, the local and systemic treatment is similar to that employed for arterial embolism (p. 86), except that no attempt is made to remove the clot (thrombectomy), since such an approach causes only temporary improvement, inasmuch as a fresh thrombus would invariably develop in the same site shortly thereafter. Another objection to thrombectomy is that in the case of arteriosclerosis obliterans, subsequent repair of the artery is made more difficult and, at times, even impossible.

If the severity of the clinical picture is such as to require immediate reestablishment of local circulation to preserve the integrity of the limb, then a thromboendarterectomy (p. 164) or insertion of a prosthesis (p. 157) should immediately be performed. Under such circumstances, arteriography is necessary to assess the extent of the disease process, the adequacy of arterial inflow, and the extent of the distal 'runoff'.

References

1   Abramson, D.I.: Diagnosis and treatment of peripheral vascular disorders (Hoeber-Harper, New York 1956).
2   Abramson, D.I.: Circulatory diseases of the limbs: a primer (Grune & Stratton, New York 1978).
3   Anderson, W.R.; Richards, A.M.: Evaluation of lower extremity muscle biopsies in the diagnosis of atheroembolism. Archs Path. *86:* 535 (1968).
4   Brenowitz, J.B.; Gregory, J.; Edwards, W.S.: Diagnosis and treatment of peripheral atheromatous emboli, J. cardiovasc. Surg. *19:* 499 (1978).
5   Fogarty, T.J.; Cranley, J.J.; Krause, R.J.; et al.: A method for extraction of arterial emboli and thrombi. Surgery Gynec. Obstet. *116:* 241 (1965).
6   Haimovici, H.: Peripheral arterial embolism: a study of 330 unselected cases of embolism of the extremities. Angiology *1:* 20 (1950).
7   Inman, W.H.W.; Vessey, M.P.; Westerholm, B.; et al.: Thromboembolic disease and the steroidal content of oral contraceptives. Br. med. J. *ii:* 203 (1970).

6 Spontaneous Chronic Occlusive Arterial Disorders: Aortoiliac Arterial Occlusive Disease and Arteriosclerosis Obliterans

Spontaneous chronic occlusive arterial disorders are the most common conditions affecting the arterial tree of the lower limbs, particularly in elderly people. Of the entities in this group most often seen in clinical practice are atherosclerosis affecting the vessels of the lower limbs, designated as arteriosclerosis obliterans, and the same pathologic process found in the abdominal cavity, termed aortoiliac arterial occlusive disease. Although the site of the obstruction in the latter condition is in the vascular tree proximal to the lower limbs, many of the symptoms and signs associated with it are located in the buttocks, thighs, legs, and feet.

The present chapter is devoted primarily to a discussion of the above two entities and associated complications because of their high incidence in the patient population. Thromboangiitis obliterans and Mönckeberg's sclerosis, also falling into the category of spontaneous chronic occlusive arterial diseases, are considered only in the sections in this chapter devoted to the differential diagnosis and prognosis of arteriosclerosis obliterans (pp. 104, 110). The various types of treatment of the spontaneous chronic occlusive arterial disorders are all found in chapter 8.

General Consideration of Atherosclerosis

Since arteriosclerosis obliterans and aortoiliac occlusive arterial disease affect primarily people in middle and late life, and since the mean age of the population continues to rise, it can be anticipated that the incidence of these disorders will also increase. The gravity of the situation is further enhanced by the progressive lengthening of life expectancy of diabetic patients through therapeutic means, thus resulting in exposure of the vascular tree, particularly the microcirculation, to longer periods of predisposing factors responsible for degenerative diseases of blood vessels. Finally, the absence of any specific curative or prophylactic measures for the control of atherosclerosis also contributes to the greater number of patients with arteriosclerosis obliterans now being seen in clinical practice.

Etiologic Factors and Pathogenesis

Atherosclerosis is a progressive disorder which is caused by a variety of factors and which gradually or, less frequently, rapidly narrows the caliber of the arterial tree in various portions and organs of the body, including the lower limbs. The disease has its origin in the continuous remodeling of the arterial wall associated with body growth and development. It is generally found in patients between the ages of 40 and 80 years. However, when diabetes mellitus coexists, the atherosclerotic process may be present in a much younger age group (from 8 to 40 years). No one category of individuals is affected to a much greater extent than others; nor is there any striking sex predisposition.

Etiologic Factors. No view regarding the mechanisms involved in the development of atherosclerosis has gained universal acceptance. One proposes that there is an error in the metabolism of fat and other lipids, this then being responsible for the formation of atheromatous plaques (p. 97). Extensive vascularization of the wall of large arteries has also been suggested as an etiologic agent, as well as the deleterious effects of prolonged stress and strain to which the arterial tree is exposed during the life of the individual (a reflection of the natural aging process). The tendency for atherosclerotic plaques to form at bends and bifurcations of arteries, sites subjected to great strain and distortion from the moving blood, would be in accord with the latter view. Systemic hypertension has likewise been implicated as an etiologic factor on a hemodynamic basis, as well as because of its injurious action on endothelial cells, followed by atherosclerosis [14]. A coagulation defect in the blood has been proposed to explain the common finding of arterial thrombosis in atherosclerosis.

It has recently been suggested that high-density lipoproteins may exert a protective influence against atherosclerosis by returning excess cholesterol and other fats to the liver for disposal. Unlike other lipoproteins, of which 50% or more by weight may be pure cholesterol, high-density lipoproteins consist largely of protein of the type which has been shown to promote the removal of cholesterol from cells in culture. The possibility has therefore been offered that a similar activity by these substances could prevent the characteristic formation of 'foamy cells' caused by fat deposition in smooth muscle cells. The latter stage of the atherosclerotic process is followed by entrance of low-density lipoproteins into the smooth muscle cells by the process of pinocytosis and then the breakdown of these substances into protein and triglyceride components by the intracellular action of lysosomal enzymes. Since the cholesterol cannot be transported from the cells, it remains in the cytoplasm, the fatty droplets accumulating in this site, a change which is responsible for the foamy appearance. Of interest in regard to the above theory is the finding that moderate intake of alcohol may cause a drop in the blood level of low-density lipoproteins and a rise in high-density lipoproteins. However, the data are by no means clear-cut enough to warrant therapeutic attempts to alter blood lipid levels by increasing alcohol intake.

Basis for Morphologic Changes. The histologic abnormalities of atherosclerosis have always been considered to be degenerative in nature. However, recently studies have been reported which do not support this view, suggesting instead that the condition is primarily a disease of smooth muscle proliferation, followed by invasion of the damaged intimal layer by blood-borne monocytes that convert to macrophages [8]. Associated with these alterations is an accumulation of connective tissue matrix, including collagen, proteoglycans, and elastin fibers, as well as large amounts of lipid. A number of factors have been proposed as etiologic agents in the production of injury to the endothelium [6, 16].

Other mechanisms have also been implicated in the genesis of atherosclerosis, although in many instances, definitive data supporting the different views are lacking. Among these are a deficiency in prostacyclin (a prostaglandin) in the arterial wall [17] and the importance of blood platelets in the pathogenesis of the condition [5]. Certain other blood components may enhance proliferation of smooth muscle cells, an action responsible for arterial narrowing.

Pathology
Morphologic Changes. The earliest visible lesions in atherosclerosis are minute yellow flecks, usually seen in the intima of the aorta, the microscopic changes consisting of swelling of the ground substance and the formation of metachromasia and minute lipid droplets. However, these fatty streaks are generally considered of questionable importance as precursors of atherosclerosis, for although some of them are transformed into plaques, others regress.

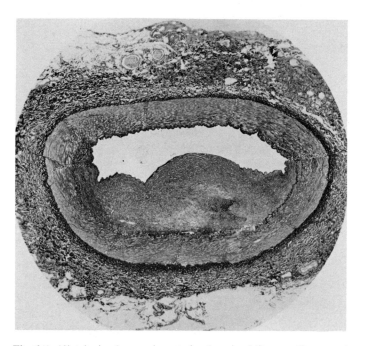

Fig. 6/1. Histologic changes in arteriosclerosis obliterans. Cross-section of a small artery demonstrating an atherosclerotic plaque occluding two thirds of the lumen. Reproduced from ref. [2] with permission.

Another type of change which appears to be much more important in the genesis of atherosclerosis is the fibromusculoelastic lesion which at first takes the form of thickening of the intima and proliferation of smooth muscle cells and connective tissue, with lipid deposits developing later. In the final state of atherosclerosis, the thickness of the intima may exceed that of the media.

The most typical manifestation of atherosclerosis is the atheroma. This lesion affects not only the arterial intima, but also the medial and adventitial coats [13]. It is most prevalent in large and medium-sized arteries and may extend into smaller vessels, particularly in the presence of hypertension and diabetes. Grossly, it consists of a raised yellowish mass that extends beyond the endothelial surface into the lumen (fig. 6/1).

Histologic examination of the atheroma reveals it to consist of proliferating endothelial cells, lipid-rich macrophages (foam cells), fibroblasts, lymphocytes, polymorphonuclear leukocytes, and accumulations of lipid materials. Structurally, there is a dense collagenous cap which is covered by endothelium on the luminal surface and which overlies and partially encases a necrotic lipid-rich core [13]. Foam cells are found most consistently around the periphery of the central lipid core but may also be observed on the surface of the collagenous cap, particularly toward the edges of the lesion. Associated alterations are medial thinning, due to atrophic loss of smooth muscle cells, and adventitial changes, including fibrosis, increased vascularity, and generally a mononuclear infiltrate of predominantly lymphocytes.

Because of distortion of the intima produced by protrusion of the plaque, secondary thrombosis is favored. The latter process may ultimately result in complete occlusion of the lumen. Such a response may also follow sudden hemorrhage into the plaque, a predisposition which exists in atherosclerosis. Subsequently recanalization of the thrombosed segment may take place, allowing a small quantity of blood to flow through new vascular channels lined with endothelium. Another facet may be erosion and ulceration of the atheromatous plaque, with superimposed buildup of a thrombus locally. Plaque rupture may also release necrotic debris originating in the lesion, resulting in cholesterol microembolization to distant arteriolar beds (p. 83).

Location of the Atheromatous Lesion in the Arterial Tree. In arteriosclerosis obliterans, the pathologic process is found in the common femoral artery and its two branches (superficial and deep femoral), the popliteal artery and its two branches (anterior and posterior tibial vessels), the dorsal pedal artery in the foot (a continuation of the anterior tibial artery), and the peroneal artery (a branch of the posterior tibial artery).

In aortoiliac arterial occlusive disease, the same type of atherosclerotic alteration exists in the abdominal aorta, proximal to or involving its bifurcation, and in the common, external, and internal (hypogastric) iliac arteries. The pathologic lesion generally first affects the iliac vessels and then progresses proximally to cause partial or complete occlusion of the aortic bifurcation. Much less often, the changes are first found in the abdominal aorta, below the origin of the inferior mesenteric artery, and then they spread downward into the iliac arteries. Generally the thrombosis is slowly progressive, with the atherosclerotic process appearing one decade earlier than expected if found elsewhere.

Of clinical significance is the fact that atheromatous alterations in the large arteries of the abdomen may frequently be associated with similar pathologic processes in the arterial tree of the lower limbs. This adversely affects prognosis with regard to the viability of the feet and seriously complicates the surgical therapeutic approach to the problem.

It is necessary to point out that several other types of pathologic change cause occlusion of the aortic bifurcation and hence must be differentiated from atherosclerosis. One of these, found primarily in men in the third and fourth decades of life, is characterized by sharply localized occlusive lesions in the aortic bifurcation, associated with little or no systemic pathologic alterations. Generally, the final complete obstruction of the vessel is caused by a very advanced fibrotic reaction. First described by *Leriche* [10] in 1940, it now bears his name – Leriche's syndrome. However, this designation has also been loosely applied to aortic bifurcation occlusions, regardless of the etiologic agent. Besides Leriche's syndrome, the same clinical manifestations may result from syphilitic aortitis, inflammatory disorders of the peritoneum, the sequelae of deep X-ray therapy, hypercholesterolemia, Marfan's syndrome, dissecting hematoma, and congenital absence of iliac arteries.

Clinical Manifestations

Arteriosclerosis developing in the arterial tree in the lower limbs may exist for a long time before symptoms appear. This is due to the fact that the occlusive process generally progresses at such a slow pace that sufficient time exists for the formation of an adequate collateral circulation. Only when there is an acceleration of the rate of occlusion of main vessels or a reduction in the efficiency of the secondary circulation will clinical manifestations of the disorder become evident locally.

Symptoms

For the most part, the complaints of patients with aortoiliac arterial occlusive disease and arteriosclerosis obliterans are the same, since their cause is identical: ischemia of exercising muscles, peripheral nerves, and skin. However, because the levels of occlusion in the two conditions are different, so are the locations of some of the symptoms, a point which will be emphasized in the following discussion.

The complaint which generally compels the patient with chronic arterial insufficiency of the lower limb to seek medical aid is intermittent claudication (p. 5). This symptom usually progresses in severity and may in some individuals significantly interfere with their life-style and ability to perform daily physical chores and remain gainfully employed. In aortoiliac arterial occlusive disease, intermittent claudication characteristically is located in the buttock or thigh, although at times it may be limited to the calf. In the patient suffering from arteriosclerosis obliterans, the symptom is usually experienced in the calf, although it may also be present in the small muscles of the foot and in the thigh. Because the block is never high enough to affect the blood supply to the muscles of the buttock, pain is not noted in this site.

Fortunately, ischemic neuropathy, another symptom found in chronic arterial insufficiency of the lower limbs, is experienced in only a relatively small number of patients with this condition. In contrast to intermittent claudication, which is present only during physical exercise and controlled by rest, this complaint appears when the patient lies down in preparation for sleep. As already noted (p. 14), he is able to get relief by sleeping in a chair, but he soon develops a severe degree of dependency edema which further reduces blood flow through the cutaneous microcirculation and thus markedly increases vulnerability to the development of ischemic ulcers or gangrene. Regardless of the site of obstruction in the vascular tree, the neuritic symptoms are present most often in the toes and less frequently in the foot proper. Generally, the severity of the complaints is not as great in aortoiliac arterial occlusive disease as in arteriosclerosis obliterans.

Finally, in the terminal stage of either entity, the patient may begin to suffer from another rest pain, that associated with impending or existing ulceration and/or gangrene (p. 18), particularly of the toes or heel. This is also an ischemic type of rest symptom, being exaggerated both by walking and by lying down. The complaint is experienced in the vicinity of the ischemic lesion and its intensity is related primarily to the patient's threshold level for pain and to the extent and severity of the ulcer or patch of gangrene. The symptoms are the same for aortoiliac arterial occlusive disease and arteriosclerosis obliterans.

Signs

Generally, when intermittent claudication of a moderate degree is the only presenting complaint in a patient with arteriosclerosis obliterans, the physical findings in the involved limb are as follows: a minor reduction in cutaneous temperature of the toes; a slight decrease in intensity of the normal pink color of the skin or a slight cyanosis or pallor when the limb is in the horizontal position; dryness and scaliness of the skin of the foot, particularly the heel; absent or reduced pulsations in the common femoral, popliteal, posterior tibial, and dorsal pedal arteries; and corresponding changes in the oscillometric readings at the various levels on the lower limbs. The appearance of the toenails and hair growth on the toes may be normal or somewhat altered, depending upon the efficiency of the existing local collateral circulation. The plantar pallor test (p. 27) may be positive despite the fact that skin color in the horizontal position does not seem to be altered. There may be a delay in venous filling time (p. 62) and in return of color in the foot on placing the lower limb in dependency after having been elevated for several minutes (p. 62). Dependent rubor may develop if this position is maintained.

In the case of aortoiliac arterial occlusive disease, the physical findings are, for the most part, similar to those described above for arteriosclerosis obliterans, except for a few minor differences. For example, pulsations in the common femoral artery in the groin are generally absent bilaterally or occasionally significantly reduced, with no pulsations felt distally. In those instances in which pulsations are still present in the groin, they are usually associated with bruits in this site and in the lower anterior segments of the abdomen, over the location of the external iliac arteries. Oscillometric readings are generally zero at the level of the thigh and distally. A common early sign in the male patient who has bilateral involvement is an inability to have or maintain an erection, due to a reduction of blood flow through the hypogastric artery and hence to the arteries and venous plexuses of the penis.

Complications of Chronic Arterial Insufficiency of Lower Limbs

Both aortoiliac arterial occlusive disease and arteriosclerosis obliterans are associated with serious complications which may place the lower limb, particularly the foot, in jeopardy.

Total Arterial Thrombosis. Sudden spontaneous complete thrombosis of a main arterial channel in chronic occlusive arterial disease is usually superimposed upon a gradually occluding vessel and hence the process may have little deleterious effect, provided the previous prolonged state of chronic anoxia had acted as an effective stimulus for the production of an adequate collateral circulation. In the absence of such a response, rapid and complete occlusion of a critical artery may be followed by the appearance of nutritional changes similar to those which follow sudden occlusion of a critical artery by an embolus (p. 81). (For further discussion of arterial thrombosis, see p. 88.)

Spontaneous Noninfected Aneurysm. A relatively common complication of atherosclerosis of the abdominal aorta and its main branches is arterial aneurysm. The lesion is due either to general dilatation of the involved vessel, associated with leakage or rupture, or to stenosing arteriosclerosis, unassociated with either of the latter complications. In the stenotic type [11], the aneurysm is rarely apparent clinically, often being detected only by aortography.

The development of an arterial aneurysm in arteriosclerosis obliterans occurs as a result of weakening of the inner coats of the affected segment of vessel. This true type of lesion is observed more frequently in the popliteal artery than in any other site in the lower limbs, with involvement of the femoral artery being next in frequency (fig. 6/2). The condition is diagnosed on the basis of the presence of a pulsating mass, with a thrill and a bruit over the lesion being rather inconstant. The symptoms of a stable uncomplicated arterial aneurysm are generally of a minor degree, and hence the condition may go unrecognized unless all peripheral pulses are routinely examined.

With rapid growth of the aneurysmal sac, symptoms may develop, due to the appearance of complications of the condition. First, there may be pain locally, caused by compression of neighboring structures, particularly peripheral nerves, by the enlarging mass. Thrombosis of the associated main vein may also occur, producing swelling of the limb distally and the other signs and symptoms of occlusion of a collecting vein (p. 260). If the portion of artery from which the aneurysm arises becomes thrombosed, due to propagation of the clot in the sac, then the clinical manifestations will depend upon the rate of obstruction and the role of the vessel in supplying blood to distal tissues (fig. 6/2). Acute occlusion of a critical channel, like the popliteal artery, produces severe symptoms and signs of ischemia, frequently resulting in death of distal structures. Internal and external bleeding may follow progressive distention and thinning and then destruction of the wall of the aneurysm. Finally, the clot in the sac may be responsible for repeated showers of peripheral arterial emboli, ultimately causing a marked degree of ischemia of distal tissues and even gangrene.

Primary Cryptogenic Mycotic Aneurysm. This condition, a very serious complication of arteriosclerosis obliterans, results from the deposition of antibiotic-resistant organisms in or on an atherosclerotic plaque [4]. Because of its rather recent emergence as a clinical entity, the possibility has been raised that it is related to the widespread use of antibacterial agents and the subsequent development of resistant strains of bacteria. These con-

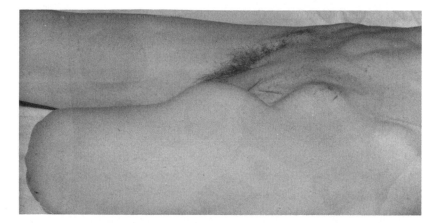

Fig. 6/2. Multiple aneurysms of the left femoral artery in a patient with arteriosclerosis obliterans. As a consequence of propagation of the clot in the lesions into the parent vessel, the latter became completely obliterated, resulting in the need for an above-knee amputation.

sist of salmonella, pneumococci, and staphylococci, in each case the organisms being responsible for a suppurative arteritis. The atherosclerotic plaque in the vessel wall becomes infected, either through septic microemboli that pass into local vasa vasorum or by surface implantation via the blood stream [7]. Due to the inflammatory process which follows, there is extensive necrosis of the plaque, resulting in weakening of the wall of the vessel or even rupture. With movement of free blood into the involved tissues, generally a false aneurysm forms locally which then becomes secondarily infected, followed by further spread of the necrotic process.

Because the onset of the condition is insidious, early recognition of primary cryptogenic mycotic aneurysm is usually not made, particularly since most of the symptoms and signs are of a general rather than of a local nature. Usually the patient, who is an older individual suffering from arteriosclerosis obliterans, begins to develop malaise, occasional bouts of fever and chills, and a progressive feeling of weakness [4]. In support of the diagnosis is a positive blood culture demonstrating the presence of staphylococci or salmonellae. Once the lesion ruptures, there is no longer any difficulty in identifying the cause for the findings. A soft tissue swelling develops in the course of one of the main arteries of the lower limbs, with the lesion progressing in size and manifesting the pulsatile character of a spontaneous arterial aneurysm. (For a discussion of atherothrombotic or cholesterol microembolism, a complication of ulceration of atheromatous plaques in the abdominal aorta associated with aortoiliac arterial occlusive disease, see p. 83.)

Ischemic Ulcers and Gangrene. A chronic occlusive arterial disease like arteriosclerosis obliterans, in itself, rarely limits blood flow to a point incompatible with viability of the tissues of the foot. However, as soon as inflammation is superimposed, as a result of infection or injury destroying the continuity of the skin, the vascular reserve may now no longer be able to meet the increased metabolic demands resulting from such a complication and, as a consequence, ischemic trophic changes may develop. In the formation of these lesions, the coexistence of diabetes plays a significant role (p. 117).

In both aortoiliac arterial occlusive disease and arteriosclerosis obliterans, when trophic changes occur spontaneously, they are usually found in the most distal portions of the limb, the toes, dorsum of the foot (fig. 6/3c), and the heel. Of course, trauma to any part of a lower limb with compromised circulation may be responsible for the appearance of an ischemic ulcer in the injured site. (For further discussion of ischemic ulceration and gangrene, see p. 40.)

Differential Diagnosis of Aortoiliac Arterial Occlusive Disease
The differential diagnosis of aortoiliac arterial occlusive disease includes consideration of entities characterized by pain in the buttocks and thighs simulating intermittent claudication in these sites. Among such disorders are herniated lumbar disk and intermittent ischemia of the cauda equina producing neurogenic claudication, entities discussed in detail on pages 12 and 13. Other conditions which may mimic intermittent claudication of aortoiliac arterial occlusive disease are arthritis of the hip, postphlebitic syndrome manifesting venous claudication (p. 289), carcinoma of the prostate with metastasis to the pelvis, and peripheral neuropathy due to diabetes (p. 120) or other disorders.

Differential Diagnosis of Arteriosclerosis Obliterans
Thromboangiitis Obliterans (Buerger's Disease). The main difficulty encountered in the differential diagnosis of arteriosclerosis obliterans is its similarity to thromboangiitis obliterans, a condition which in recent years has become a rare clinical entity in the USA, although being diagnosed with

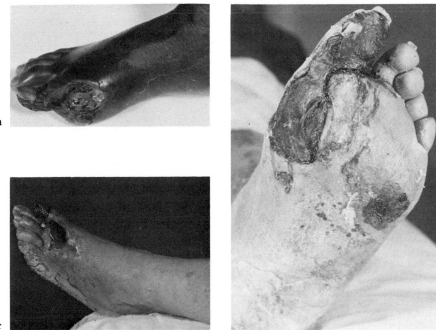

Fig. 6/3. Examples of varying degrees of trophic changes in the foot in patients with a markedly compromised local circulation due to arteriosclerosis obliterans. **a** Ulceration on the medial aspect of the foot resulting in the destruction of the great toe. **b** Extensive gangrene of the big toe and adjoining portion of foot, involving primarily the plantar surface. **c** Superficial necrosis on dorsum of foot.

increasing frequency in the Far East and elsewhere in the world [9, 15]. However, there are certain physical findings and laboratory data which are helpful in making the distinction. These are discussed below, as well as the similarities between the two disorders.

Thromboangiitis obliterans is a generalized vascular disorder with the predominant changes occurring in the extremities. It primarily affects young men and is characterized by remissions and exacerbations. Whereas at one time it was believed that the disease affected only Jews of Slavic extraction, this view has been found to have no basis. No causative agent has been established, although several have been proposed, among which is tobacco smoking.

The clinical picture of thromboangiitis obliterans resembles that of arteriosclerosis obliterans. In both, the initial symptom may be intermittent claudication of the muscles of the lower extremities, although the location of the symptom may be different. In thromboangiitis obliterans, it is generally experienced in the small muscles of the foot and in the calf and rarely above the level of the knee [15], whereas in arteriosclerosis obliterans, it is not infrequently present in the thigh, as well as in the leg and foot. Ischemic neuropathy in the toes may be present in both conditions, and in the far-advanced cases, ulceration and gangrene as well.

However, there are a number of clinical findings which differentiate thromboangiitis obliterans from arteriosclerosis obliterans, among which are the following [3]: (1) In thromboangiitis obliterans, the onset of the signs and symptoms of arterial insufficiency of the extremities occurs at a relatively young age (average of 28 years), whereas in arteriosclerosis obliterans (without coexisting diabetes), the individuals are very much older (average of 58 years). (2) All patients with thromboangiitis obliterans smoke, with production of ulcers and gangrene in a large number during the period in which this habit is continued (fig. 6/4) and rarely during abstinence. In the case of arteriosclerosis obliterans, trophic lesions have occurred in individuals who abstained or who never smoked. (3) Inflammatory involvement of the superficial veins, in the form of migratory thrombophlebitis, occurs repeatedly in about 40% of the patients with thromboangiitis obliterans (fig. 12/4), whereas this condition has not been reported in arteriosclerosis obliterans. (4) In thromboangiitis obliterans, obstruction of the brachial, radial, and ulnar arteries in the upper limbs is present in a relatively large percentage of cases [9], and in approximately 15%, ulcers and/or gangrene develops on the fingers and hand (fig. 6/4b), whereas the latter changes are rarely, if at all, observed in arteriosclerosis obliterans. (5) In thromboangiitis obliterans, arteriographic examination of the upper extremities may reveal occlusive lesions in the brachial, radial, and ulnar arteries, findings not noted in arteriosclerosis obliterans. (6) In thromboangiitis obliterans, arteriographic study of the lower extremities generally demonstrates stenosis or complete occlusions of the popliteal artery and anterior and posterior tibial arteries (fig. 6/5a, b) and rarely of more proximal vessels [15]. In contrast, in arteriosclerosis obliterans, obstructive lesions may be found in the aortic bifurcation and the common iliac, external iliac, common femoral, and superficial (fig. 6/5c, d) and deep femoral arteries, as well as the distal vessels in leg and foot. In the latter condition, also, the arteries demonstrate irregular and eccentric filling defects and segments of complete

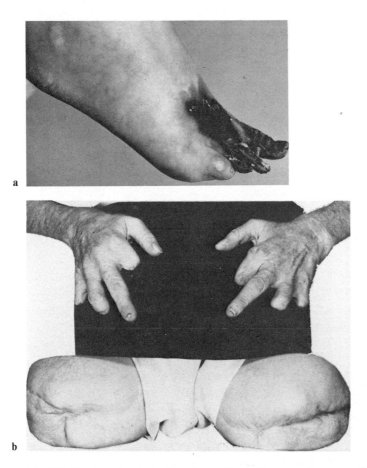

Fig. 6/4. Trophic changes in thromboangiitis obliterans. **a** Gangrene of the right foot involving four of the toes and extending onto the foot proper. **b** Loss of fingers on both hands and of both lower extremities due to extensive gangrene of the four limbs. Both patients persisted in smoking despite the progression of the necrotic process. Reproduced from ref. [1] with permission.

occlusion (fig. 6/5c, d). Visualization of the vessels below the block is frequently observed as a result of the movement of contrast material through the profuse network of collateral channels generally found bridging the obstructed portion of artery. In contrast, in thromboangiitis obliterans, the arteries show narrowing but not the filling defects, although sites of complete occlusion may be present. For the most part, the vessels are less tortuous than in arteriosclerosis obliterans.

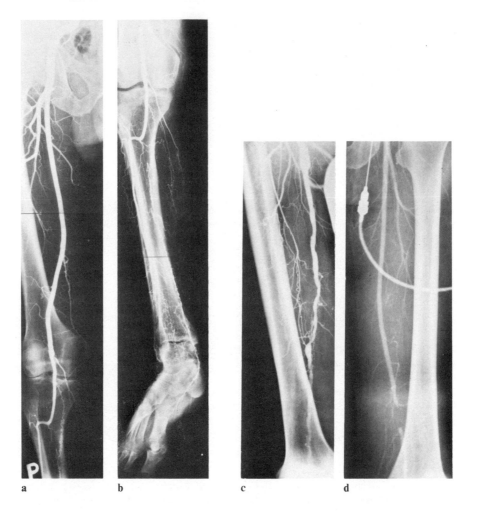

a b c d

Fig. 6/5. Diagnostic arteriographic changes. **a, b** Changes observed in thromboangiitis obliterans. **a** Common, deep, and superficial femoral arteries in the thigh demonstrate normal contour and no signs of involvement. **b** Popliteal artery appears to be normal, but the posterior tibial artery is completely occluded at its origin. The anterior tibial artery demonstrates a total obstruction in its lower two thirds. Collateral vessels are noted in the leg and foot. **c, d** Changes observed in arteriosclerosis obliterans. **c** Irregularities, stenoses, and complete occlusions noted in the superficial femoral artery. The distortion of the lumen is the result of projection of atherosclerotic plaques. Numerous collateral vessels are present in the thigh. **d** Total occlusion of the superficial femoral artery in its passage through Hunter's canal in the lower third of the thigh. The distal portion of the vessel is visualized through flow in the collateral vascular tree.

Mönckeberg's Sclerosis. Although this disorder is considered to be a chronic occlusive arterial disorder, there is considerable question as to whether it, by itself, is responsible for any significant impairment of local circulation and, hence, whether it causes any clinically identifiable difficulties. Typically, there is gross deposition of calcium in the media of large muscular arteries, which is readily visualized by means of soft tissue X-ray technique. At first it was generally considered to be part of the aging process and quite distinct and independent of the atherosclerotic process (p. 96). However, some evidence has been presented to support the view that the calcification which occurs in or along elastic fibers and along internal elastic lamella constitutes the earliest form of plaque formation and hence is an integral part of the atheroma [12]. It is difficult to state whether the pathologic process develops in muscle cells of the media or whether the primary event is a proliferative or degenerative change in the intercellular connective tissue, followed by calcium deposition. The latter, in turn, is considered to lead to destruction and replacement of muscle cells.

In any event, medial calcification does not materially reduce the size of the lumen of the involved vessel and hence is not responsible for the development of symptoms of local arterial insufficiency, such as intermittent claudication or rest pain due to ischemic neuropathy. Nor are ischemic ulcerations or gangrene ever present in the condition. Furthermore, examination of the limb reveals no signs of impaired local circulation, with skin color and temperature, hair and nail growth, and sweating pattern all being normal. The amplitude of the pulsations in the posterior tibial and dorsal pedal arteries in the foot may be reduced somewhat because of the damping effect the deposition of calcium in the media of the vessels has on this factor. Similarly, and for the same reason, the oscillometric readings at the level of the ankle may be decreased to low normal levels. It is also important to note that in Mönckeberg's sclerosis, there are no signs of generalized atherosclerosis elsewhere, of the type frequently found in arteriosclerosis obliterans.

Nonvascular Conditions. There are a large number of orthopedic, neurologic, and metabolic clinical entities characterized by pain in the feet and legs which may be mistaken for intermittent claudication due to arteriosclerosis obliterans. For this reason, they must be considered in the differential diagnosis of the latter disorder. Since they are all described in detail on pages 9–12, there is no need to discuss them any further.

Prognosis

Aortoiliac Arterial Occlusive Disease and Arteriosclerosis Obliterans

In the case of the patient suffering from either aortoiliac arterial occlusive disease or arteriosclerosis obliterans, the outlook depends, in great part, upon the degree of atherosclerotic involvement simultaneously present in vital organs elsewhere, particularly in the heart, brain, and kidneys, rather than upon the severity of the occlusive changes in the lower limbs. Only rarely does death result from the latter, as for example when a major amputation is required to manage extensive gangrene in a patient who is a poor candidate for any type of anesthesia and surgical procedure.

Since the pathologic process in the blood vessels of the lower limbs is progressive, the appearance of nutritional disturbances will eventually depend upon the efficiency of the collateral circulation. If the latter continues to grow at a rate which is sufficient to offset the slow occlusion taking place in a major arterial trunk, then ulcers or gangrene will never be observed. Of course, if the existing equilibrium is destroyed, as by trauma to the extremity, then they may develop.

The great majority of people suffering from either aortoiliac arterial occlusive disease or arteriosclerosis obliterans will, therefore, be able to lead a fairly normal life, except for some difficulty in walking, provided that they abstain from smoking and pay strict attention to the local care of their feet. However, as a group, longevity is significantly reduced because of reasons already noted. The cause of death is primarily cardiovascular diseases and, much less often, cerebrovascular disorders. (For contribution of diabetes to the prognosis of aortoiliac arterial occlusive disease and arteriosclerosis obliterans, see pp. 112, 117.)

Thromboangiitis Obliterans

Thromboangiitis obliterans has a good prognosis provided the patient stops smoking and never reverts back to this habit. At the same time, he must take meticulous care of his feet. Under such conditions, the pathologic process no longer appears to progress and walking distance will increase as the development of collateral vessels is stimulated at the same time that no further occlusion of main arterial channels occurs. Moreover, in most instances, ulcers or gangrene will not form on the feet and old ones may heal. Of course, severe trauma to the limb may still result in the appearance of new trophic lesions.

If the patient with Buerger's disease continues to smoke, there is little question that more and more vessels in the four extremities will be obliterated, with a very good possibility that ulcers and gangrene will appear. Generally, no therapeutic response can be expected with either medical or surgical programs under such circumstances, the final available measure to control the severe pain being minor or major amputation of a limb or limbs. Since the pathologic occlusive process eventually also affects critical vessels in the heart, brain, and gastrointestinal system, among other organs, longevity may be markedly reduced by progression of ischemia in such sites.

References

1   Abramson, D.I.: Diagnosis and treatment of peripheral vascular disorders (Hoeber-Harper, New York 1956).
2   Abramson, D.I.: Vascular disorders of the extremities (Harper & Row, Hagerstown 1974).
3   Abramson, D.I.; Zayas, A.M.; Canning, J.R.; Edinburg, E.: Thromboangiitis obliterans: a true clinical entity. Am. J. Cardiol. *12:* 107 (1963).
4   Blum, L.; Keefer, E.B.C.: Clinical entity of cryptogenic mycotic aneurysm. J. Am. med. Ass. *188:* 505 (1964).
5   Constantinides, P.: Importance of the endothelium and blood platelets in the pathogenesis of atherosclerosis. Triangle *15:* 53 (1976).
6   Constantinides, P.; Robinson, M.: Ultrastructural injury of arterial endothelium. 1. Effects of pH, osmolarity, anoxia, and temperature. Archs Path. *88:* 99 (1969).
7   Duncan, S.M.; Cooley, D.A.: Surgical considerations in aortitis. Part II: mycotic aneurysms. Texas H. Institute J. *10:* 329 (1983).
8   Edwards, P.A.; Fogelman, A.M.: Current concepts of the pathogenesis of atherosclerosis. Pract. Cardiol. *7:* 131 (1981).
9   Hirai, M.; Shionoya, S.: Arterial obstruction of the upper limb in Buerger's disease: its incidence and primary lesion. Br. J. Surg. *66:* 124 (1979).
10 Leriche, R.: De la résection du carrefour aortico-iliaque avec double sympathéctomie lombaire pour thrombose artéritique de l'aorte. Le syndrôme de l'oblitération termino-aortique par artérite. Presse méd. *48:* 601 (1940).
11 Martin, P.: On abdominal aortic aneurysms. J. cardiovasc. Surg. *19:* 597 (1978).
12 Pareira, M.D.; Handler, F.D.; Blumenthal, H.J.: Aging processes in the arterial and venous system of the lower extremities. Circulation *8:* 36 (1953).
13 Schwartz, C.J.; Erhart, L.A.; Gerrity, R.G.: Atheroma: a review. Hosp. Med. *13:*18 (1977).
14 Schwartz, S.M.: Hypertension, endothelial injury, and atherosclerosis. Cardiovasc. Med. *2:* 991 (1977).
15 Shionoya, S.; Ban, I.; Nakata, Y.; et al.: Involvement of the iliac artery in Buerger's disease: pathogenesis and arterial reconstruction. J. cardiovasc. Surg. *19:* 69 (1978).
16 Stemerman, M.B.: Atherosclerosis: the etiologic role of blood elements and cellular changes. Cardiovasc. Med. *3:* 17 (1978).
17 Szczeklik, A.: Prostacyclin and atherosclerosis. Triangle *19:* 61 (1980).

7 Spontaneous Chronic Occlusive Arterial Disorders: The Diabetic Foot and Leg

General Considerations

The podiatrist should always view the foot of a diabetic patient with great circumspection and some misgivings if he or she is contemplating performing an elective therapeutic measure on it. When arteriosclerosis obliterans coexists, such a combination is an absolute contraindication to any podiatric surgical approach.

Since the advent of insulin in 1921, ketoacidosis is no longer the predominant cause of death in diabetes mellitus, and instead serious vascular problems affecting critical organs have assumed this role, with the disease currently ranking fourth in mortality in the USA. Such a situation has developed because of the survival of many patients who would have died without insulin, thus permitting them to live long enough to become candidates for the various types of vascular disorders associated with this disease.

Diabetes mellitus is not a single disorder but an assortment of primary and secondary entities that have in common an impairment of carbohydrate metabolism, as manifested by an increased fasting plasma glucose level. That the predisposition of this disorder is genetically determined, there is little doubt.

In this chapter, an attempt is made to formulate a basis for the better understanding of those vascular manifestations of diabetes mellitus that are clinically apparent in the foot and leg and that collectively have been referred to as the diabetic foot.

Basis for Accelerated Atherogenesis in Diabetes

The question as to whether diabetes mellitus has a significant etiologic role in, or influence on, the natural course of arteriosclerosis obliterans has not been fully answered. It is generally accepted, however, that in the presence of diabetes mellitus, atherogenesis is markedly accelerated [6], an advanced stage of this process being found even in the very young diabetic patient. As a general rule, atherosclerosis in the lower limbs and elsewhere appears a decade earlier in the diabetic patient than in the nondiabetic individual, and it is responsible for a more severe degree of vascular insufficiency. Some of the factors which have been implicated in the rapid development of atherosclerosis under such circumstances are briefly discussed below.

Role of Abnormal Cholesterol and Lipid Metabolism. Accelerated atherogenesis in diabetes has been attributed to the abnormal cholesterol and lipid metabolism found in this disorder [10]. Of interest in this regard are the findings that such alterations are frequently reversed when the diabetic state is controlled with insulin, with the result that hyperlipemia in the treated patient is neither so common nor so marked as has been supposed. Moreover, since a cause-and-effect relationship has not been proved, the theory that alterations in cholesterol and lipid metabolism are the prime cause of arteriosclerosis in diabetes must await much more intensive study before being considered seriously.

Role of Insulin Production. It is possible that insulin may be the link between diabetes and arteriosclerosis. For it has been shown that this substance interferes with the action of other hormones in activating a fat-hydrolyzing lipase normally present in the endothelial lining of the arterial wall. Since the fat hydrolyzing lipase has the function of initiating mobilization and removal of fat, the inhibiting effect of insulin may result in fat accumulation in the form of atheromatous plaques. The fact that the diabetic may demonstrate periods in which the circulating insulin level is abnormally high may be of importance in this regard. For example, exogenous insulin has been found to be present in excess of requirements for some time after its administration. Moreover, in the case of the individual who develops diabetes in the later decades, initially the endogenous insulin level in the blood stream is often higher than normal, even though the material secreted by the pancreas at this stage is not very effective in glucose metabolism.

Role of Serum Glucosamine and Total Protein-Bound Serum Polysaccharide Levels. It has been found that glucosamine and total protein-bound polysaccharides are significantly elevated in the serum of diabetic patients with well-established, detectable degenerative vascular disease, whereas values are normal in those in whom abnormal change in blood vessels are absent. The significance of such findings must await further investigation.

Role of Deranged Arterial Wall Metabolism. There is some speculation as to the relationship between blood glucose levels and the formation of sorbitol as a causative factor in atherosclerosis. When glucose levels are high, sorbitol, a product of glucose metabolism, is enzymatically formed. In this regard, increased activity of the enzymes involved in sorbitol metabolism has been identified in the aortic wall, resulting in changes in intimal metabolism that predispose to atheroma formation.

Role of Pathologic Changes in Vasa Vasorum of Large Arteries. The typical changes in the microcirculation associated with diabetes (p. 116) may also affect the vasa vasorum (arterioles) supplying the walls of large arteries, thus rendering them more susceptible to plaque formation. Involvement of small arteries by the same process could also contribute to a more rapid production of arteriosclerotic changes, since the resulting alterations would constitute an increase in local peripheral resistance, thus placing a greater load on main arteries.

Pathophysiology
Changes in the Microcirculation. Physiologic examination of the cutaneous microcirculation of diabetics has revealed dilatation of the entire length of the capillary, including its venular end. In the great percentage of cases, immature capillary plexuses are present. Venous congestion is another frequent finding. A possible explanation for such changes is that a high pressure exists in the terminal vessels.

Alterations in Capillary Permeability. It is widely accepted that in the diabetic, there is an increase in permeability of the capillary wall, thus making such an individual prone to hemorrhagic and nonhemorrhagic bleb formation following even mild pressure to the skin. This view is supported by studies using fluorescence techniques, all of which have demonstrated a considerable degree of leakage as compared with normal capillary vessels. Such a situation exists despite the fact that thickening of the basement membrane commonly noted in the capillary bed of the diabetic (p. 116) would be expected to counteract this tendency.

Capillary Fragility. This response in the skin of diabetics with vascular manifestations is significantly increased. As a consequence, subcutaneous hemorrhages are not uncommon. Such an abnormal trait may also contribute to the development of hemorrhagic blisters and hemorrhages under calluses, responsible, in part, for the initiation of neurotrophic ulcers.

Pathology

Vascular abnormalities in diabetes are found in all segments of the arterial tree (macroangiopathy) and of the microcirculation (microangiopathy) and consist of both chemical and morphologic alterations. The pathologic changes can be divided into the following categories: (1) lesions of large arteries which usually resemble the atheromatous process (p. 97); (2) nonatheromatous intimal proliferation of the walls of small terminal arteries, such as the digital vessels, resulting in narrowed lumens due to thickened walls, and (3) arteriolar and capillary microangiopathy. Most of the vascular difficulties found in the diabetic foot can be attributed to stenosis or complete obstruction of the terminal arteries and vessels of the microcirculation, although involvement of large arteries also plays a significant role in the development of a compromised local circulation.

Chemical Changes in Vascular Wall. Of interest with regard to the pathologic alterations in diabetes is the observation that chemical analysis of brachial and femoral arteries from patients with this condition revealed 3 times as much cholesterol and 7 times as much calcium in these structures than was found in vessels from nondiabetic persons. Such data support the view that primary calcinosis of the media is a fairly common change in the diabetic. In some instances, the abnormality is of such magnitude as to produce active ossification of the arterial wall, particularly in the case of the blood vessels of the lower extremities. Preceding the deposition of the calcium, there are destructive alterations in the muscular and elastic layers of the media, similar to the changes noted in Mönckeberg's sclerosis (p. 109).

Large Artery Involvement. In the juvenile diabetic, atheromatous lesions start in early childhood and progress throughout his life, being favored by good nutrition. Although with routine staining the histologic appearance of the abnormalities in the intima is the same as in the nondiabetic individual with atherosclerosis (p. 96), special stains have identified some of the infiltrates in the vessel wall to be mucopolysaccharide in nature.

The location of the atherosclerotic process in the large arteries of the lower limbs is significantly influenced by the coexistence of diabetes. For example, in the young diabetic with arteriosclerosis obliterans, the brunt of the pathologic changes falls on the smaller, more distal main vessels, such as the popliteal and the anterior and posterior tibial arteries, thus resembling the location of the pathologic changes observed in thromboangiitis obliterans (p. 106). Such alterations are in contrast to those observed in the nondiabetic individual with arteriosclerosis obliterans, in whom there is often involvement of the proximal major vessels, such as the aortoiliac, common femoral, deep femoral, and superficial femoral arteries, as well as of the distal arterial tree.

Microangiopathy. The changes in the microcirculation (arterioles, capillaries, and venules) in diabetes are considered to be characteristic and unique to this disorder [16] but not necessarily pathognomonic of it [19]. The pathologic changes in the capillaries consist of accumulations of fine and, to a lesser extent, more mature collagen fibers, distributed in a focal manner, the deposits appearing as thickened basement membranes.

The process is extensive and is found in a variety of tissues, including the skin and muscle of the lower limbs. It has also been observed in prediabetics [16], suggesting that it precedes laboratory manifestations of carbohydrate intolerance as reflected in elevated blood sugar levels. In fact, the possibility has been raised that microangiopathy is a consequence of a metabolic disorder associated with insulin deficiency. However, opposed to such a view is the reported finding that thickening of the basement membrane of capillaries also occurs with normal aging in nondiabetics (although rarely to the extent seen in those with long-standing diabetes), thus indicating that this process is not specific for diabetes. The relationship of microangiopathy to the appearance of clinical vascular manifestations of diabetes has not been established.

The degree of hypertrophy of the basement membrane, which can be quantitated by electron microscopic techniques, cannot be clearly correlated with such factors as age or weight of the patient or with the duration or severity of the associated carbohydrate abnormality. However, with regard to the latter factor, there is some evidence to support the pathogenetic role of excessive blood sugar, each incremental rise in the level appearing to increase the likelihood of cardiovascular events occurring. Augmented vascular pressure also seems to contribute to diabetic angiopathy. In this regard, it has been noted that basement membrane thickening is exaggerated in the lower limbs of diabetics, where the venous pressure is the greatest, thus raising the resistance to blood flow through the capillaries. It is possible that microangiopathy follows injury to the endothelium of the microcirculation, increasing vessel permeability and leading to a proliferation of connective tissue (basement membrane thickening).

In general, the average basement width in the capillaries of the diabetic is greater than twice that found in normal subjects (800–2,000 Å). This striking accumulation of basement membrane material presents as a thick red ring in the vascular wall when stained by periodic acid-Schiff reagent (PAS) and is said to be PAS-positive. It is composed of glycoprotein, a specialized form of collagen material containing a carbohydrate content of about 9% [2]. The inner surface of the basement membrane serves as a 'scaffold' for parenchymal cells and its outer side fastens the vessel to surrounding connective tissue. The origin of the materials making up the basement membrane and the reason for their increased deposition in diabetes to cause a thickening of this structure remain a mystery.

Associated with the changes in basement membrane are endothelial proliferation and localized weakening of the vessel wall. The latter abnormality may be the precursor of capillary microaneurysms commonly observed in diabetes, especially with foot angiopathy.

Vascular and Neurologic Abnormalities of the Diabetic Foot

As a general rule, it can be stated that patients suffering from diabetes for at least 10 years (regardless of the age of onset) are likely to have some clinically significant atherosclerosis (and hence symptoms and signs of local vascular insufficiency), as well as other manifestations of the disorder. However, the rate of development of the various conditions differs from individual to individual [9]. Rather than considering them to be complications of diabetes, these entities should be viewed as concomitants of the disease, produced by the interaction of insulin deficiency and hyperglycemia with other risk factors in ways which are not well understood [13].

The vascular and neurologic changes observed in the diabetic foot present in a wide variety of ways, ranging from peripheral neuropathy to wet gangrene with spreading cellulitis. Some are responsible for considerable morbidity and mortality.

Possible Etiologic Mechanisms Responsible for Clinical Vascular Manifestations of Diabetes
A number of factors have been proposed as being responsible for the increased incidence of severe disorders of the vascular tree in the lower limbs noted in diabetics. These include: (1) a greater degree of atherosclerosis of large arteries due either to onset of this state at an earlier age or to an

accelerated rate of progression; (2) increased terminal small artery or arteriolar disease; (3) a variation in the pattern of occlusive disease resulting in greater interference with tissue perfusion; (4) less-effective development of collateral circulation; (5) changes in capillary permeability, causing interference with diffusion of respiratory gases, nutrients, or metabolites; (6) increased viscosity of the blood; (7) sensory and autonomic neuropathy producing either an adverse vascular response or an increased incidence of trauma to, or neglect of, lesions in the foot, and (8) a marked vulnerability to infection (see below). As has already been stated (p. 116), no clear-cut evidence exists to implicate the increased thickness of the basement membrane of capillaries in the development of clinical vascular manifestations of diabetes. However, none of the enumerated mechanisms can be eliminated from consideration, although it must also be emphasized that evidence in support of the importance of some of them is either unconvincing or nonexistent.

Ischemic Factor. A number of the above states may be responsible for the development of local ischemia. The hypoxia and acidosis associated with the latter, in turn, further increase the viscosity of the blood serum and cause rigidity of the red blood cells, alterations which aggravate the ischemia by contributing to the already existing impairment of perfusion through the tissues. The resulting stasis in the microcirculation, together with the increased thrombogenic and decreased fibrinolytic activity found in the blood of diabetics, favors thrombosis and complete occlusion of vessels. All of these processes predispose to loss of viability of local structures and to the end stage of gangrene. Of interest in this regard is the report indicating that patchy gangrene of the foot or isolated necrosis of toes occurs in 67% of diabetics, as compared with 18% of nondiabetics [8], suggesting a greater localization of occlusions in the arteries of the feet of diabetics.

Contribution of Infection. Equally important in the production of nutritional disturbances in the diabetic foot is the fact that diabetes undermines the natural defenses of the body and the resistance of tissues to infection. Moreover, the disorder encourages cutaneous inflammation, probably through dehydration, altered immunologic capacity of tissue cells, and an abnormal state of cellular nutrition. However, the total quantity of cellular exudate resulting from tissue injury does not approach that of healthy controls. There is likewise a delayed leukocyte migration to the site of tissue injury, a finding which may be related to subnormal handling of infection at the cellular level. Also of importance is the finding in untreated decompensated diabetics of extreme reductions in plasma levels of fibronectin, a complex glycoprotein. Loss of this large molecule has been associated with prolonged wound-healing, altered bone and connective tissue metabolism, and increased susceptibility to infection.

Among other factors contributing to the greater vulnerability of the diabetic foot to inflammation and infection is damping of sensory perception due to a frequently coexisting neuropathy. Such a situation causes the patient to become insensitive to minor trauma, nontreatment of which results in extension of the destructive process.

However, it is necessary to point out that there is some evidence to support the view that a diabetic who is well controlled with insulin is no more susceptible to infection than a non-diabetic [12]. The advent of antibiotics has also helped to manage infections in diabetes and thus reduce the mortality and morbidity due to bacterial invasion.

Intermittent Claudication

As in the case of arteriosclerosis obliterans and for the same reasons, intermittent claudication (p. 7) may be present in the diabetic lower extremity. The etiologic agent is an inadequate arterial circulation to the muscles locally, due to stenosis or complete occlusion of arteries supplying the limb. Because the symptoms are frequently located in the foot, they may mimic complaints originating in orthopedic alterations in arches or joints locally. (For treatment of intermittent claudication, see p. 141.)

Peripheral Neuropathy

Peripheral neuropathy, a relatively common finding in both the insulin-dependent and noninsulin-dependent diabetic patient, may occur at any stage of the disease, even subclinical. It is usually bilateral and more frequently affects the lower than the upper limbs. It is found primarily in middle-aged and elderly individuals.

Pathogenesis. The mechanism responsible for the development of peripheral neuropathy in diabetes is not well understood. Microangiopathy affecting the vasa nervorum of peripheral nerves (p. 116) has been considered to be an etiologic agent in the asymmetric type of neuropathy (p. 120), but even under such circumstances, there does not seem to be diffuse involvement of these vessels. Infarction in the involved nerves has also been reported [15]. In the case of the symmetric type of neuropathy (see below), the possibility has been advanced that there is no relationship between nerve involvement and vascular alterations. Instead, the etiologic agent has been considered to be either a specific nutritional deficiency or abnormal carbohydrate or fat metabolism. In this regard, recently it has been demonstrated that decrements in motor nerve conduction velocity could be highly correlated with the degree of fasting hyperglycemia in untreated patients with noninsulin-dependent diabetes. Moreover, the nerve conduction velocity figures improved when the blood sugar was therapeutically lowered. Such results suggest that symmetric peripheral neuropathy is directly related to a metabolic defect secondary to insulin deficiency. In summary, it is likely that both vascular and metabolic effects are important in the pathogenesis of diabetic neuropathy.

Pathology. The essential morphologic lesions in peripheral neuropathy are demyelination (degenerative changes in the Schwann cells) and a lesser degree of involvement of the axons of small fibers of peripheral nerves and of dorsal nerve roots, with secondary alterations in the spinal cord. Sensory, motor, or autonomic nerves may thus be affected, with pathologic changes being either isolated or present in several nerves, often symmetrically.

Clinical Manifestations. Peripheral neuropathy cannot be considered a single clinical entity, with the symptoms and signs varying considerably depending upon which nerves are affected. The different syndromes include: distal symmetric polyneuropathy involving both motor and sensory functions; autonomic neuropathy, causing autosympathectomy of the lower limbs, and proximal painful mononeuropathy (asymmetric peripheral neuropathy), resulting in asymmetric dysfunction of a major nerve trunk.

Asymmetric peripheral neuropathy usually has a sudden onset, characterized by pain and motor weakness. In the lower limb, there may be multiple involvement of the femoral, sciatic, or obturator nerve and, as a result, the condition often is confused with lumbar disk disease. The clinical picture usually stabilizes, followed by functional recovery in weeks, months, or years, related to the rate of regeneration and remyelination of the affected axons.

Distal symmetric polyneuropathy, the most frequently encountered type of diabetic neuropathy, characteristically has an insidious slow onset and progressive course. The symptoms are generally first experienced in the toes, with the condition spreading in a roughly symmetric fashion to involve the proximal portions of the lower limbs in a 'stocking-glove' type of sensory change. The abnormal neurologic changes cannot be identified with any particular nerves.

An early symptom in peripheral neuropathy is severe pain in the lower limb, which represents degeneration and hence irritation of nociceptive sensory nerve fibers. Symptoms may also take the form of paresthesias of the toes, fleeting lancinating sensations, and a subjective sense of burning or coldness in the foot. All of these are prone to nocturnal exacerbation. As the process continues to progress to the point of interfering with the transmission of afferent impulses to the spinal cord, numbness or 'deadness' replaces the noxious sensations.

Associated physical findings are marked loss of vibration sense perception (using a standard 128 tuning fork), especially in the toes; absent ankle jerks; absent or reduced patellar reflexes, and cutaneous hypersensitivity progressing to diminution and then loss of sensory perception (pain and fine touch) and reduced awareness of joint position as stimulation of neurons by the pathologic process is followed by degeneration of these structures. Neurogenic atrophy of the small muscles of the foot may be an early finding (fig. 7/1a, b), leading to deformity (p. 124). However, as a general rule, the motor nerves are much less heavily damaged than are the sensory components. Paralleling the degree of clinical alteration in the peripheral mixed nerves is a continued slowing of sensory and motor nerve conduction velocities as determined by laboratory testing. Roentgenographic studies will frequently reveal medial artery calcification.

With initial irritation of the sympathetic fibers in the peripheral mixed nerves, early signs of increased sympathetic tone appear, in the form of coldness, cyanosis, hyperhidrosis, and even edema of the foot. As the process advances to a stage of nonfunction due to total degeneration of the fibers, autosympathectomy replaces the findings of exaggerated tone. Now the limb is warm and well-colored, and the skin is dry, fissured, and susceptible to cracking. The peripheral pulses are bounding, and the oscillometric readings at various levels on the lower limb are high normal, changes which, naturally, are only observed when there are no atherosclerotic occlusions in the large arteries. Studies exist indicating that in the autosympathectomized foot, the blood flow pattern is altered, in the sense that there is arteriovenous shunting, either through preexisting normal arteriovenous anastomoses or through an abnormal capillary bed. Such bypassing of the normal capillary bed will obviously impair tissue oxygenation. This concept is supported by the finding in the autosympathectomized foot of abnormal sonograms (Doppler blood-velocity profiles) and increased venous oxygenation of blood in the dorsal foot veins [5, 7]. Distention of the latter vessels may be quite prominent even when the limb is elevated, suggesting that there are an augmented blood flow and an elevated blood pressure in them. (For the treatment of peripheral neuropathy, see p. 170.)

Differential Diagnosis. Although generally leg pain in diabetics is ascribed to underlying peripheral neuropathy, in some instances this symptom is due to the mental depression that may exist in such individuals. It is usually bilateral, aching in character, unremitting, and intensified at night [13]. Increased sensitivity of the skin frequently causes even a light touch to be painful or uncomfortable. The most severe pain is usually located in the thighs, but it may also be present in the entire limb. An important differential diagnostic point is that regression of the symptom occurs in response to administration of antidepressant drugs, such as the tricyclic, tetracyclic, and monoamine oxidase inhibitor groups, relief usually being experienced within 7–20 days following the onset of therapy. On the other hand, agents purported to act on peripheral nerves (e.g. phenytoin and Carbamazepine) are generally unsuccessful in controlling the pain. (For the differentiation of peripheral neuropathy from ischemic neuropathy and from other conditions which may mimic it, see p. 5.)

Neurotrophic Ulcer

The neurotrophic ulcer is a relatively common vascular entity in the diabetic patient also suffering from peripheral neuropathy (p. 119), although it may be found in other conditions in which there is interference with transmission of afferent impulses, such as peripheral neuropathy associated with chronic alcoholism, syphilis, syringomyelia, poliomyelitis, spinal cord compression, and myelodysplasia. Of interest is the observation that many patients with severe neurotrophic foot ulcers tolerate such lesions for long periods of time before they eventually seek medical attention [18], probably because of the lack of associated local pain.

Pathogenesis and Pathology. The neurotrophic ulcer is most often seen in the hypalgesic foot, demonstrating loss of sensation and rarely in one suffering from hyperesthesia. Generally, as a result of thinning out of the fat pads over the metatarsal arch in the foot, callosities are formed as space replacements; the neurotrophic ulcer then develops due to continuous pressure of the callosities on a devitalized dermal area. Calluses also form because of tight, poorly fitting shoes and muscular imbalance. Likewise of

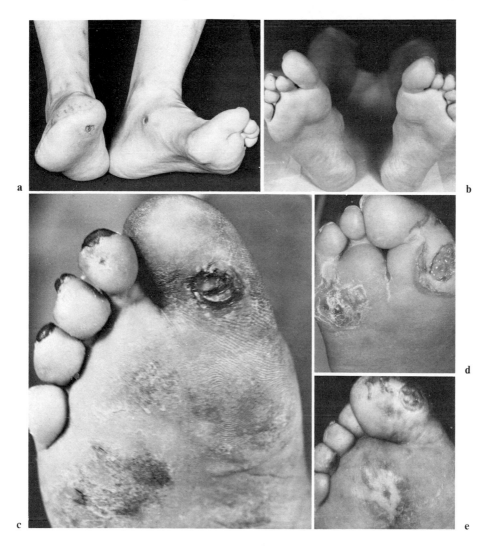

Fig. 7/1. Complications of diabetes. **a, b** Marked atrophy of small muscles of the feet due to peripheral neuropathy, associated with tingling and burning in toes and areas of hypesthesia and anesthesia of the feet. **c–e** Neurotrophic ulcers on plantar surface of feet over metatarsal heads in patients with diabetic peripheral neuropathy. In **c** and **e,** gangrenous plaque present on great toe. Reproduced from ref. [1] with permission.

importance in the formation of a neurotrophic ulcer are changes in the dynamics of the foot, leading to overloading of the forefoot (see below), and dryness of the skin, which follows autosympathectomy due to the associated peripheral neuropathy.

Clinical Manifestations. The neurotrophic ulcer in the diabetic patient is commonly found under hard areas of a callus on the plantar surface of the foot, located either at the base of the great, third, or fifth toe, over a metatarsal head (fig. 7/1c–e), or on the heel, all high pressure areas. The lesion usually starts with the appearance of erythema, and then the site becomes swollen and fluctuant, followed by the formation of a true abscess. This generally opens outward, with drainage of thin and malodorous seropurulent material. The ulcer may appear to be small, but frequently it undermines rather extensively below the skin. It may have a deep funnel-like base extending as far as the underlying bone. In advanced cases, there may be widespread destruction of the metatarsal heads, with multiple areas of suppurative osteomyelitis. Under these circumstances, bone sequestrums may be extruded through the base of the ulcer. The evolution of the lesion is often chronic, showing very little tendency to spontaneous healing.

The diagnosis of a diabetic neurotrophic ulcer is made on the basis of marked destruction of soft tissues and even of bones of the foot associated with practically no pain, the presence of a good circulation in the main arteries of the foot in most instances, and the existence of peripheral neuropathy manifested by impaired or absent vibration sense perception and other sensory changes and a decrease or loss of the ankle jerk. In the presence of an adequate local arterial circulation, frequently there are roentgenographic signs of rarefaction, lysis, or destruction of bone in the site of involvement. (For the treatment of the neurotrophic ulcer, see p. 171.)

Muscle Imbalance

The anatomically distorted foot frequently found in diabetic patients, especially when combined with rheumatoid arthritis, is due to local imbalance of the intrinsic muscles deprived of adequate sensory input (particularly proprioception) and motor impulses as a result of peripheral neuropathy. Consequently, cavus formation, foot drop, elevation of the arch, rocker-bottom foot, hammering of toes, clawed toes, subluxation of metatarsophalangeal joints, and prominence and protrusion of metatarsal heads may all occur. The loss of proprioception and pain sensation, together with the motor abnormalities, causes a redistribution of pressure during standing

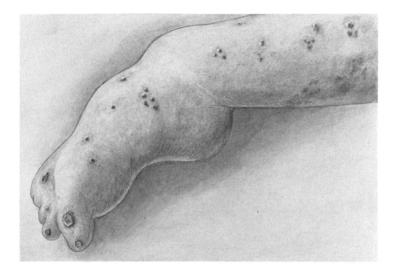

Fig. 7/2. Drawing of changes produced by neurotrophic arthropathy of ankle joint (Charcot's joint), producing marked distortion of the foot.

and walking. As a result, the pressure under metatarsal heads of diabetic patients with peripheral neuropathy may rise in excess of 20 kg/cm² on walking [4], as compared with 10 kg/cm² or less in the normal foot [11]. Such alterations in dynamics significantly increase the risk of painless trauma to the foot and hence the production of a neurotrophic ulcer (p. 122).

Neurotrophic Arthropathy
(Neuropathic Joint Disease; Charcot's Joints)
Neurotrophic arthropathy is a form of chronic progressive degenerative arthropathy of one or more peripheral joints in the lower limbs associated with various neurologic disorders. The clinical result is the production of a deforming, primarily painless or nearly painless joint disorder, frequently affecting the structures of the foot (fig. 7/2).

Etiology and Incidence. Charcot's joints usually develop in people past the age of 40 years. Diabetic taboneuropathy is now the main cause of the condition, although at one time it was syphilis. Other etiologic agents are syringomyelia, chronic alcoholism, poliomyelitis, spinal cord compression, hereditary sensory neuropathy, peripheral nerve section, and leprosy.

Pathogenesis and Pathology. Common to all the neurologic conditions responsible for the development of neurotrophic arthropathy is a loss of proprioceptive and/or pain sensation. Such an abnormality, in turn, leads to relaxation of supporting structures and chronic instability of the involved joint. At the same time, the foot is deprived of protective reactions to minor traumas of daily physical activity and subjected to unusual stresses because of the underlying neurologic disease. As a consequence of these factors, a type of premature severe degenerative joint disease develops.

The pathologic changes in neurotrophic arthropathy are similar to those observed in the ordinary degenerative joint disease. Common findings are fibrillation and erosion of lining cartilage, destruction of menisci, formation of loose bodies, and finally marginal osteophytic growth [14]. However, the latter alteration is more extensive than encountered in ordinary degenerative joint disease, perhaps because of the hypermobility of the Charcot's joint. Proliferation of cartilage occurs in the zone of provisional calcification beneath the articular surface, followed by calcification and, in areas, dense bone formation. Intra-articular complications may develop, in the form of subluxations, dislocations, and fractures of articular facets, epicondyles, or condyles.

Clinical Manifestations. The symptoms and signs associated with neurotrophic arthropathy are generally insidious in their onset. The first finding may be an enlargement of a single joint in the foot, associated with some discomfort, disproportionately mild compared with the changes noted in the involved structure. Another early sign is instability of the affected joint (fig. 7/2). At other times, the syndrome may appear with dramatic suddenness. A careful neurologic examination invariably reveals the presence of some type of peripheral nerve disorder which interferes with afferent nerve impulse transmission. In most instances, local arterial circulation is normal. (For the treatment of neurotrophic arthropathy, see p. 173.)

Roentgenography. X-ray examination of the foot is very helpful in determining the degree of joint damage, although in the early stage, there may only be a nonspecific effusion. Later, there are invariably extensive destructive and hypertrophic changes, including marked erosion of articular cartilage and fragmentation of subchondral bone [14]. Free bodies may be present in the joint space and chip and compression fractures are common. The portions of the foot most characteristically affected are the ankle, the astragalotibial joint, the tarsometatarsal joint and the metatarsophalangeal joint. Involvement of combinations of these structures is commonly noted. With progression of the condition, there may be complete disintegration of the osseous structures, especially the tarsal and proximal ends of the metatarsals. The shafts of the latter often become tapered and may fracture. Less new bone formation is noted in the foot than is the case with lesions elsewhere. In fact, in many instances, callus development is noticeably absent. Lysis and absorption of bone generally proceed steadily despite therapy.

Nutritional Lesions in the Diabetic Foot

Because of the frequent presence in the diabetic foot of such etiologic factors as ischemia, peripheral neuropathy, and vulnerability to infection in varying degrees (p. 118), it is not uncommon to find local ulceration or gangrene to be the first presenting clinical manifestation in individuals suffering from diabetes (fig. 7/3). This is in contrast to those with arterial insufficiency of a lower limb due to arteriosclerosis obliterans, in whom intermittent claudication generally precedes the appearance of trophic changes by years; or, as in the case of a great majority of such persons, ulcers or gangrene may never develop.

In the diabetic foot, even a minor break in the continuity of normal skin, as in the course of dealing with an ingrown toenail, may be followed by the appearance of an area of devitalized tissue which quickly becomes moist and odorous due to the liquifying effect of a superimposed secondary infection (wet gangrene). At the same time, mummification of the necrotic structures is delayed. Inflammation may spread rapidly through the lymphatics and along tendon sheaths and tissue planes to involve a considerable portion of the extremity. If unchecked by intensive antibacterial agents, there may be marked systemic reactions which place the patient's life in jeopardy. Roentgenograms of the involved foot may demonstrate the presence of bone necrosis and osteomyelitis. Medial calcification of such vessels as the digital arteries may also be noted.

If the diabetic is also suffering from occlusion of large arteries due to arteriosclerosis obliterans, the clinical picture may be different. The signs of inflammation are minimal, for an adequate blood supply is required for such a response. Secondary infection is generally not as marked as in the case of the diabetic foot with normal arterial circulation. Moreover, the signs of bone rarefaction, lysis, or necrosis, as determined by X-ray examination, will not be found. (For the treatment of nutritional lesions in the diabetic foot, see p. 145.)

Fig. 7/3. Nutritional changes in the diabetic foot. Varying degrees of gangrene and ulceration of the toes are noted.

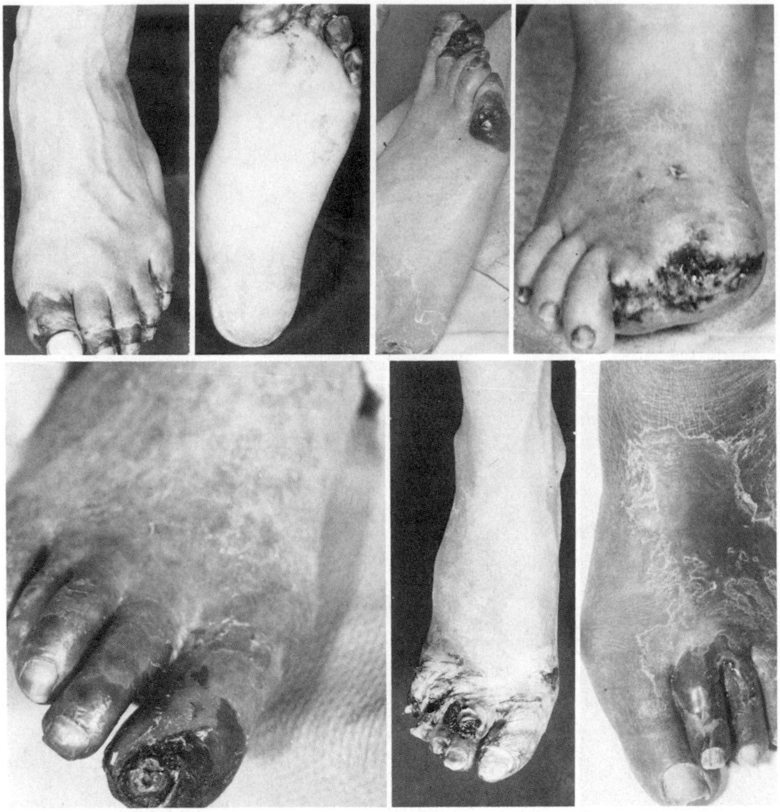

Dermopathy

A number of cutaneous abnormalities are associated with diabetes mellitus, possibly due to microangiopathy in the cutaneous microcirculation.

Necrobiosis Lipoidica Diabeticorum. This is a skin disorder associated with diabetes (although also found in nondiabetics) in which characteristic cutaneous lesions are present on the anterior surface of the legs and, less often, elsewhere on the lower limbs (fig. 7/4). These consist of oval, firm, yellow plaques with an atrophic waxy telangiectatic surface. The condition

a   b   c

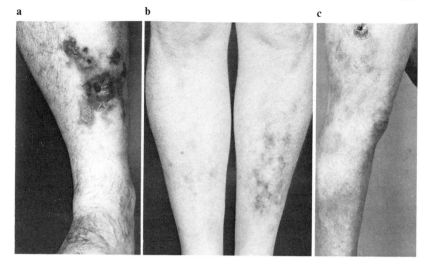

Fig. 7/4. Clinical manifestations of necrobiosis lipoidica diabeticorum, a complication of diabetes mellitus.

initially resembles erythema induratum and, later, complications of venous stasis. Biopsy of a lesion generally reveals necrobiosis of the derma, with palisading-like infiltrates and chronic obliterative arteriolitis. A cortisone-stress glucose tolerance test is usually positive. Occasionally the lesion will ulcerate.

The condition is usually found in female patients who are insulin-dependent. In most instances, the lesions appear in sites of previous trauma on the legs. As they slowly heal, generally in a period of many months, they become pink and are covered with a thin layer of skin.

Skin Spots. These are cutaneous lesions tending to appear on the extensor surface of the lower limbs of diabetic patients [3]. The early lesions are usually less than 1 cm in diameter, multiple, and painful. The typical change consists of an erythematous indurated area with a central papule. Crusting develops initially, and as the lesion slowly heals, it becomes covered with atrophic scar tissue. Skin spots represent areas of microinfarction producing longitudinal superficial necrosis of the skin. They are evidence for the presence of diabetic microangiopathy.

Prognosis

Although approximately 75% of all deaths attributed to diabetes results from the vascular alterations common to this disorder, atherosclerotic involvement of the arterial tree in the lower limbs plays only a relatively minor role in this regard. Nevertheless, ischemia of the foot is still the commonest cause of morbidity in diabetes. Its treatment is difficult and frequently unrewarding, resulting in the need for a minor or major amputation. There is no question that the likelihood that arterial disease of the lower limbs will lead to such an outcome is significantly increased in the presence of diabetes. Such a possibility is enhanced, in part, by the higher incidence of trauma to, and neglect of lesions on, the foot, secondary to peripheral neuropathy, and by the development of less effective collateral circulation.

References

1   Abramson, D.I.: Circulatory diseases of the limbs: a primer (Grune & Stratton, New York 1978).
2   Beisswenger, P.G.; Spiro, R.G.: Studies on the human glomerular basement membrane: composition, nature of carbohydrate units and chemical changes in diabetes mellitus. Diabetes 22: 180 (1983).
3   Binkley, G.W.: Dermopathy in the diabetic syndrome. Archs Derm. 92: 625 (1965).
4   Boulton, A.J.M.: Detecting the patient at risk for diabetic foot ulcers. Practical Cardiol. 9: 135 (1983).
5   Boulton, A.J.M.; Scarpello, H.B.; Ward, J.D.: Venous oxygenation in the diabetic neuropathic foot: evidence of arteriovenous shunting? Diabetologia 22: 6 (1982).
6   Colwell, J.A.; Lopes-Virella, M.; Halushka, P.V.: Pathogenesis of atherosclerosis in diabetes. Diabetes Care 4: 121 (1981).
7   Edmonds, M.E.; Roberts, V.C.; Watkins, P.J.: Blood flow in the diabetic neuropathic foot. Diabetologia 22: 9 (1982).
8   Goldenberg, S.; Alex, M.; Joshi, R.A.: Nonatheromatous peripheral vascular disease of the lower extremity. Diabetes 8: 261 (1959).
9   Jialal, I.; Welsh, N.H.; Joubert, S.M.: Vascular complications in non-insulin-dependent diabetes in the young. S. Afr. med. J. 62: 155 (1982).
10 Kannel, W.B.; Dawber, T.R.; Friedman, G.D.: Risk factors in coronary heart disease: evaluation of several lipids as predictors of coronary heart disease. Framingham study. Ann. intern. Med. 66: 888 (1964).
11 Lippmann, H.I.: Must loss of limb be of consequence of diabetes mellitus? Diabetic Care 2: 432 (1979).
12 Malins, J.: Clinical diabetes mellitus, pp. 267–268 (Eyre & Spottiswoode, London 1968).

13   Pecoraro, R.E.; Porte, D., Jr.: What is diabetes mellitus? Vasc. Diag. Ther. *3:* 9 (1982).

14   Rodnan, G.P.; Maclachlan, M.J.; Brower, T.D.: Neuropathic joint disease (Charcot's joints). Bull. rheum. Dis. *9:* 183 (1959).

15   Ruff, M.C.; Asbury, A.K.: Ischemic mononeuropathy and mononeuropathy multiplex in diabetes mellitus. New Engl. J. Med. *279:* 17 (1968).

16   Siperstein, M.D.; Norton W.; Unger, R.H.; Madison, L.L.: Muscle capillary basement membrane width in normal, diabetic and prediabetic patients. Trans. Ass. Am. Physns *79:* 330 (1966).

17   Turkington, R.W.: Depression masquerading as diabetic neuropathy. J. Am. med. Ass. *243:* 1147 (1980).

18   Walsh, C.H.; FitzGerald, M.G.; Solar, N.G.: Association of foot lesions with retinopathy in patients with newly diagnosed diabetes. Lancet *i:* 878 (1975).

19   Yodaiken, R.E.: The basal lamina (basement membrane) of diabetic capillaries; in Davis, The microcirculation in diabetes, vol. 8, pp. 37–54 (Karger, Basel 1979).

8 Spontaneous Chronic Occlusive Arterial Disorders: General Principles of Therapy

Despite recent technical advances in the use of vascular prostheses, the great majority of patients suffering from chronic occlusive arterial disorders of the lower limbs must still be treated by conservative measures, a point of view which, unfortunately, is not always adopted by the podiatric and medical professions. Since presently it is not possible to control or slow the progressive nature of atherosclerosis by medical or surgical means, all that can be hoped for in the management of this state is the establishment of conditions most favorable to the formation of a new collateral circulation and enlargement of an already existing one. At the same time, attempts should be made to eliminate or minimize all agents or factors which could conceivably retard the development of such a system of vessels. Of the greatest importance, the skin of the lower limbs must be protected from injury. Intermittent claudication, which is invariably an early symptom of chronic occlusive arterial disorders, has no direct influence upon the viability of the limb, for it is never associated with necrosis of the involved muscles and is experienced only during physical activity. Nevertheless, it is a nuisance, an inconvenience, and a deterrent to walking and hence also requires treatment.

Numerous medical and surgical programs have been proposed as therapy for the vascular manifestations of diabetes mellitus, arteriosclerosis obliterans with and without diabetes, and aortoiliac arterial occlusive disease. Those to be described below are applicable to the management of these disorders, as well as of thromboangiitis obliterans except for a few measures. No special therapeutic program is indicated for Mönckeberg's sclerosis since symptoms and signs of impaired local arterial circulation are absent in this disorder. In fact, it is questionable as to whether the patient with this condition should even be made aware of its presence, since this may cause him to become preoccupied with the circulation in his lower limbs and thus to magnify minor nonvascular complaints into what he believes are vascular difficulties of major consequences.

General Care of the Skin of the Lower Limbs

Foot Hygiene

The primary aim of the conservative therapeutic program is to maintain the continuity and viability of the skin of the lower limbs. For this purpose, meticulous care of the feet is essential. To accomplish such a goal, a number of simple procedures must be initiated for all patients with a chronic occlusive arterial disorder of the lower limbs, regardless of the stage of the disease. The same holds true for the individual suffering from diabetes mellitus in conjunction with arteriosclerosis obliterans or from diabetes alone (p. 168). There is no question that the proper care of the feet saves many more lower limbs than does any other type of treatment, medical or surgical, for this program is very effective in preventing the appearance of ulcers and gangrene.

The various rules that the patient must follow are presented to him in the form of a printed list of directions (table 8/I), so as to act as a daily reminder of the significant role that he must play in the success of the program. To emphasize this attitude, a considerable portion of the first office visit should be devoted to the subject. Also stressed are the possible serious consequences of neglecting even one of the rules.

Topical Care of Skin. The feet should be washed daily using lukewarm water and a bland, nonalkaline, nonmedicated soap and then, after meticulous drying of the skin, particularly between the toes, an alcohol compound or a mild astringent should be applied to toughten the superficial tissues. This is followed by the use of a lubricating substance, such as a lanolin cream or ointment, to prevent dryness, cracking, or fissuring of the skin, especially of the heel. The material should not be allowed to spread between the toes in the web, so as to prevent maceration in this site.

The patient is instructed to cut his nails only after the feet have been soaked in lukewarm water for 10–15 min to soften the tissues. He should trim the nails straight across and even with the toes, using sharp clippers to remove a small portion each time not too close to skin and repeating the procedure fairly often. At no time should he attempt to cut down into the corners of the nail in contact with the skin, nor should he dig into the nail bed or around the cuticle. Finally, he should be advised to file off sharp edges using an emery board. If the patient finds this task onerous, because of failing eyesight or obesity which interferes with his reaching the toes readily, a member of his family should take it over. Or he should visit his

Table 8/I. Foot hygiene for lower limbs with compromised arterial circulation and/or diabetes

---

(1) Carefully wash your feet daily in tepid (80–93 °F) water with face soap and then dry them carefully, especially between the toes, using a clean soft towel. Do not rub the skin. Apply a small quantity of a face cream containing lanolin to the feet to replace the natural oils removed by the bath, being particularly careful to cover the skin of the heels. Do not allow any of the cream to get into the web between the toes since this would soften the tissues and predispose them to athlete's foot. Such a program helps prevent dryness, scaliness, and cracking of the skin, all changes which could initiate ulcers. Placing small strands of lamb's wool between the toes may help prevent accumulation of moisture in the web. Socks or stockings should be changed daily.

(2) You should have your toenails trimmed by a competent person who is aware of the fact that you have lack of local circulation and/or diabetes. It is helpful in cutting the nails with a clipper or nipper to soften them by first soaking them for 15 min in lukewarm soapy water. They should be cut straight across, and the corners should not be cut down. The trimming should be done in a very good light.

(3) Never expose your feet and legs to any type of concentrated heat, such as a hot water bottle, electric heating pad, heat cradle, hot foot bath, hot body bath, short-wave diathermy, infrared lamp, ultraviolet light lamp, and ultrasound. Even when the treatment is ordered by a physician for some other local condition, such as arthritis, refuse to allow it. Otherwise, there is a good possibility that a third-degree burn will develop, followed by gangrene. For the same reason, you should be careful not to get a sunburn on the legs and feet.

(4) You should always wear square-toed or round-toed shoes of soft leather, large enough but not too large, which cause no pressure on the toes or on any bunions you may have. Break in new shoes slowly by wearing them for only short periods of time (0.5 h) at the beginning and then gradually increase the duration every day thereafter. It is a good practice routinely to examine your shoes before you put them on, looking for nailheads or nailpoints extending through the insole, wrinkling of the lining, or a pebble under the insole.

(5) Never apply corn plasters or other corn remedies to corns and calluses; also, never attempt to cut them. Instead, take pressure of shoes off corns, bunions, or calluses, using pads or larger shoes. Your podiatrist should be very helpful in this respect. If any other treatment is necessary, he or she will only attempt minimal surgical procedures (steps which are absolutely essential to make you more comfortable), being fully aware of the dangers associated with a more extensive approach in view of your circulatory problem.

(6) Never apply any strong antiseptic drug or caustic, like tincture of iodine, Lysol, or carbolic acid, to your feet in the treatment of an abrasion or a cut since such a step may be followed by the formation of a nonhealing ulcer. Instead, use alcohol, fresh hydrogen peroxide, or Betadine solution. If a sore is to be covered by a sterile bandage, the adhesive tape used to keep the gauze in place should not be permitted to come in direct contact with the skin. This precaution applies to all types of adhesive material, even when composed of paper.

(7) Be careful not to get athlete's foot. In this regard, never walk without wearing shoes or bedroom slippers, whether in the house or outside. This step will also prevent

Table 8/I (continued)

---

stubbing of your toes or stepping on tacks or other objects which could inflict injury to your feet. Even a minor bruise on the sole may be responsible for the development of a non-healing, incapacitating ulcer.

(8) Seek medical or podiatric aid immediately after you discover any type of blister, infection of the toes, athlete's foot, ingrowing toenails, or trouble with bunions, corns, or calluses. Do not attempt to treat the difficulty yourself. If you have trouble examining your feet, especially the soles, you should have a member of your family routinely inspect them very carefully (once a week). Of importance is to look for chafed spots, pressure points, blisters (to which you are especially susceptible), cracks between toes, and excessive dryness and scaliness of the legs and feet, particularly the heels.

(9) When outdoors in the winter, always keep your feet warm by using wool socks and wool-lined or fur-lined boots. At the same time, protect your whole body from the cold by wearing heavy underwear, a heavy coat, and warm mittens. If the outside temperature drops below 0 °F, do not leave your home. Never find yourself in a situation during the winter months when you have to wait longer then 15 min for public transportation or for help for your disabled automobile, for a longer period of exposure may result in frostbite of the feet. At night, before retiring, it is a good practice during the winter months to cover your feet with loose-fitting bed socks or oversize, heavy wool socks.

(10) *Never smoke cigarettes, cigars* or a *pipe* or use tobacco in any other form.

---

podiatrist more frequently, the latter being aware of the fact that an impaired local arterial circulation exists and that only minimal but meticulous treatment is indicated.

Control of Fungal Infections. Athlete's foot, usually presumed to be due to keratinophilic fungi, may also be caused by bacteria, yeasts, and other types of fungi [50], a factor which must be taken into consideration when treating the condition. The fungi generally responsible for tinea pedis are: *Trichophyton rubrum, Trichophyton mentagrophytes, Epidermophyton floccosum,* and *Candida albicans,* a yeastlike fungus. The most prevalent are *T. rubrum* and *T. mentagrophytes.*

The patient suffering from a chronic occlusive arterial disorder of the lower limbs must be made aware of the seriousness of developing dermatophytosis in the web between the toes, for such a condition may act as a portal of entry of bacteria and the formation of a penetrating ulcer which generally extends into the foot proper and may even require a minor or major amputation (fig. 8/1a).

The most important factor in prophylaxis with regard to dermatophytosis is scrupulous hygiene of the feet (p. 133) and the routine application of a fungicidal powder, cream, or spray, such as Desenex, Tinactin, or Lotrimin cream, between the toes. The patient should wear protective rubber slippers when using a shower in a hotel room or gymnasium and should reapply a fungicidal powder immediately afterward, first drying carefully between the toes.

In the acute but uncomplicated stage of dermatophytosis caused by *T. rubrum,* the feet are treated with a hardening agent like aluminum subacetate, 20% (Burow's solution), twice a day for 20 min, followed by the application of a mild antifungal cream such as triacetin cream (Enzactin Cream). With such therapy, the redness, scaling, and cracking should be controlled within a week. If there is considerable crusting, the abnormal material can be removed with a 3% Vioform cream. All socks previously worn should be boiled and the shoes should be discarded if at all feasible in order to avoid reinfection from fungi which might still be present in the lining.

In chronic cases of dermatophytosis, stronger antifungal creams should be used, such as tolnaftate solution, haloprogin, miconazole [38], or Verdefam. All of these are effective treatments, being given twice a day; the cream is rubbed into the lesions until it disappears. Generally, the chronic phase of dermatophytosis can be controlled with such management over a period of 3–8 weeks. If this does not occur, the fungicidal antibiotic, griseofulvin, is added to the program, being given orally in a dosage of 500 mg twice a day after meals. It is necessary to point out that this medication may be responsible for overgrowth of nonsusceptible organisms, particularly *Candida.*

Secondary infection with streptococci is common with *T. mentagrophytes* and when present produces an acute inflammatory state, associated with lymphangitis, fever, chills, and malaise, a state requiring intensive treatment. The patient should immediately be placed at complete bedrest, with the involved toes separated by halves of small corks. The feet should be soaked for 20 min daily in solutions of either potassium permanganate (1:8,000 and later 1:4,000 concentration), silver nitrate (0.125–0.25%), or a combination of copper sulfate and zinc sulfate in a saturated solution of camphor (Alibour solution). If the systemic responses are not quickly controlled, antibiotics, such as tetracycline, erythromycin, or potassium phenoxymethyl penicillin (V-cillin K), should be administered in a dosage of 250 mg 4 times a day for 5 days. The podiatrist must be alert to the appearance of an allergic response to the medications, a not uncommon complication of the therapy.

Management of Other Local Nonvascular Lesions. It is very important to emphasize to the patient with impaired arterial circulation to the lower limbs that he should never attempt to treat ingrown toenails, corns, calluses, or bunions. Instead these should always be managed by a podiatrist or physician who is aware of the existence of compromised local blood flow and hence will cautiously perform a minimum of surgical therapy on the lesions. It should also be pointed out to the patient that the application of a keratolytic agent, in the form of a corn plaster or medicated pad, to a corn may lead to ulceration or even gangrene (fig. 8/1b). Whenever possible, means to remove pressure from lesions produced by such a force should be instituted rather than repeated surgical therapy, an approach which carries a definite element of risk. An oval of soft foam rubber, 0.25 inches (0.635 cm) thick and notched at one end to fit between the affected toes will usually relieve pressure on soft corns in this location. A piece of lamb's wool wrapped around the toe is an even simpler pad. A printed explanation of the reason for the development of corns is likewise helpful in obtaining the patient's cooperation in controlling a situation which may at times be disabling and certainly dangerous if improperly treated.

In the presence of even minor injuries to the feet, such as abrasions or a superficial cut, the patient should be instructed to apply alcohol, fresh hydrogen peroxide, or Betadine to the site and warned against the use of concentrated tincture of iodine, Lysol, phenol, or other strong chemicals, any one of which may cause severe burns of the skin. The involved site should then be covered with sterile gauze, taking care that the adhesive tape used to keep the bandage in place does not come in contact with the skin. The latter precaution should also be followed by the podiatrist during subsequent treatments, for direct application of the tape to skin may lead to irritation and maceration of underlying tissues and actual denudation when the material is forcefully removed. Such responses may be followed by ulceration and gangrene in previously unaffected sites.

Protection from Noxious Agents

Precautions against Injury. The feet must be protected from all mechanical trauma, since an injury thus sustained may be responsible for the development of blisters, ulceration, or gangrene (fig. 8/1c, d). The patient should wear only well-fitting shoes with a straight last, snug but not tight, preferably made of soft leather and adequately contoured to avoid pressure areas. The soles should be thick. If deformities of the feet exist, as in the case of the diabetic foot (p. 124), it may be necessary to have the shoes custom-made. For the individual who performs work that could conceivably cause injury to the feet, protective shoes, reinforced with metal covering on the tips are indicated. Or he should seriously consider changing his occupation to more sedentary work.

Precaution against Heat. The patient with arterial occlusive disorders of the lower limbs should be made aware of the great danger resulting from the application of heat in any form to the feet and legs, since this may precipitate a burn which frequently necessitates amputation (fig. 8/1e). The podiatrist, too, should never use direct heat in any form, including shortwave diathermy, ultrasound, and ultraviolet light, among others, in the treatment of inflammation superimposed upon an ischemic ulcer or gangrene or in the control of coexisting disorders of joints. The deleterious effects of raising tissue temperature in a limb with a compromised local arterial circulation are discussed in detail on page 197.

Precaution against Cold. In the winter months, the lower limbs should be kept warm through the use of woolen socks and full-length woolen underwear, and exposure of the body to cold should be reduced to a minimum. Also, if the patient must go outdoors in a cold environment, he should wear shoes with a warm lining of wool or synthetic material, or he should cover his shoes with fur-lined boots ('stadium boots' or overshoes). At all times the rest of the body should also be warmly clad; otherwise, reflex vasoconstriction will occur in the toes.

When the environmental temperature falls to below 0 °F (–17.8 °C), it is advisable for the patient to remain indoors, since, under such circumstances, if a situation arises which compels him to be inactive in the cold for even a short period of time, he may develop frostbite of the affected limb or limbs (fig. 8/1f). Because of such potentially serious consequences, if at all feasible, the patient with a chronic occlusive arterial disorder of the lower limbs should seek residence in a uniformly warm climate, with very little humidity.

The basis for the deleterious vascular effect of a low environmental temperature is the existing significant decrease in peripheral blood flow resulting from the pathologic occlusive process in the leg and foot, thus reducing the efficiency of the only available mechanism for conveying heat to the tissues. Further aggravating the situation is the normal marked vasoconstriction of the cutaneous circulation elicited by cold. As a result of both

a b c

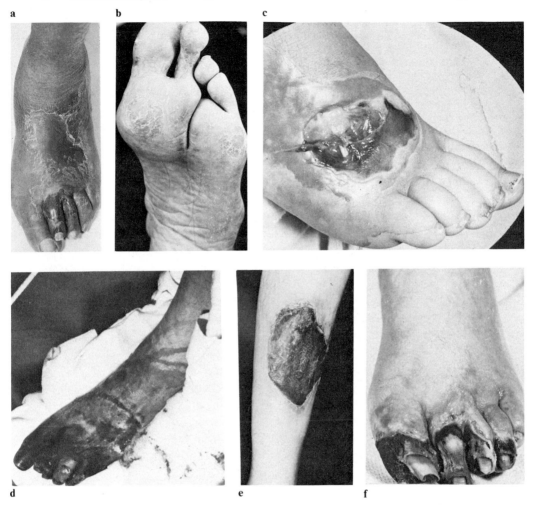

d e f

Fig. 8/1. Nutritional disturbances in feet of patients with impaired arterial circulation in the lower limbs (due to arteriosclerosis obliterans or to diabetes), resulting from trauma or improper local care. **a** Gangrene of two toes at their base caused by a staphylococcic infection whose portal of entry was dermatophytosis of web of toes. **b** Surgical amputation of a gangrenous fourth toe in a diabetic with good local circulation, following treatment of a corn with a medicated corn plaster. **c** Nonhealing indolent ulceration on dorsum of the foot of a patient with arteriosclerosis obliterans due to a heavy object falling on limb. **d** Gangrene of entire foot due to a heavy tool falling on it. **e** Third-degree burn produced by application of a heating pad to the leg following occlusion of the femoral artery by an embolus. Limb was subsequently amputated. **f** Gangrene of the toes (frostbite) in a patient with arteriosclerosis obliterans, precipitated by a short period of exposure to a moderately low environmental temperature. Reproduced from ref. [1] with permission.

factors, the fall in temperature is great enough to permit cold injury to develop locally. (For a discussion of the deleterious effects of cold on the cutaneous circulation, see p. 319.)

Abstinence from Smoking. The evidence that tobacco smoking has a permanent deleterious effect upon the circulation in the lower limbs of patients with arteriosclerosis obliterans and causes progression of the occlusive process is not as clear-cut as in the case of thromboangiitis obliterans. Nevertheless, such individuals should be advised to abstain, on the basis that smoking is a potent vasoconstricting stimulus which affects the cutaneous circulation and thus decreases the nourishment to the skin, making it more vulnerable to the development of ulcers and gangrene. However, although such a measure undoubtedly contributes to maintaining the circulation to the skin at the highest possible level of efficiency, it does not always prevent the appearance of nutritional changes, as is almost invariably the case in thromboangiitis obliterans. For reasons which are not clear, there may be a resulting increase in claudication distance in some patients with arteriosclerosis obliterans but only after several months of abstinence.

Systemic Measures
Attempts to Slow the Atherosclerotic Process. Considerable difference of opinion exists regarding the value of lowering a relatively normal level of serum lipids by whatever means so as to prevent or slow the development of atherosclerosis. Less controversy is present in the case of patients demonstrating hyperlipoproteinemia and xanthomatosis, and in such individuals, trials of hypolipemic therapy are indicated [7].

Management of Associated Systemic Conditions. Certain systemic disorders adversely affect oxygen delivery to the tissues of the lower limbs and hence reduce the amount available for the satisfaction of their metabolic needs. In the case of the patient with a chronic occlusive arterial disorder, such a situation contributes materially to an already existing local ischemia and, therefore, it is essential to manage the secondary condition. For example, if a moderate or severe anemia is present, it should be dealt with through the administration of iron in some form. If heart failure exists, it should be controlled in order to increase the efficiency of the heart in delivering blood to peripheral tissues. It is apparent, also, that any chronic lung disorder which interferes with oxygenation of the blood in the pulmonary vascular bed requires intensive therapy. Interestingly enough, attempts to drop a coexisting significantly elevated blood pressure rapidly by medical means may adversely affect the state of circulation in the limb with a compromised blood flow. Evidently reducing the head of pressure in the vascular tree results in a decrease in perfusion of blood through stenotic vessels in the lower extremities, thus untowardly influencing the amount available to the tissues locally.

Medical Management of Specific Clinical Manifestations

Control of Intermittent Claudication
The first and frequently only therapeutic program required for the patient with aortoiliac occlusive arterial disease or arteriosclerosis obliterans, complaining only of intermittent claudication, is a conservative approach (p. 154). Measures should be directed toward increasing walking distance, at the same time that the various steps for maintaining viability of the skin (p. 133) are scrupulously adhered to and abstinence from smoking is carried out. It should be stressed to the patient that intermittent claudication produces no serious consequences [37] (other than changing his lifestyle by acting as a deterrent to normal physical activity) and that its presence in no way indicates that ulcers and gangrene will follow. Such reassurance is very helpful in properly preparing him for the exercise program (see below), as well as in supporting his peace of mind. There is no point, however, to make mention of the fact that longevity in the patient suffering from intermittent claudication is significantly reduced because of the high incidence of atherosclerotic disease in critical organs that may coexist in such an individual.

Physical Activity. Early in the disease, it is most important to impress the patient with the fact that he must make an effort to exercise daily, for a life of physical inactivity generally leads to disuse atrophy of the muscles of the lower extremities which further limits his ability to ambulate. Moreover, such a situation is responsible for mental deterioration and adoption of the role of an incurable invalid, an attitude which is entirely unwarranted.

Generally, graded exercises should be initiated in the hope that the gradually increasing load placed on the arterial system locally will act as a stimulus for the further growth of collateral vessels, thus resulting in improvement in the ability to walk [25, 30, 35, 47]. To accomplish this goal, the patient should continue walking for about a half-block after intermittent claudication is experienced, even though the pain builds up in intensity. He than rests, and when the symptom has completely disappeared, the exercise is continued, again into the period in which pain is present. After several months on such a program, the patient will usually find that he can now walk the extra half-block without pain. At this point, he should again increase his walking distance by another half-block and continue the regimen, gradually augmenting his capacity to ambulate without experiencing pain. No attempt should ever be made to lengthen the period of walking with pain much beyond a half-block. Theoretically at least, under such circumstances, irreversible changes could develop in the active muscles as a result of a relatively prolonged severe state of local acute ischemia. It is well to remember that in the type I diabetic, exercise may cause a moderate decrease in plasma glucose and, in some individuals, even symptomatic hypoglycemia; in others, there may be an increase in plasma glucose [46].

If intermittent claudication is experienced primarily in the calf muscles, exercise training on a stationary bicycle ergometer has no therapeutic value. For, any beneficial metabolic changes that might follow such a program would be limited to the thigh muscles utilized in this type of physical work. Since these are minimally involved in walking, little or no beneficial effect on such an activity would therefore be expected from training on a bicycle ergometer.

Physical Adjustments and Aids. Early in his disease the patient becomes aware of the fact that when utilizing the pace to which he had previously become accustomed, he is unable to carry out many of his daily chores without great inconvenience because of having to stop repeatedly to obtain relief from his symptoms. Hence, he soon learns that by materially reducing his rate of walking, he is able to cover a much greater distance without difficulty, although requiring a longer period of time to reach his destination. Unfortunately, as indicated above, such a program has no beneficial effect on permanently lengthening claudication distance, but still, under certain circumstances, it is necessary for the patient to make such an adjustment to physical activity. Many individuals use canes in order to reduce the weight placed on the involved extremity; others have found that if they walk stiff-legged, without bending their knees or contracting the calf muscles to any degree, the onset of pain is also delayed, provided that the intermittent claudication is located in the upper portion of the leg. Weight reduction, if the patient is obese, will also be helpful in allowing him to walk a little further without pain, at the same time, possibly helping to control factors responsible for the development of atherosclerosis. Another measure that may be helpful is the use of lifts placed on the heel of the shoes, since such a step modifies the gait and causes the patient to use the thigh muscles instead of the gastrocnemius muscle to throw his feet forward. External short leg braces that restrict or eliminate ankle motion may also increase walking ability. Naturally, any biomechanical fault in the feet should be treated.

In the past, such procedures as intermittent venous occlusion, Paevex boot, Sanders' oscillating bed, and Buerger's postural exercises (p. 208) have all been given extensive clinical trials for the treatment of intermittent claudication. However, for the most part, they have been discarded since objective evidence was never available to indicate that they had any value in increasing claudication distance or that they were responsible for an augmentation in muscle blood flow in the lower limbs.

Principles of Drug Therapy. Many medications have been proposed as therapy for intermittent claudication, but very few have withstood critical evaluation. Since alpha-receptor effector end organs are rarely found in the walls of blood vessels directly supplying voluntary muscles, alpha-receptor end organ blocking agents (p. 147) have little if any effect on altering muscle circulation. Hence, they have no role as therapy for the patient with arteriosclerosis obliterans whose sole complaint is intermittent claudication. Also to take into consideration is the fact that such medications are expensive to administer on a long-range basis and may be associated with adverse reactions (p. 148).

The only drugs which theoretically are of potential value in increasing claudication distance are agents which stimulate beta-receptor end organs, for these structures are present in relatively large numbers in the walls of blood vessels to muscles. Among the medications used clinically for this purpose are nylidrine hydrochloride (Arlidin) and isoxysuprine hydrochloride (Vasodilan). Although both have been reported to double resting muscle blood flow, they do not appear to have a significant beneficial effect on increasing claudication distance, probably because a 20-fold augmentation is required to take care of the markedly elevated metabolic needs of exercising muscles. Of clinical interest is the reported observation that the current widespread use of beta-blockers [propranolol hydrochloride (Inderal), atenolol (Tenormin), metoprolol tartrate (Lopressor), and others] for various types of cardiac difficulties and hypertension at the same time causes a reduction in walking ability in patients who also have arteriosclerosis obliterans and experience intermittent claudication. The relative importance of such an adverse response must await further study.

Systemic Measures. A number of other steps have been proposed for the purpose of favorably influencing blood flow dynamics in the muscle of the lower limbs and hence of increasing walking ability. Of value in this regard is to place the patient on a low-fat, low-cholesterol, high-complex carbohydrate, high-fiber diet [25], together with weight reduction if he is obese. Theoretically, medical means to reduce blood viscosity would also be indicated.

Medical Management of Ischemic Neuropathy

The medical therapeutic program for the management of the severe symptoms of ischemic neuropathy (p. 14), found in the terminal stage of arteriosclerosis obliterans, is frequently ineffective. Nevertheless, this approach should be attempted before considering more heroic measures. For the most part, the steps are similar to those outlined for the treatment of peripheral neuropathy of the lower limbs associated with diabetes mellitus (p. 170).

Other measures which may reduce the severity of the pain in the feet on lying down in bed in preparation for sleep are: elevation of the head of the bed (about 6–8 inches; 15.24–20.32 cm) to increase arterial inflow into the lower limbs; removal of the weight of the bedclothes from the lower limbs by appropriate means; use of oversize woolen socks to contain whatever heat is delivered to the feet by the limited local blood flow; and application of heat to the abdomen and chest to produce reflex or indirect vasodilatation in the feet (p. 200). The use of narcotics to control the pain must be approached only with great care, for individuals suffering from ischemic neuropathy are readily prone to addiction.

As a last-resort medical measure, it may be necessary to permit the patient to sleep in a chair, with his feet in dependency. Such a position invariably causes immediate relief from all neuritic symptoms, but, unfortunately, when assumed for any period of time, it is responsible for the development of dependency edema. Contributing to the magnitude of the response is the existing ischemia of the walls of the cutaneous and subcutaneous capillaries, resulting in greater permeability in them and encouraging an even more rapid transudation of fluid from the blood into the tissue spaces. As a consequence of the further compressive effect of the local edema on the microcirculation, the latter is mechanically obstructed, thus exaggerating the already existing severe ischemic state of the tissues locally and predisposing them to the development of trophic changes – ulcers and gangrene. (For surgical management of ischemic neuropathy, see p. 153.)

Medical Management of Nutritional Lesions
Except prossibly in the presence of a rapidly progressing occlusive process in the cutaneous vessels, the circulation to the skin rarely falls to a point incompatible with viability of this structure. It is only when inflammation due to infection or other noxious agents is superimposed or injury destroys the continuity of the skin that the vascular reserve becomes unable to cope with the elevated metabolic demands resulting therefrom and hence ischemic trophic lesions develop. In the presence of the latter, the therapeutic program described on pages 133 and 141 must be modified somewhat and other measures introduced. The goals of treatment when ischemic ulceration or gangrene appears to be developing or already exists in the foot are: (1) to prevent extension of the destructive process to contiguous relatively normal tissue; (2) to facilitate demarcation of necrotic from viable structures; (3) to control local infection and prevent or treat systemic responses due to absorption; and (4) to institute measures which encourage growth of granulation tissue in, and epithelialization of, the site of the lesion after removal of all nonviable material by debridement or following spontaneous separation. The achievement of such aims does not require sequential steps but rather the institution of several therapeutic approaches at almost the same time.

Restriction of Physical Activity. Walking should be reduced to a minimum so as to decrease pain associated with stretching of inflamed structurcs and to prevent spread of the local infection into surrounding tissues, the lymphatic system, and the blood circulation. Another objection to ambulation under these circumstances is that it causes dilatation of the vessels in the small muscles of the foot, with resulting greater ischemia of the skin in the vicinity of the lesion due to shunting of available blood supply into areas of increased metabolic activity. If walking is essential, crutches should be utilized in order to remove the weight of the body from the involved lower limb.

It is necessary to point out, however, that the patient should not remain in bed for prolonged periods of time, for such a situation is responsible for a drop in blood pressure and the development of a state of deconditioning (p. 332). Instead he should be permitted to sit in a chair with the lower limbs in dependency for a good portion of the day. Also, repeated exercises of the remaining three unaffected limbs should be carried out under the supervision of a physical therapist or a nurse competent in the field of rehabilitation medicine. If the patient is at home, the exercise program can be carried out under the supervision of a member of the family who has received instruction in this regard.

Local Care of Lesion. This aspect of therapy is most important in healing ulcers or gangrene. When large quantities of secretion and purulent material exist, it is necessary to cleanse the wound daily using a lukewarm footbath containing a small quantity of tincture of green soap (1 teaspoonful in a basin of lukewarm water) or, if available, with immersion in a whirlpool bath maintained at around 32 °C (90 °F). After each soaking, the entire limb should be dried carefully, particularly between the toes, and the lesion should be covered with sterile gauze and a bandage, with adhesive tape being placed only on the latter.

If necrotic tissue partly or completely covers an ulcerated area, this material should be carefully removed by debridement and without a local anesthetic, preferably immediately after a period of soaking to soften the nonviable material. For the actual procedure, small clippers (tissue nippers with one flat side) are necessary. In every instance, only obviously devitalized structures are removed; if performed properly, no bleeding or pain is elicited. Such an approach helps prevent the growth of bacteria and thus facilitates formation of granulation tissue and epithelialization of the lesion.

If the commonly found heavy, adherent eschar does not respond to simple debridement, then it is advisable to utilize a proteolytic enzyme like Elase ointment or Dakin's solution, applied to the lesion several times daily. It is necessary to point out, however, that these substances should be used with a great deal of caution, for, in some instances they may cause maceration of surrounding, apparently normal, structures.

Since ischemic tissue walls off infection very poorly (with the result that the exudate tends to burrow deeply), it is necessary to keep sinus tracts open in order to facilitate drainage. This is accomplished by probing the tracts, to break up repeatedly forming fibrous partitions, and irrigating them with a watery solution of an appropriate antibiotic. Also of value is daily immersion in a whirlpool bath.

Local Measures to Increase Blood Flow. Since healing of a trophic change requires a considerable increase in local circulation over that necessary for the resting metabolic needs of the tissues, it is essential to achieve an augmentation in blood flow by medical means if this is possible. The only mechanism available is dilatation of small vessels and collateral channels not affected by the pathologic process. This may be accomplished by the topical application of a 2% nitroglycerin ointment (Nitrol ointment). The drug is a myovascular relaxant, acting directly upon the circular muscle fibers in the blood vessel wall. It is applied in the following manner: A strip of the ointment, equal to the maximum circumference of the involved digit, is squeezed onto a piece of paper (part of the kit), along an edge of its long length. Then the paper is wrapped around the toe so that the medication covers its entire base. The material is left in place for about 1 h to permit full absorption of the nitroglycerin to take place through the intact skin and produce vasodilatation of the underlying digital arteries and their main branches. At the end of this period of time, the ointment base is removed. The measure is repeated 3 times daily in the hope that it will facilitate demarcation of necrotic material from viable tissue, thus contributing to local healing. At night, the lesion is cleansed with a mild antiseptic and covered with sterile gauze. In some patients, repeated applications of the nitroglycerin ointment may elicit a nitrate headache which can generally be controlled with aspirin.

Systemic Measures to Increase Local Blood Flow. Orally or parenterally administered vasodilator drugs have had extensive clinical trial as therapy for nutritional lesions of the foot. The rationale for their use is that the resulting increase in blood flow may be helpful in delimiting and preventing extension of the lesion. The vasodilating effect of these medications is transitory and so frequently repeated administration is necessary.

In contrast to the situation in muscle vessels (p. 143), alpha-adrenergic receptor end organs are extensively found in association with cutaneous arteries, thus suggesting that alpha-receptor blocking agents, such as phenoxybenzamine hydrochloride (Dibenzyline) and tolazoline hydrochloride (Priscoline) would be effective in increasing blood flow to the skin of the toes by preventing vasoconstrictor impulses from reaching these end organs and liberating norepinephrine locally. However, because circulating blood follows the pathway of least resistance, there is a strong tendency for the resulting increased local blood flow to be diverted from the tissues suffering from the more severe state of ischemia into surrounding structures in which the compromised circulation is much less marked and, as a consequence, a greater degree of vasodilatation exists. Also contributing to a reduced perfusion to affected structures is the fact that alpha-receptor blocking agents are given orally or parenterally, thus producing a generalized vasodilatation in normal vascular beds and a drop in systemic blood pressure, especially in the upright position (orthostatic hypotension). Such a response further reduces the head of pressure in the stenotic vessels supplying the affected structures and hence decreases the rate of local blood flow.

Under certain circumstances, the alpha-receptor blocking agents may have a therapeutic effect. For example, if an element of vasospasm is superimposed on the organic occlusive process, then they may cause a significant increase in local circulation. Also, it is possible that even in the face of severe terminal artery and microcirculation disease, these agents may still have a vasodilating action on the newly formed and unaffected collateral vessels, thus augmenting local cutaneous circulation in the vicinity of the lesions.

Alpha-adrenergic receptor blocking agents should be administered with caution in patients with marked cerebral or coronary arteriosclerosis or renal damage. Nasal congestion is a very common adverse reaction to these drugs, as well as miosis. Inhibition of ejaculation may also occur. Because of the possibility of orthostatic hypotension, if feasible, the patient should be at bedrest when receiving them.

A number of myovascular relaxants, like cyclandelate (Cyclospasmol), have also been used in an attempt to increase cutaneous blood flow in the vicinity of an ulcer or gangrene. Such drugs act directly on the circular smooth muscle fibers in the blood vessel wall, relaxing them and thus causing local vasodilatation. As in the case of alpha-receptor blocking agents (see above), cyclandelate should be used with extreme caution in patients with severe coronary or cerebral atherosclerosis because of the possibility that compromised blood flow in involved organs may be further exaggerated by shunting of blood into normal structures in response to the vasodilator action of the drug.

The therapeutic effect of orally or parenterally administered myovascular agents can be expected to be of little consequence as vasodilator drugs. This is in contrast to their strong action in this regard when applied directly to the skin of the affected digit, as in the case of the use of nitroglycerin ointment (p. 147).

In summary, it can therefore be stated that orally or parenterally administered vasodilator drugs, which unquestionably increase cutaneous circulation in the toes of a normal limb, have a limited application as therapeutic agents in the management of the ischemic ulcer or gangrene in the patient with arteriosclerosis obliterans. In the presence of an intact skin of the foot and leg, cutaneous vasodilator drugs play no role as therapy.

Other Systemic Measures. Having determined by appropriate culture and sensitivity studies the bacterial agents responsible for the inflammatory state of the lesion (p. 299), the proper antibacterial medications are administered to the patient either orally or parenterally. However, it must be recognized that such a measure cannot be expected to produce a dramatic response in controlling the local infection since the compromised arterial circulation works against the development of a significantly high therapeutic concentration of the antibiotic in the tissues surrounding the lesion. Nevertheless, such a step should still be carried out.

A very difficult problem encountered in most patients with arteriosclerosis obliterans who are suffering from ulcers or gangrene of the foot is how to control the associated pain. As already emphasized, the severity of this symptom varies markedly depending upon the level of the patient's threshold for pain and the degree and extent of involvement of the structures of the foot. It is frequently necessary to resort to the administration of large quantities of narcotics for this purpose.

Attempts to Facilitate Deposition of Granulation Tissue and Epithelialization. After all necrotic tissue has been removed and infection is controlled, the next step is the topical application of substances which may help accelerate the healing process, such as crude coal tar, 5%, chlorophyll ointment (Chloresium ointment), White's A and D ointment, and vitamin A ointment. Although it is questionable as to whether any of the stimulating medications have any direct therapeutic action on clean ulcers, they do help protect the delicate newly forming tissues from the irritation of a dry dressing. It is also necessary to decrease the frequency with which the lesions are cleansed and dressed, since this will reduce the possibility of manipulation causing injury and thus inhibiting the rate of healing. Some evidence is available to support the view that healing of ulcers, particularly in diabetics, is facilitated by the oral administration of zinc sulfate [21].

Role of Percutaneous Transluminal Angioplasty

Originally proposed by *Dotter and Judkins* [18] in 1964, percutaneous transluminal angioplasty has been used extensively in the vascular clinics in Europe [55] for the treatment of stenotic lesions in the arterial tree supplying the lower limbs. In contrast, this procedure has only recently begun to be studied in the USA, the delay probably being due to skepticism prevailing in vascular circles regarding the physiologic rationale for its application. Nevertheless, currently much more attention is being paid to the method, and numerous papers are appearing in the American literature reporting very favorable results with its use.

Technique and Basic Principles of the Method. The procedure involves nonsurgical dilatation of stenotic peripheral arteries or, on occasion, the creation of a new lumen in a completely occluded vessel, using a balloon-tipped or double lumen catheter inserted intraluminally under local anesthesia. With more recent technical improvements and refinements, the original balloon catheter of *Dotter and Judkins* [18] has been replaced by the dilating polyvinyl chloride balloon coaxially mounted near the tip of a standard cardiovascular double-lumen catheter (Grüntzig balloon catheter) [24]. This instrument is introduced into the artery and guided under fluoroscopy, being preceded by a guide wire. Also utilized are balloon catheters made of polyethylene and of reinforced polyurethane. These allow higher dilating pressures to be used with less tendency for expansion of the balloon beyond its intended maximal diameter [34]. Coagulation of the blood is reduced during the treatment period by a single dose of heparin, for the intra-arterial catheter decreases blood velocity and laminar flow and elicits turbulence, all factors which are conducive to intravascular clotting. After application of the distending force for about 8 s, an angiogram is obtained to determine whether the desired extent of widening of the arterial lumen has been achieved.

Originally, the rationale for the treatment was considered to be dilatation of the involved segment of artery, due to lateral compression and remodeling of the atheromatous material against the intact vessel wall by the central expanding force supplied by the distending balloon, with simultaneous release of fluid constituents of plaque [22]. However, recently this theory has been questioned and other possibilities have been proposed [11, 54]. One of these rejects the view that a semisolid structure like an atherosclerotic plaque can be flattened against the wall of an artery to any appreciable degree because the material is incompressible. Instead, it is suggested that balloon dilatation causes an increase in outside diameter of the vessel resulting from overstretching of arterial layers [12].

In support of the above concept is electron microscopic evidence of intimal disruption (cracking) and widespread destruction of vascular muscle cells, with or without stretching or fragmentation of elastic fibers, immediately after balloon dilatation. Later there are further fragmentation and lysis of damaged muscle cells and movement of macrophages into the traumatized area. At about 1 week after the procedure, myofibroblasts appear in the area and, at 2 months, extensive collagen deposition (scar formation) occurs. The marked overstretching and destruction of muscle cells may result in muscular paralysis and inability of the segment of vessel to respond to vasodilators or vasoconstrictors, thus maintaining it in a permanently dilated state. In fact, follow-up angiography obtained months or years after the procedure was performed have demonstrated that the segment of lumen subjected to dilatation was actually wider than the diameter noted immediately after the procedure [54].

Clinical Results. Regardless of which explanation applies, the reported studies indicate that the early success rate of percutaneous transluminal angioplasty compares favorably with that of vascular reconstructive procedures in several groups of patients [23, 49]. However, it must be kept in mind that generally the procedure cannot be expected to produce results, in terms of patency, that are as durable as those of surgery, for it is a more localized procedure than the bypass graft which circumvents the entire diseased segment of vessel [34]. Naturally, it in no way influences the relentless progression of the atheromatous process, so that other lesions will undoubtedly develop proximally or distally to the now-dilated portion of vessel, thus predisposing to new areas of complete occlusion, as is also the case for bypass surgery (p. 162).

Besides use of percutaneous transluminal angioplasty as an alternative approach to bypass surgery, it appears especially to have a definite role in the case of the patient, usually a diabetic, who has ischemic neuropathy or is facing loss of a limb due to distal ischemic gangrene. Many of the individuals falling into such a category (a salvage situation) are elderly, suffering from multiple medical problems and hence poor candidates for extensive vascular surgery. Percutaneous transluminal angioplasty is feasible and applicable under such circumstances since no general anesthetic is required and the entire procedure can be performed in a relatively short period of time, with the hospital stay being limited to 1 or 2 days. Moreover, there is no risk of lack of wound-healing, a possibility which not infrequently plagues the vascular surgeon and may completely reverse the outcome of a previously successful operation. However, it is necessary to point out that the patency rate for diabetics is only about 50%, as compared with almost 90% for nondiabetics [22].

As in vascular surgery (see below), patient selection for percutaneous transluminal angioplasty is critical, for the procedure is far from applicable to all situations. For example, total iliac or femoral artery occlusions which are more than 5 cm long should not be considered for the procedure. Other factors influencing a successful outcome are the age of the obstruction, as related to the duration from the onset of clinical manifestations, and the quality of the distal 'runoff'. If impenetrable luminal fibrosis exists, the procedure is not technically possible, the same applying to the presence of extensive calcium deposits in the atheromatous material.

There are some serious complications associated with percutaneous transluminal angioplasty. These include conversion of a stenotic lesion into a complete occlusion of an artery; liberation of peripheral arterial emboli composed of fragments of intimal tissue, particularly in the case of involvement of the common iliac artery; dissection of the arterial wall by the catheter when recanalization fails because of inability to penetrate dense connective tissue; and perforation of the arterial wall by the guide wire and catheter.

Surgical Management of Clinical Manifestations

This section deals with a critical evaluation of the various surgical procedures which have for their aim an augmentation in arterial blood flow to the leg and foot. However, no attempt is made to describe the operative techniques in detail, since such information is not applicable to the podiatric care of a patient. If, on occasion, it is required, excellent monographs on the subject are available. To be considered below are venous and artificial graft-bypass procedures, thromboendarterectomy, and lumbar sympathectomy.

The role of surgical therapy in arteriosclerosis obliterans has still not been clearly defined. For example, there is a growing body of opinion supporting the view that reconstructive vascular approaches should be limited to those patients who require an immediate increase in blood flow to a foot in order to prevent irreversible ischemic changes or to salvage one in which ulceration or gangrene already exists and is extending despite intensive conservative therapy. In general, it can be stated that approximately 10% of individuals suffering from chronic occlusive arterial disorders of the lower limbs are proper candidates for some type of surgical therapeutic procedure. In order to identify the latter group of individuals, it is necessary to follow certain rigid guidelines which can be separated into two categories (see below and p. 156).

For the diabetic with arteriosclerosis obliterans requiring an immediate increase in blood flow to maintain viability of a foot, the decision to utilize a surgical approach for this purpose involves even more considerations and a greater circumspection than in the case of a local compromised circulation alone.

General Considerations Regarding Choice of Candidates for Revascularization Procedures

The aim of this section is to emphasize those factors which determine whether a patient requires insertion of a vascular prosthesis or a thromboendarterectomy. In order to enlarge upon and clarify the various aspects that must be taken into consideration, examples of these situations are presented below.

In Presence of Rapid Progression of Occlusive Process. If a patient who for years has suffered only from intermittent claudication now also begins to complain of rest pain in the foot on lying down in bed (ischemic neuropathy) or rest pain in toes associated with discoloration and coldness of the involved digits (impending gangrene), either set of clinical changes indicates that rapid progression of the occlusive process has occurred in the arterial tree, without adequate time for an effective collateral circulation to develop. Because neglect of the presence of such symptoms and signs may result in the need for an amputation, every effort should be made immediately to initiate measures to increase local blood supply. Another situation requiring the same therapeutic approach is a rapid deterioration of walking ability in an individual who previously manifested stable claudication. This alteration in the clinical picture is again a reflection of a rapidly progressing atherosclerotic occlusion in large arteries, with a good possibility of the development of acute severe local ischemia and necrosis in the foot if left untreated.

To cope adequately with the above conditions, a surgical reconstructive procedure is essential regardless of the age of the patient; otherwise, an operation will still be required, but it will be an amputation of a lower limb, causing the individual either to assume a wheelchair existence or to rely upon an artificial limb for ambulation. Of course, if the elderly patient has associated cardiopulmonary involvement or serious disorders elsewhere, he may be a very poor candidate for any type of anesthetic and surgical procedure and, under such circumstances, the choice must be the one which is least hazardous to his life.

In Presence of Intermittent Claudication Only. Whether surgical management is indicated for the patient whose sole complaint is pain on walking has still not been settled [14, 26, 35]. In this situation, a number of practical factors must be taken into consideration in the final decision. These include the age of the individual and whether he is gainfully employed and, if so, the type of occupation. For example, if he has a job which involves considerable walking during the course of the day, as is the case for a salesman carrying a sample case to his customers or for a private detective following a suspect, it is obvious that an inability to cover even a short distance without experiencing pain that forces him to stop and rest will significantly interfere with his duties.

Moreover, the person with intermittent claudication who has the potential of injuring his lower limbs during the course of a working day by tools falling on them (as may be so for the plumber, the electrician, or other types of artisans) is always in jeopardy with regard to the maintenance of viability of the skin of his feet even when using protective shoes.

For all of the above individuals, a reconstructive vascular procedure is definitely indicated in order to increase claudication distance and help protect the feet from developing ulcers or gangrene following an injury to them. Again, of course, there must be no associated disorders which contraindicate any type of surgical approach.

A question which must be addressed deals with the management of stable intermittent claudication alone in older persons who have retired from their occupations and in younger individuals who are still employed but are not inconvenienced in their job by their difficulty in walking. Most patients who are no longer working have no need to reach a specific destination in a certain period of time and hence can adjust their pace so as to experience a minimum of discomfort while walking. The fact that they no longer must follow a rigid schedule helps them to accommodate readily to their affliction. Most importantly, as previously emphasized, many older people with arteriosclerosis obliterans, as manifested only by intermittent claudication, may also suffer from atherosclerosis of critical organs, including the heart, kidneys, and brain. These coexisting disorders make such individuals poor candidates for a prolonged period of anesthesia required in order to perform the various complex procedures on the arterial tree in the abdomen and/or lower limbs. Another point to consider is that such a surgical approach under these circumstances falls into the category of an elective operation. Finally, because of the different complications associated with vascular reconstructive surgery (p. 162), the desired goal may not be achieved, or if initially there is a successful outcome, the increased blood flow may not persist due to thrombosis of the prosthesis, thus making the patient vulnerable to the appearance of trophic changes in the foot. For, during the period in which the graft is delivering blood to distal tissues, no stimulus exists for growth of a collateral system. With its sudden occlusion, a state of ischemia may therefore develop in the foot. Such a sequence of events has been responsible for the not infrequent situation of a patient entering the hospital for the surgical management of intermittent claudication and subsequently being readmitted for a major amputation.

In summary, it can be stated that surgical correction for intermittent claudication is generally not performed except in the most disabling cases. This is because the long-term risk of limb loss in patients solely with such a complaint is small [29].

Because of all the above-enumerated potential risks and adverse responses associated with reconstructive surgery in the elderly patient suffering only from intermittent claudication, it is inadvisable and even foolhardy to attempt such an approach on them. Instead, this group, which comprises the great percentage of individuals suffering from arteriosclerosis obliterans, should be treated conservatively (pp. 133, 141).

Of course, there are always some exceptions to the above rule, such as the person who has always hiked long distances in his youth and middle age and now finds that he is only able to cover several short blocks before he has to stop and rest to obtain relief from his pain. This physical handicap will generally have a severe psychologic impact on his morale and he may begin to show rapid signs of mental deterioration because of his fear of becoming a physical invalid. To counteract such a situation, the possibility of a vascular reconstructive procedure should be offered to the patient. At the same time, he should be made aware of the risks associated with the operation and be fully cognizant of the fact that it is not essential for preserving the limb, its purpose being mainly to increase his walking ability. Naturally, he must be in a physical condition capable of withstanding any complications or adverse reactions to the surgery.

Another controversial aspect of the problem of determining which patient suffering only from stable intermittent claudication is a proper candidate for a reconstructive vascular procedure is the level of the occlusion in the arterial tree. It is felt by many workers in the field that if the block is below the groin, in the femoropopliteal segment of the arterial tree, a prosthesis or thromboendarterectomy is not indicated. Instead, conservative therapy should be instituted. Of course, again if the patient demands surgery and is fully aware of all the risks involved, the procedure should be carried out. As a general rule, if intermittent claudication has existed for less than 6 months, it is advisable to postpone any surgical intervention until the efficiency of the developing collateral circulation can be evaluated and demonstrated clinically.

Summary. The possibility of being able to satisfy one or several of the following goals must be considered when deciding upon a proper candidate for a reconstructive vascular procedure: (1) preventing or averting development of nutritional changes; (2) if these already exist, attempting to heal them; (3) controlling the symptoms of ischemic neuropathy; (4) offsetting the deleterious effects of a rapidly progressing occlusive process, as reflected in a sudden marked worsening of the clinical picture; (5) contributing to the ability of the patient to be gainfully employed; and (6) fulfilling the desires of the occasional patient, psychologically affected by intermittent claudication, to be able to walk greater distances without pain. (For the questionable role that vascular reconstructive procedures play as a preliminary to podiatric surgery, see p. 344.)

Technical Considerations Regarding Choice of Candidates for Revascularization Procedures

Having satisfied the general criteria, as listed above, it is now necessary to ascertain whether the pathologic changes in the artery to be treated are such that the insertion of a graft or a thromboendarterectomy has a good possibility of significantly increasing blood flow to the foot. To obtain this information, it is necessary to perform contrast angiography (p. 72). Such a procedure supplies pertinent data regarding operability and the selection of the site and the type of surgical approach to utilize.

Although knowledge concerning the technical information derived from contrast angiography is not as important to the podiatrist as being acquainted with the criteria for selection of subjects for vascular reconstructive procedures, nevertheless, a brief review of this subject is considered to be useful and appropriate. The points of interest to the vascular surgeon, as visualized in the angiogram, are as follows: (1) the size of the involved artery; (2) the location and length of the primary occlusion; (3) the presence of stenosis or complete occlusion of other vessels; (4) the state of the arteries proximal to the primary involvement (the 'run-in'); (5) the state of the vessels beyond the obstructed artery (the 'runoff'); and (6) the extent of the available collateral circulation.

The length of the thrombosed segment is important in determining whether to perform a thromboendarterectomy, if the involvement is limited to an inch (ca 2.5 cm) or so of artery, or insert a venous or artificial prosthesis, if the occlusion extends for significantly more than this distance. If, on the other hand, a vessel like the superficial femoral artery is occluded in its entire length, the possibility of achieving a successful outcome with a venous graft is markedly reduced because of the extensive involvement.

If a vascular prosthesis is to remain patent for any period of time, two factors must be present: an adequate 'run-in' and, most importantly, a comparable 'runoff' (fig. 8/2a, b). In other words, there must be a good head of pressure and blood flow in the artery or arteries feeding the vascular prosthesis and an effective arterial tree distally to distribute the blood flow to the tissues of the leg and foot. Absence of either condition (fig. 8/2c, d) will result in occlusion of the graft in a short period of time. It is this situation which is responsible, in great part, for the failures associated with vascular reconstructive surgery. As a general rule, the patient demonstrating extensive disease of the arterial tree in a lower limb is a poor candidate for any type of reconstructive vascular surgery.

For the above reasons, every individual who has been subjected to a bypass procedure or a thromboendarterectomy must be under the medical supervision of his physician or the vascular surgeon for the remainder of his life. Through such careful observation, rapid obliteration of a prosthesis or a thromboendarterectomized segment of artery can quickly be identified and steps necessary to remedy this serious state instituted immediately. (For management of an occluded vascular prosthesis, see p. 162.)

Vascular Prostheses

At present, insertion of a vascular graft in an attempt to reestablish local circulation is generally accepted as the most effective surgical approach to the problem. As a result, this procedure has been subjected to intensive clinical trial.

Graft Materials. A large number of different substances have been used as vascular prostheses. In the case of blocks in the abdominal arteries, bifurcated tubes of Edwards woven Teflon or of Cooley double-velour Dacron are the most commonly used prostheses [33].

For grafts below the groin, the one of choice is an autologous reversed venous graft (fig. 8/3). Venous grafts in situ have also been considered and studied since they have a great advantage over the former type, provided

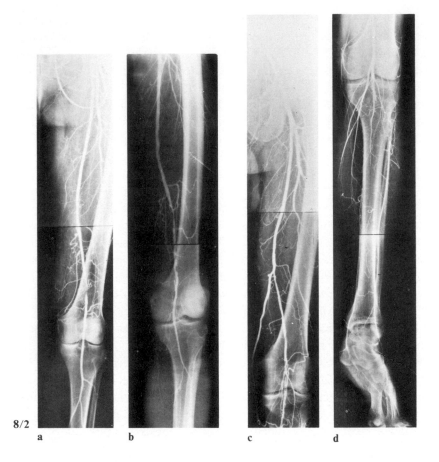

8/2

a   b   c   d

Fig. 8/2. Contrast arteriograms demonstrating findings which either support or negate the possibility of reconstructive vascular surgery. **a** Single short complete block present in the superficial femoral artery in its course through Hunter's canal. The proximal and distal segments of the vessel show no other signs of atherosclerosis. The distal 'runoff' is excellent, with the popliteal and its branches being clearly visualized. On the basis of the anatomic findings, a venous bypass graft or possibly a thromboendarterectomy is practical, provided an essential need to increase local blood flow exists. **b** Several stenoses are visualized in the lower portion of the superficial femoral artery. The proximal segment of the vessel demonstrates minor changes in the wall. The 'runoff', in the form of a well opacified apparently normal popliteal artery and its branches, appears to be adequate. On the basis of the changes, a fairly long venous femoropopliteal bypass graft is indicated, provided the clinical picture satisfies the criteria listed on page 153. **c, d** Arteriograms, obtained from the upper and lower portions of the lower limb of the same patient, demonstrate findings in the arterial tree which are not amenable to any type of reconstructive vascular procedure. There is a high complete block in the superficial femoral artery, with

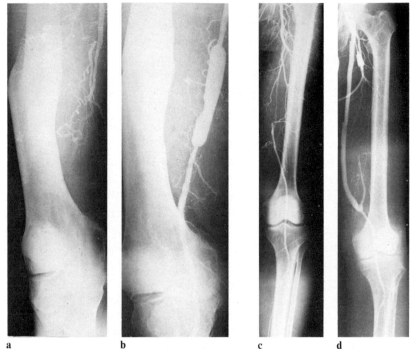

8/3

  a   b   c   d

no visualization of an effective 'runoff' in the leg. The popliteal artery and its branches are not visualized, indicating blocks in them and, instead, there is an extensive development of collateral channels. However, if a salvage procedure is being considered essential for the maintenance of viability of the foot, then a long artificial graft from the proximal segment of the superficial femoral artery to either the opacified posterior tibial artery at the ankle or the midsection of the anterior tibial artery is a possibility.

Fig. 8/3. Insertion of vascular prostheses in patients with arteriosclerosis obliterans. **a** Arteriographic demonstration of a complete block in the superficial femoral artery. **b** Visualization of an end-to-end patent reversed venous graft, with distal vessels now being opacified. **c** Arteriographic demonstration of a complete block of the superficial femoral artery in its middle portion and extending for some distance distally. The lower segment of artery below the occlusion is opacified through blood flow in the collateral vessels. **d** Visualization of a patent reversed venous graft, with distal vessels being opacified for some distance down the leg. Reproduced from ref. [2] with permission.

the technical problems associated with destroying the venous valves can be overcome. Artificial prostheses when inserted into the arterial tree below the groin have little possibility of remaining patent for any period of time and hence should not be used unless no other option is available.

Recently human umbilical cord vessels [15, 16] and expanded poly-tetrafluoroethylene prostheses [9, 52] have been proposed for patients who were otherwise faced with loss of a limb and in whom graft materials were either unavailable or unsuitable. Much more extensive trials with these substances are necessary in order to evaluate them properly as substitutes for the conventional graft materials. Thus far, evidence has appeared to indicate that intimal hyperplasia is a complication of polytetrafluoroethyl-ene graft, as it is of saphenous vein and other substitutes [20], an alteration which is responsible for graft thrombosis. However, the patency rates for this type of material have been found to be better than those accomplished with alternative conduits and approach the patency rates obtained with autogenous saphenous vein [9, 10].

Operative Techniques. The usual type of anastomosis for the abdomi-nal arteries is an aortic bifurcation graft, with the upper limb attached end-to-end or end-to-side to the distal segment of the abdominal aorta and the distal two limbs anastomosed each to a patent common femoral artery. If only one common iliac artery is occluded or stenosed, the proxi-mal end of a single stretch of graft is anastomosed to the vessel above the block and the distal end is attached to the common femoral artery on the same side.

In the case of occlusions in the arterial tree in the lower limbs, below the level of the groin, the most common procedure is a superficial femoral-popliteal bypass graft (fig. 8/3b, d). The upper anastomosis generally is an end-to-side attachment at a point above the block in the superficial femoral artery and the lower anastomosis is an end-to-side attachment to a patent popliteal artery.

A number of other types are used for overcoming blocks in the arterial tree in the lower limbs. One of these is the cross-over femorofemoral anas-tomosis used when the circulation in one limb is significantly and seriously reduced, whereas that in the other is still adequate. This approach is effec-tive only if there are no definite stenoses in the femoropopliteal system in the affected limb, since these could interfere with perfusion of blood even in the face of an increase in proximal perfusion pressure in the common femo-ral artery resulting from the bypass. The procedure is primarily of value when blocks exist in an unilateral common or external iliac artery which are not amenable to a surgical approach.

A potential danger associated with the cross-over femorofemoral by-pass procedure is that too great a quantity of blood will be shunted away from the donor limb, in the event that its distal vascular tree is somewhat involved, thus placing its structures in jeopardy. As a general rule, cross-over femorofemoral bypass grafts should not be performed if the donor iliac artery approaches 50% stenosis. It is of interest that no signs of progression of atherosclerotic changes have been noted in the vessel years after the procedure was performed. Among other infrequent surgical approaches is axillary-femoral artery bypass graft using an artificial prosthesis. Rarely does the latter remain patent for any significant period of time.

Salvage Procedures. In certain instances when conservative therapy has not been successful in healing an ulcer or a patch of gangrene on the distal segment of toes or extension of the process has occurred, it may be of value to attempt a salvage procedure in place of a major amputation in order to control the situation [43, 45]. Under such circumstances, an anastomosis may be indicated between the lower segment of a patent superficial femoral artery and a patent segment of a tibial artery at the level of the ankle, using a long artificial vascular prosthesis. Even though such an operation may only result in a temporary increase in local circulation before thrombosis occurs, this may be sufficient to prevent progression of a necrotic lesion and facilitate demarcation of viable from nonviable structures, thus permitting healing of the lesion. Once the latter occurs, the metabolic needs of now intact skin can readily be met by even a markedly reduced local blood flow, should the graft become occluded. As a result, the limb may be preserved, although a portion of a toe or toes may have to be sacrificed.

In order to carry out a successful salvage operation, it is necessary to determine whether a patent segment of posterior tibial or dorsal pedal artery is present at the level of the ankle. Such information is obtained by attempting to fill the vessels of the lower segment of leg and the foot with radiopaque material in the course of performing a pedal arteriogram, a modification of the conventional technique (p. 73). Under such circumstances, the portion of patent vessel is opacified by contrast media entering it via the collateral vessels.

Attention should be called to the fact that anatomic visualization of an open distal segment of tibial artery does not mean that blood flowing through it ordinarily contributes significantly to the delivery of nutrition to the foot. However, following a successful long graft operation, the high perfusion pressure in the superficial femoral artery is now transmitted to the blood in the patent distal segment of tibial artery, with the result that a high level of perfusion pressure is established in the vessels of the foot and local nutritional needs are again satisfied.

Conditions Influencing Patency of a Bypass Graft. A number of factors may be responsible for lack of success in maintaining graft patency; these include: technical operative errors [28]; poor judgment in choice of patients for the procedure, such as insertion of a prosthesis despite visualization of a poor 'runoff' by angiography; progression of the atherosclerotic process in distal vessels, leading to spontaneous thrombosis; a similar development in proximal vessels; infection of the graft; and thrombosis of a venous graft due to valve cusp fibrosis. It is again emphasized that in no way does the increased blood flow through the vascular prosthesis retard or interfere with the progressive atherosclerotic process occurring in the local arterial tree.

Besides being responsible for occlusion of grafts, certain complications of reconstructive procedures may seriously endanger the life of the patient. These include hemorrhage from the anastomoses, actual separation of an anastomotic junction, and infection in the bed of the prosthesis and in a thrombus filling the graft itself. Delayed healing in the operative sites may also pose a serious problem.

A number of other types of complications may develop early in the postoperative period. If the groin is the operative site, there is the possibility for the development of a lymph fistula because of the large accumulation of lymph channels and lymph nodes in this region. A common complication of a femoropopliteal bypass procedure is the early postoperative appearance of swelling of the entire limb, frequently also the result of damage to the lymph channels and nodes in the groin. This change may persist for weeks and months after the operation. Both the lymph fistulas and the swelling are difficult to control.

Management of Occluded Prostheses. When grafts fail early in the postoperative period (first 30 days), immediate operation is advisable to correct an overlooked technical error. In the period from 6 months to 2 years, when occlusion of the prosthesis results from graft stenosis due to smooth muscle proliferation [13], early reoperation and patch grafting are justified even if the patient is asymptomatic. Identification of such a situation can be determined by frequent physical examinations and noninvasive physiologic monitoring.

Late graft failures (after 2 years) may result from graft degeneration [6, 53], anastomatic true and false aneurysms [3], narrowing at the site of distal anastomosis, and infection [27]. These complications may be corrected by further reconstructive surgery designed to bypass new atherosclerotic lesions causing stenosis or complete closure of the vessel or to deal with other abnormal vascular difficulties. It is necessary to emphasize, however, that the second or third attempt to perform a revascularization procedure can rarely be expected to be as successful as the first operation [8].

Evaluation of Procedure. Despite the great number of adverse conditions capable of producing thrombosis of vascular prostheses, long-term follow-ups of reversed saphenous vein grafts for advanced femoropopliteal disease have revealed that about 50% of them will remain patent and without arteriographic evidence of degeneration up to 15 years [17]. However, there are also many other reports indicating a much shorter period of patency, with only 50% of the prostheses being operative after 3 years or less [39].

Bypass Procedures for Diabetics with Arteriosclerosis Obliterans. For such individuals, it is essential to keep in mind that in the case of those who fall into a younger age group, the atherosclerotic process may be located in the distal portion of the arterial tree in the lower limbs: the popliteal artery and its main branches, the anterior and posterior tibial arteries. Such a situation makes the conventional type of procedure technically inapplicable. Moreover, no 'runoff' into the foot may exist under such circumstances, primarily because of the frequently associated diffuse obliteration of the terminal arterial bed (p. 115). All of these factors are responsible for a more serious prognosis than is present in nondiabetics with arterial insufficiency, in whom slow occlusion of the proximal larger arteries usually elicits the formation of adequate collateral circulation distally in the leg and foot.

Despite the above theoretical objections, numerous studies have appeared in the literature supporting the view that diabetics with arterial insufficiency of the foot are good candidates for revascularization procedures. The latter include femoropopliteal, femorotibial, and femoroperoneal bypasses. In general, the revascular operation is successful in 30–40% of diabetic patients, which is much less than is the case for patients with arteriosclerosis obliterans alone.

Thromboendarterectomy

Since the advent of vascular prostheses, thromboendarterectomy has assumed a much less important role as a means of increasing blood flow to the limb suffering from arteriosclerosis obliterans.

Technique. The method consists of the production of a cleavage plane between the diseased intima (with attached intraluminar thrombus, internal limiting membrane, and media) and the external limiting membrane and adventitia of the artery. The separation is accomplished by means of a stripper inserted through an incision in the vessel, followed by removal of the core of loosened material reamed out by the instrument. The procedure is performed using a number of different techniques: the oscillating endarterectomy instrument, carbon dioxide gas endarterectomy, eversion endarterectomy, and semiclosed endarterectomy, among others.

Indications for Thromboendarterectomy. Ideally, the method is primarily applicable to small segments of stenotic lesions in large-calibered channels, such as the abdominal aorta and its main branches. For the procedure to be effective, the obstruction must be produced by a thrombus which is nonorganized or only minimally organized; moreover, there must be absence of calcification of the arterial wall. If a long stretch of occlusion is treated in this manner, the incidence of rethrombosis is high.

The advantage of the procedure is that no foreign material is introduced into the body, as is the case when an aortic bifurcation graft is used. Moreover, the operation is completed in much less time than is the case for the insertion of a prosthesis, and damage to the existing circulation is not as great. However, there may be more postoperative complications (p. 165).

When utilized for blocks below the level of the groin, as for superficial femoral-popliteal obstructions, thromboendarterectomy is much less successful than in the case of abdominal vessels. However, it has frequently been used for occlusions of the deep femoral artery (profundaplasty) [51], since the atherosclerotic process is generally limited to this short vessel and does not involve its extensive and rich branchings. As a result, the procedure is effective in reestablishing circulation to the leg and foot via the now patent deep femoral artery, its terminal branches, and those of the popliteal artery with which there are numerous communications. In order to enlarge the lumen of the deep femoral artery, a venous patch is frequently inserted in the arteriotomy incision. In a sense, the vascular network arising from the deep femoral artery can be considered to be a natural bypass between the common femoral and the popliteal arteries in the event of obliteration of the full length of the superficial artery, a situation in which insertion of a long stretch of vascular prosthesis or a thromboendarterectomy would probably end in failure.

Thromboendarterectomy is only infrequently used in the diabetic with arteriosclerosis obliterans because in many instances the blocks are located in the popliteal and tibial arteries, sites which do not readily lend themselves technically to such an approach. Moreover, in those individuals in whom the main occlusions are in more proximal vessels, such as the common and superficial femoral arteries, there are generally associated blocks in the 'runoff' distally. Under such circumstances, thromboendarterectomy of the proximal lesions would be expected to have little effect on increasing nutritional circulation to the foot.

Complications. Thromboendarterectomy may be associated with a number of serious adverse consequences. Among these are: (1) rethrombosis; (2) aneurysmal dilatation of the weakened arterial walls; (3) inadequate closure of the arteriotomy incision due to the poor state of the remaining wall, leading to serious hemorrhage; (4) peripheral emboli composed of fragments of intimal tissue; (5) dissection of the arterial wall by the catheter; (6) occlusion of critical arteries arising below the obstruction by compression of the clot against their orifices as the catheter is passed; and (7) perforation of the arterial wall by the guide wire and catheter. The basis for rethrombosis is either the aggregation of platelets, deposits of fibrin, or accumulation of material left by the procedure. In some instances, there is postoperative fibrosis, causing constriction of the lumen which predisposes to thrombus formation.

Evaluation of Procedure. Considerable debate exists regarding the role of thromboendarterectomy as a means of revascularizing a lower limb. Some workers believe that excellent results with regard to preservation of a limb can be expected from the operation, although it cannot be regarded as a substitute for other methods of direct femoropopliteal revascularization [5, 51]. Others are of the opinion that it does not restore walking capacity completely, although it may improve trophic lesions of the limb [4]. Another evaluation is that in the presence of both aortoiliac and femoropopliteal disease, thromboendarterectomy by itself is not sufficient to control the impairment of circulation.

The theoretical objections to the use of vascular prostheses in diabetics with arteriosclerosis obliterans (p. 163) apply equally to thromboendarterectomy. Nevertheless, several clinical studies are available indicating that beneficial effects may result from such a therapeutic approach in this group of patients.

Lumbar Sympathectomy

The role of lumbar sympathectomy as therapy in arteriosclerosis obliterans is debatable. In recent years, the procedure has been significantly downgraded as a treatment tool. It consists of the surgical removal of the first three lumbar paravertebral sympathetic ganglia on one side and, if indicated, two on the other, leaving the first ganglion intact.

On theoretical grounds, the operation would appear to have some application, since it produces loss of vasoconstrictor tone to a limb in need of greater local circulation. In contrast to the response to vasodilator drugs (p. 147), the procedure has no effect on vasomotor control over the rest of the body and hence there is no undesirable lowering of systemic blood pressure or local perfusion pressure. As a result, there is an increase in blood flow into the limb, provided that the arterial tree is still capable of dilating on removal of vasomotor tone. However, experimental studies have shown that the marked augmentation in circulation persists only for a few weeks, after which there may be a slight permanent increase. Also of importance in the evaluation of the procedure is the fact that the changes in blood flow are primarily in the cutaneous vascular tree of the foot, particularly the digits, with only minor alterations occurring in the skin of the leg and no significant, if any, increase in muscle circulation. Hence, the operation does not contribute to a lower level of amputation when extensive gangrene of the foot requires removal of a limb. Nor is it useful in the treatment of intermittent claudication. Because the increase in blood flow is not permanent, it is not indicated as a prophylactic measure to prevent the appearance of ulcers or gangrene.

Lumbar sympathectomy, therefore, has limited therapeutic application. It may contribute to a successful outcome after amputation of a gangrenous toe provided an element of vasospasm exists, a situation which is rarely the case in arteriosclerosis obliterans. It may help control the rest pain of ischemic neuropathy, and for this reason, it has a role in the case of the patient who is not a candidate for a graft procedure or thromboendarterectomy.

Lumbar sympathectomy is rarely of value in diabetics who are also suffering from arteriosclerosis obliterans. This is because in those who also have peripheral neuropathy, autosympathectomy may already exist as a result of destruction of the peripheral mixed nerves containing the sympathetic fibers; hence, the operation would contribute nothing further. Moreover, since diabetes frequently affects the terminal blood vessels, removal of sympathetic control over this type of vascular bed, particularly in the presence of diabetic microangiopathy, will not cause any significant increase in local blood flow. When peripheral neuropathy does not exist, in some patients, lumbar sympathectomy may relieve rest pain [19] and help control small ulcerations of the toes or foot proper. It may also facilitate healing of an operative site after amputation of a toe when only diabetes exists. Lumbar sympathectomy plays some role as a therapeutic procedure in thromboangiitis obliterans, since this disorder is frequently associated with an element of superimposed vasospasm. Hence, it may contribute to the control of local ulceration or gangrene of the foot and may be responsible for healing of an operative site following amputation of a toe. In contrast, reconstructive vascular procedures are of little value in this condition, since the occlusive process is almost invariably located in the popliteal artery and distally and not in the common or superficial femoral vessels.

Therapy for Complications of Aortoiliac Arterial Occlusive Disease and Arteriosclerosis Obliterans

Spontaneous Noninfected Aneurysms
Lesions of Abdominal Aorta. Because of the low incidence of catastrophic complications of the stenotic type of abdominal aortic aneurysm, conservative management is frequently indicated unless surgery is demanded by associated limb ischemia [39]. This approach is in contradistinction to therapy for the general dilatation of the abdominal aorta which almost always requires surgical intervention to prevent leakage or rupture, except when very serious contraindications to an extensive operative procedure exist.

Lesions in Arterial Tree of Lower Limbs. For a spontaneous aneurysm of the main arteries in the lower limbs, the proper therapeutic program generally involves excision of the lesion and reconstruction of arterial continuity by end-to-end anastomosis if feasible or by insertion of a vascular prosthesis. It is preferable to perform the necessary procedure before complications of the aneurysm develop, for otherwise their presence may make the technical approach to the problem much more difficult, thus materially reducing the possibility of a successful outcome.

Primary Cryptogenic Mycotic Aneurysms

Since primary cryptogenic mycotic aneurysms are associated with high mortality and morbidity from hemorrhage and overwhelming sepsis, early intensive treatment is essential. Appropriate high doses of antibiotics should be instituted immediately and then the patient should be subjected to ligation of the involved artery and excision of all infected tissue and foreign bodies, followed by reconstruction of vascular continuity if possible. However, it is necessary to point out that vein grafts, vein patches, suture repair, and Dacron graft replacement are frequently associated with re-bleeding and persistent infection requiring secondary procedures to control such complications. In any case, antibiotic therapy is continued for 6 weeks postoperatively. (For the treatment of atherothrombotic and cholesterol emboli, another complication of atherosclerosis of the arterial tree, see p. 87.)

Therapeutic Programs Specifically for Diabetics with or without Arteriosclerosis Obliterans

Besides the therapies to be discussed in this section (which apply almost exclusively to the diabetics), all the treatment programs already considered in the present chapter are also useful for the patient suffering from diabetes or from this disorder in conjunction with arteriosclerosis obliterans.

Local Care of the Feet

In fact, meticulous care of the feet of the diabetic is even more important than in the case of the individual with arteriosclerosis obliterans alone. It is also necessary to keep in mind that diabetics are notorious for the formation of calluses and corns. Hence, it is essential that shoes be properly fitting and soft and that they do not exert undue pressure in any area. Keratolytic agents like corn plasters should, of course, never be utilized for the treatment of the corns and calluses. The diabetic is particularly susceptible to the deleterious effects of heat, in part, because he may also be suffering from peripheral neuropathy and therefore has lost sensation in the involved foot. As a result, he is unable to determine the actual intensity of topically applied heat.

For the above reasons, the diabetic should be very careful in determining the temperature of the water used for a shower or a bath or, if unable to, because of peripheral neuropathy present also in the hands, should rely on the opinion of others for this purpose. With such a step, the possibility of thermal injuries should be significantly reduced. Moreover, the patient should never walk barefooted in order to prevent mechanical and thermal trauma and should avoid prolonged exposure to the sun since such an agent may be responsible for the development of a second or third degree burn. The most important factor in the treatment of the diabetic foot is the acceptance by the patient that this condition exists so that he can take the necessary precautions. Denial of the problem, a response that is not uncommon in the group of diabetics with peripheral neuropathy, may frequently lead to the development of serious complications and the need for numerous hospitalizations. Hence, in-depth explanation of his difficulty to the patient and discussion of the risks associated with noncompliance with simple prophylactic measures are essential approaches to therapy.

Control of Blood Sugar Level

The role of an elevated blood sugar level in the production of vascular abnormalities in diabetes has not been fully elucidated [48]. There is some evidence that poor control of the hyperglycemic state accelerates the process, whereas good control prevents, minimizes, or postpones the appearance of the vascular changes. However, it should be emphasized that poor therapy does not invariably lead to their production; nor does proper treatment necessarily guarantee immunity from them. With regard to the formation of large artery disease, excellent control of adult-onset diabetes may act as a deterrent, although such a possibility has by no means been conclusively proved [32].

With regard to microangiopathy, there is some evidence that advances in the capability to monitor metabolic control, as well as the evolution of techniques for more physiologic insulin delivery (insulin pumps), may slow down the rate of development of this vascular change [36]. However, there is some evidence that many of the microangiopathic complications associated with diabetes are genetic in nature and actually precede the development of hyperglycemia.

Also of importance in the elucidation of the problem is the fact that meticulous control of the hyperglycemia is not without hazard, particularly with relation to the onset of hypoglycemia and its attendant adverse reactions. Furthermore, the above statements are only tentative, since no documentation exists concerning the vascular benefits of lifelong precise control of diabetes. Finally, accurate minute-to-minute maintenance of a normal blood glucose level is not feasible under present conditions.

Therapy for Peripheral Neuropathy

General Measures. Enough evidence exists to support the belief that good control of hyperglycemia in the diabetic is advisable in the management of peripheral neuropathy (p. 120). Other measures are proper hygiene, adequate nutrition, and physical therapy to maintain range of motion of the joints in the affected limb. In the presence of foot drop, the ankle joint and foot should be properly protected with a foot-drop brace in the hope that spontaneous improvement will subsequently occur.

Drug Therapy. As a general rule, an intensive course of thiamin chloride by mouth (200 mg 4 times daily) is indicated. If such a program is continued for several months, some return of vibration sense perception can be expected. No adverse effects have been noted from prolonged use of this medication. Another drug which has been reported as having a beneficial effect is phenytoin sodium (Dilantin), 0.1 g 3 times a day for several months. If improvement is equivocal, then two courses of phenylbutazone (Butazolidin), 200 mg twice a day, may be given for 5 days each, in conjunction with Dilantin. Prednisone, 10 mg 3 times a day, may also be utilized at the same time, Vitamin B_{12}, 1,000 μg daily for a week and 3 times a week thereafter for a relatively long period of time, has also been suggested. Other medications which have had clinical trials with apparently some success are promethazine hydrochloride (Phenergan) and clofibrate (Atromid S). Recently a potent aldose-reductase inhibitor (Sorbinil) has been reported to be effective in treating symptomatic somatic and autonomic neuropathies [31]. A single 250-mg dose of the drug was found to produce substantial relief of pain, beginning on the third or fourth day of treatment, especially in patients with muscle atrophy (amyotrophy). Improvement in nerve conduction velocity was noted in some of the treated patients.

Since very severe pain may be present in diabetic peripheral neuropathy, attempts have to be made to control the symptom with medication.

However, it is important to avoid the administration of narcotics in large doses so as to prevent addiction, and hence, if at all feasible, aspirin and codein should be substituted.

Therapy for Neurotrophic Ulcers

Medical Measures. The first therapeutic approach to the control of the neurotrophic ulcer in the diabetic foot with peripheral neuropathy is its prevention. Most important in this regard is the determination of pressure points under the foot. These can be identified very simply by the Harris mat or slipper-dash sock print, each of which leaves an impression of foot pressures. With such information available, attempts should now be made to redistribute the weight on the limb by the use of conventional means, thus reducing the risk of the development of calluses over metatarsal heads. Trimming of existing calluses should be routinely carried out and steps should be instituted to control cracking and fissuring of the skin of the plantar surface of the feet (resulting from a reduction or absence of sweat and sebaceous gland secretions) by the daily application of hand lotions or creams containing lanolin. The plantar surface of the feet should be routinely inspected for excoriations and superficial infections by the patient using a mirror if feasible, or if not, by a member of his family. Any break in the continuity of the skin warrants immediate and intensive treatment.

The conservative treatment of the neurotrophic ulcer is difficult and recurrences are frequent. Nevertheless, such an attempt should always be made initially. Of great importance is removal of pressure from the involved area. At first this is accomplished by bedrest which also prevents the spread of superimposed infection almost invariably found in the lesion. Later the ulcerated area is protected from weight-bearing by the use of a molded insole.

In every case, infection should be attacked aggressively. Smears should be taken as early as possible in the manner described on page 299, and the offending organism isolated. Then, on the basis of sensitivity tests, appropriate antibiotics should be used in high dosages. When bacterial cultures cannot be obtained, antibiotic therapy should be started empirically, using a wide-spectrum drug. Because of the excellent local blood supply generally present, there is no problem in building up an adequate concentration of the antibiotic in the infected tissues. Hence, in most instances the spread of the inflammation is readily controlled and localization of the lesion follows.

In conjunction with the above measures, debridement of necrotic tissue should be carefully carried out. Callus material should also be removed, until the pink edges of the ulcer are visible. All of this is performed without local or general anesthesia, following a short interval of immersion in a whirlpool bath to soften the material to be removed. It is necessary to point out that prolonged soaking of the diabetic foot in a watery solution, however, such as continuous irrigation of a wound with boric acid solution, is contraindicated, since maceration of the skin will invariably occur. Moreover, cutaneous lesions should not be covered with antibiotic ointments, particularly those located in the web between toes, because the oily base ordinarily used will have the same effect. Sinus tracts leading from the original site of involvement should be destroyed using silver nitrate applicators. If thick eschars are present over the lesion, there is no advantage to the use of local antibiotics, since these will not penetrate the necrotic material.

In those instances when it is essential for the patient to remain ambulatory in order to continue being gainfully employed, it may be necessary for him to resort to crutches even early in the treatment period or to apply a walking cast. In the case of the latter measure, first the ulcer is debrided of all devitalized structures and then covered with sterile gauze and a 0.25 inch thick felt padding. One end of a catheter is placed in proximity to the sterile dressing and the other end is directed between the web of two toes onto the dorsum of the foot and led out during application of the cast. Such an arrangment makes it possible to utilize the catheter for subsequent installation of local medications in the ulcer site. After the use of appropriate and abundant cast padding, the plaster is applied up to a level just below the knee, a rubber rocker being attached for weight bearing [44]; the latter is delayed for 24 h. Casts are reapplied at weekly intervals until healing of the ulcer is achieved. This method is not suitable if either deep sepsis or osteomyelitis exists [44].

Surgical Measures. It is necessary to point out that there are some workers [40, 41] who believe that surgical procedures should always be utilized as therapy for neurotrophic ulcers. Among the procedures that have been proposed are tenotony of the flexors of the toe or toes involved and disarticulation [42]. Lesions tend to heal fairly promptly after resection and a weight-bearing foot is obtained. Ambulation with crutches is permitted within a few days after surgery and graduated weight bearing is begun in 3 weeeks. After total healing, orthotic devices and properly fitted shoes are prescribed in order to permit a correct distribution of body weight in function.

Therapy for Neurotrophic Arthropathy

The basic principles of treatment for the involved joint suffering from neurotrophic arthropathy consist of immobilization of, and restriction of weight-bearing on, the affected structure. Surprising improvement may occur if complete immobilization of a lower limb can be provided by plaster casts.

Operative measures are usually limited to amputation or arthrodesis of a weight-bearing joint. The latter procedure, however, frequently fails because of infection, nonunion, or both. Nevertheless, in the relatively young adult, improvement following successful fusion makes the attempt worthwhile. Syme's amputation appears justified in the case of Charcot's joints of the foot.

References

1   Abramson, D.I.: Diagnosis and treatment of peripheral vascular disorders (Hoeber-Harper, New York 1954).

2   Abramson, D.I.: Vascular disorders of the extremities (Harper & Row, Hagerstown 1974).

3   Agrifoglio, G.; Costantini, S.; Zanetta, M.; et al.: Infections and anastomotic false aneurysms in reconstructive vascular surgery. J. cardiovasc. Surg. *20:* 25 (1979).

4   Agrifoglio, G.; Costantini, S.; Castelli, P.; et al.: Thromboendarterectomy for peripheral occlusive arterial disease. J. cardiovasc. Surg. *20:* 369 (1979).

5   Belcastro, S.; Azzena, G.; Pampolini, M.; et al.: Angioplasty of the profunda femoris in revascularisation of the lower extremity. J. cardiovasc. Surg. *20:* 265 (1979).

6   Berguer, R.; Higgins, R.F.: Deterioration of grafts and prostheses. J. cardiovasc. Surg. *17:* 493 (1976).

7   Brandt, R.; Blankenhorn, D.H.; Crawford, D.W.; et al.: Regression and progression of early femoral atherosclerosis in treated hyperlipoproteinemic patients. Ann. intern. Med. *86:* 139 (1977).

8   Burgess, E.M.: Major lower extremity amputation following arterial reconstruction. Archs Surg., Chicago *108:* 855 (1974).

9   Campbell, C.D.; Brooks, D.H.; Webster, M.W.; Bahnson, H.T.: The use of expanded microporous polytetrafluoroethylene for limb salvage: a preliminary report. Surgery, St. Louis *79:* 485 (1976).

10   Campbell, C.D.; Brooks, D.H.; Webster, M.W.; Diamond, D.L.; Peel, R.L.; Bahnson, H.T.: Expanded microporous polytetrafluoroethylene as a vascular substitute: a two-year follow-up. Surgery, St. Louis *85:* 177 (1979).

11   Castaneda-Zuniga, W.R.; Formanek, A.; Tadavarthy, M.; et al.: The mechanism of balloon angioplasty. Radiology *135:* 565 (1980).

12   Chin, A.K.; Fogarty, T.J.; Kinney, T.B.; Hayden, W.G.; Shoor, P.M.; Rurik, G.W.: Pathophysiologic bases for transluminal dilatation. Surg. Forum *32:* 323 (1981).

13 Clowes, A.W.: Current theories of arterial graft failure. Vas. Diag. Ther. *3:* 41 (1982).

14 Dahllöf, A.-G.; Björntorp, P.; Holm, J.; et al.: Metabolic activity of skeletal muscle in patients with peripheral arterial insufficiency. Effect of physical training. Eur. J. clin. Invest. *4:* 9 (1974).

15 Dardik, H.; Dardik, J.: Successful arterial substitution with umbilical vein. Ann. Surg. *183:* 252 (1976).

16 Dardik, I.I.; Ibrahim, I.M.; Dardik, H.: Experimental and clinical use of human umbilical cord vessels as vascular substitutes. J. cardiovasc. Surg. *18:* 555 (1977).

17 Dhall, D.P.; Mavor, G.E.: Long-term behavior of reversed saphenous vein grafts for advanced femoropopliteal disease. Surgery Gynec. Obstet. *146:* 241 (1978).

18 Dotter, C.T.; Judkins, M.P.: Transluminal treatment of arteriosclerotic obstruction. Description of a new technic and a preliminary report of its application. Circulation *30:* 654 (1964).

19 Eadie, D.G.A.: The management of arterial disease. Br. J. Hosp. Med. *3:* 337 (1970).

20 Echave, V.; Koornick, A.R.; Haimov, M.; Jacobson, J.H. II: Intimal hyperplasia as a complication of the use of the polytetrafluoroethylene graft for femoral-popliteal bypass. Surgery, St. Louis *86:* 791 (1979).

21 Engel, E.D.; Erlick, N.E.; Davis, R.H.: Diabetes mellitus: impaired wound healing from zinc deficiency. J. Am. Podiat. Ass. *71:* 536 (1981).

22 Freiman, D.B.: Percutaneous transluminal angioplasty for occlusive arterial disorders of the limbs: current status. Pract. Cardiol. *9:* 66 (1983).

23 Freiman, D.B.; Spence, R.; Gatenby, R.; Gertner, M.; Roberts, B.; Berkowitz, H.D.; Ring, E.S.; Oleago, S.A.: Transluminal angioplasty of the iliac and femoral arteries: follow-up results without anticoagulation. Radiology *141:* 347 (1981).

24 Grüntzig, A.; Hopff, H.: Perkutane Rekanalisation chronischer arterieller Verschlüsse mit einem neuen Dilatations-Katheter. Dt. med. Wschr. *99:* 2502 (1974).

25 Hall, F.A.; Barnard, R.J.: The effects of an intensive 26-day program of diet and exercise on patients with peripheral vascular disease. J. cardiac Rehabil. *2:* 569 (1982).

26 Hammarsten, J.; Holm, J.; Schersten, T.: Peripheral arterial insufficiency: experience from 229 operated limbs. J. cardiovasc. Surg. *17:* 503 (1976).

27 Hammarsten, J.; Holm, J.; Schersten, T.: Infection in vascular surgery. J. cardiovasc. Surg. *18:* 543 (1977).

28 Harjola, P.-T.: Causes of rethrombosis after arterial reconstruction. J. cardiovasc. Surg. *16:* 357 (1975).

29 Hasson, J.; Abbott, W.: Value of routine treadmill testing prior to elective surgery for peripheral arterial disease. Pract. Cardiol. *9:* 47 (1983).

30 Holm, J.; Dahllöff, A.-G.; Björntorp, P.; et al.: Enzyme studies in muscles of patients with intermittent claudication. Effects of training. Scand. J. clin. Lab. Invest. *31:* suppl. 128, p. 201 (1973).

31 Jaspan, J.; Herold, K.; Maselli, R.; Bartkus, C.: Treatment of severely painful diabetic neuropathy with an aldose reductase inhibitor: relief of pain and improved somatic and autonomic nerve function. Lancet *ii:* 758 (1983).

32 Knatterud, G.L.; Klimt, C.R.; Levin, M.E.; Jacobson, M.E.; Goldner, M.G.: Effects of hypoglycemic agents on vascular complications in patients with adult-onset dia-

betes. VII. Mortality and selected nonfatal events with insulin treatment. J. Am. med. Ass. *240:* 37 (1978).

33 Knox, R.; Charlesworth, D.: Aortic bifurcation grafts: a study of the long-term patency of two different prostheses. Vas. Diag. Ther. *3:* 19 (1982).

34 Kumpe, D.A.; Jones, D.N.: Percutaneous transluminal angioplasty: radiologic viewpoint. Appl. Radiol. *11:* 29 (1982).

35 Larsen, C.A.; Lassen, N.A.: Effects of daily muscular exercise in patients with intermittent claudication. Lancet *ii:* 903 (1966).

36 Lundbaek, K.: Diabetic angiopathy. Mod. Concepts cardiovasc. Dis. *43:* 103 (1974).

37 Lyle, C.R.; Downs, A.R.: Grafting for femoropopliteal occlusive disease. Vas. Diag. Ther. *2:* 35 (1981).

38 Mandy, S.G.; Garrot, T.C.: Miconazole treatment for severe dermatophytoses. J. Am. med. Ass. *230:* 72 (1974).

39 Martin, P.: A reconstruction of arterial reconstruction below the inguinal ligament. J. cardiovasc. Surg. *13:* 34 (1972).

40 Martin, W.J.; Weil, L.S.; Smith, S.D.: Surgical management of neurotrophic ulcers in the diabetic foot. J. Am. med. Ass. *65:* 365 (1975).

41 McCook, J.; Beauballet, P.; Llanes, P.; et al.: Surgical treatment of the perforating ulcer of the foot. J. cardiovasc. Surg. *7:* 101 (1966).

42 McCullough, C.C., Jr.: Diabetic neurotrophic ulcers of feet: surgical correction by wedge or pie resection. Missouri Med. *58:* 117 (1961).

43 Nicholas, G.G.; Barker, C.F.; Berkowitz, H.D.; et al.: Reconstructive surgery distal to popliteal trifurcation: effect on the history of arterial occlusive disease. Archs Surg., Chicago *107:* 652 (1973).

44 Pollard, J.P.; Le Quesne, L.P.: Method of healing diabetic forefoot ulcers. Br. med. J. *286:* 436 (1983).

45 Purdy, R.T.; Bole, P.; Makanju, W.; Munda, R.: Salvage of the ischemic lower extremity in patients with poor runoff. Archs Surg., Chicago *109:* 784 (1974).

46 Ruderman, N.B.; Young, J.C.; Schneider, S.H.: Exercise as a therapeutic tool in the type I diabetic. Pract. Cardiol. *10:* 143 (1984).

47 Scherstén, T.: Indications and methods of exercise training of patients with intermittent claudication. Pract. Cardiol. *8:* 45 (1982).

48 Service, F.J.; Daube, J.R.; O'Brien, P.C.; Zimmerman, R.; Swanson, C.S.; Brennan, M.D.; Dyck, P.J.: Effect of blood glucose control on peripheral nerve function in diabetic patients. Mayo Clin. Proc. *58:* 283 (1983).

49 Spence, R.K.; Freiman, D.B.; Gatenby, R.; et al.: Long-term results of transluminal angioplasty of the iliac and femoral arteries. Archs Surg., Chicago *116:* 1377 (1981).

50 Terleckyj, B.; Goldman, S.M.; Abramson, C.: Microflora of the intertriginous toe surfaces of patients with athlete's foot. J. Am. Podiat. Ass. *71:* 529 (1981).

51 Thompson, B.W.; Read, R.C.; Slayden, J.E.; et al.: The role of primary and secondary profundaplasty in the treatment of vascular insufficiency. J. cardiovasc. Surg. *18:* 55 (1977).

52 Veith, F.J.; Moss, C.M.; Fell, S.C.; Rhodes, B.A.; Haimovici, H.: Comparison of expanded PTFE and vein grafts in lower extremity arterial reconstructions. J. cardiovasc. Surg. *19:* 341 (1978).

53 Welsh, P.; Parisi, C.; Rosas, G.; Repetto, R.; Palodino, C.: Degenerative changes in autologous saphenous veins used as arterial bypass grafts. J. cardiovasc. Surg. *15:* 700 (1974).

54 Zarins, C.K.; Lu, C.T.; Gewertz, B.L.; Lyon, R.T.; Rush, D.S.; Glagov, S.: Arterial disruption and remodeling following balloon dilatation. Surg. *92:* 1086 (1982).

55 Zertler, E.; Grüntzig, A.; Schoop, W.: Percutaneous vascular recanalization (Springer, New York 1978).

9 Spontaneous Chronic Occlusive Arterial Disorders: Major and Minor Lower Limb Amputations

Even in the case of properly treated patients suffering from a chronic occlusive arterial disorder of the lower limb, a certain small number will develop necrosis of a foot or feet which becomes unresponsive to conservative therapy. This situation generally arises as a result of accelerated progression of the obliterative process in a critical artery, in the absence of a corresponding growth of collateral vessels. Under such circumstances, removal of the devitalized tissue, in the form of a major or minor amputation, is essential for the well-being of the patient. This chapter is devoted to the various problems inherent in consummating such a decision and means to deal with them.

Factors Leading to Amputation

The development of a number of local and systemic changes in the patient with a treatment-resistant ischemic ulceration or gangrene of a foot makes it imperative to consider amputation as the only option left for controlling a deteriorating and serious situation.

Extension of a Necrotic Lesion of a Toe onto the Foot Proper
Progressive Arterial Thrombosis. When an area of gangrene, initially limited to the distal portion of a toe or toes, begins to extend onto the foot itself despite intensive conservative efforts to localize and delimit the process, the possibility exists that larger arcuate arteries from which the digital vessels arise have become occluded or that proximal channels feeding these vessels have developed the same pathologic change. As progression of the necrotic lesion occurs, generally tendons, bone, and joints of the foot proper become affected, as well as overlying skin and subcutaneous tissue. When such a situation develops, the likelihood of saving the limb by conservative therapy is poor. Under certain limited conditions, a reconstructive salvage

operation (p. 161) may sometimes be helpful, but usually the proper course is a major amputation, since the gangrenous process will continue to involve more toes and distal segments of the foot.

Local Infection. A superimposed, uncontrolled infection, which at times is found in the patient suffering from both arteriosclerosis obliterans and diabetes mellitus or from the latter alone, is frequently responsible for the same sequence of events as noted when progressive local arterial thrombosis occurs (see above). Under such circumstances, extensive spread of the local necrotic process, with subsequent destruction of neighboring tissues, will result from the inflammatory state. At the same time, arterioles and capillaries in the area of involvement will become thrombosed, thus also contributing to local tissue damage. Again, further delay is no longer warranted, since at this point a conservative approach generally does not alter the ultimate outcome.

Constitutional Responses to Absorption from Gangrenous Lesion

As more and more structures are affected by ischemia and/or infection, with loss of viability, systemic signs of absorption of toxic material may be noted in the patient, including a rise in body temperature, drowsiness, apathy, and loss of appetite. Since it is not advisable to permit such a situation to persist because of the serious consequences to the physical and mental state of the patient, he should be prepared for the possibility of amputation of the affected limb.

Untoward Effects of Pain

In some individuals with a low threshold for pain, it becomes necessary to consider amputation of a lower limb due to the exaggerated response to the symptoms, rather than because of the severity of the existing nutritional lesion alone. In such a situation, it is assumed, of course, that all medical means to control pain has been found to be futile, including continued use of large quantities of narcotics. In patients of this type, such a heroic measure as a major amputation is essential to prevent further accentuation of an already existing drug addiction or even suicide. Fortunately, this situation is encountered only rarely in individuals with arteriosclerosis obliterans, but more often in those with thromboangiitis obliterans who have not abstained from smoking. At times, peripheral nerve crushing may temporarily help control the symptoms, which are then replaced by a sense of numbness of the foot and leg.

Physical and Mental Deterioration of the Patient

If conservative management of the gangrenous or ulcerative lesion on the foot has been prolonged, without any beneficial changes resulting therefrom, the physical status of the patient may begin to decline, thus making him a poor candidate for subsequent unquestionably necessary surgery. At the same time, his mental state and morale are also deteriorating because of the many adverse psychologic factors that are continuously harassing him. Such possibilities must be taken into consideration when determining the course of action for the patient with a chronic, indolent, nonhealing ulceration or gangrene of the foot.

Preoperative Goals

With the decision reached that the only course available to cope with the situation is amputation of the involved limb, it is necessary to institute a number of preliminary measures to increase the possibility of a successful outcome from such an approach.

Psychologic Preparation of Patient for Surgery

The usual response of an individual informed that amputation of a lower limb is the only available option for controlling his condition is that he would rather die than permit an approach which would have such a devastating effect upon his body image. It therefore becomes essential to use every means possible to make him adopt a realistic point of view regarding the only solution to his problem. Consummate tact, patience, and persuasiveness are frequently required to reach such a goal, provided, of course, that there is enough time for this purpose.

On occasion, however, the gangrenous process progresses so rapidly that need for immediate amputation is imperative, with the result that the patient cannot be adequately prepared psychologically. This makes the task of obtaining his consent to the procedure even more difficult. Nevertheless, in most instances, there is sufficient time to persuade him to the proper decision because of the generally protracted course of his illness, the lack of signs of improvement, the severe local pain, the deteriorating effects of bedrest, and the high costs of prolonged hospitalization. The mental anguish of relatives on observing the suffering he is enduring for no good purpose contributes to reaching the correct conclusion. Emphasized also is the obvious fact that if nothing is done, the patient will linger on for weeks and months, suffering all during this period, before death occurs.

At the same time, it is essential to emphasize to the patient that he may be able to carry out many of his previous daily activities following amputation in a fairly normal and efficient manner using a prosthesis. In this regard, it is worthwhile to have an amputee with an artificial leg discuss the matter with him and demonstrate how capably he has adjusted to his difficulty. Counseling from a psychiatrist or a medical social worker may likewise be of value. When subjected to all of the above-mentioned influences, in almost all instances the patient will reluctantly agree to the proper step.

Physical Preparation of Patient for Surgery

As soon as it becomes clear that amputation is inevitable, attempts should be taken at once to build up the physical state of the patient so as to prepare him for the life of an amputee. The first approach is to improve his general condition by means of blood transfusions, intravenous fluid, and adequate proteins and vitamins in his diet. At the same time, controlled exercises, in the form of calisthenics using the muscles of the three uninvolved extremities and the trunk, should be instituted. Attempts should also be made to prevent or reduce joint contractures proximal to the anticipated level of amputation and maintain normal range of motion with therapeutic exercises. Training should be begun in teaching the patient to transfer from the bed to the chair and then to the standing position, with weight-bearing only on the unaffected lower limb. Balance and postural exercises should also be carried out. It is likewise of value to instruct the patient in those measures which strengthen the muscles of the upper limbs used in crutch walking and to train him in this procedure utilizing only the uninvolved limb. The manner in which these steps are performed gives the examiner some insight as to the patient's potential for walking with a prosthesis following operation.

Determination of Optimal Level for Amputation

A number of factors must be considered in reaching a decision as to the proper site for amputation of a limb. The most important of these is the goal of retaining the maximum and optimum amount of tissue without seriously incurring the risk of a prolonged period of bedrest to achieve healing of the stump. This view is especially applicable to the elderly patient who generally has other infirmities for which inactivity and bed confine-

a   b   c

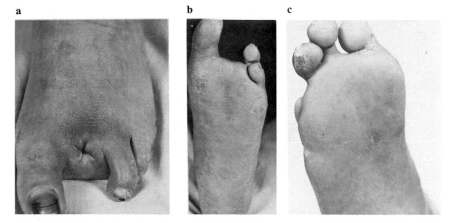

Fig. 9/1. Surgical amputation of toes in patients with diabetes and no manifestations of involvement of the large arteries in the lower extremities. **a, b** Amputation of second and third toes. **c** Amputation of fourth and fifth toes. In each instance complete healing of the operative site resulted. All patients demonstrated normal pulsations in dorsal pedal and posterior tibial arteries in involved feet. Reproduced from ref. [1] with permission.

ment are detrimental [2]. Another pertinent point to take into account is that such an individual generally also responds poorly to a second anesthetic and an amputation at a higher level when such a course is required because of lack of satisfactory healing of, or uncontrolled infection in, the initial operative site.

The following discussion is limited to topics pertaining specifically to amputations in patients with an underlying chronic or acute occlusive arterial disease in the lower extremities and has no bearing on the treatment of a limb with a normal circulation that has sustained extensive trauma, thereby requiring a similar surgical approach.

Consideration of Foot and Ankle Amputations. The benefit derived from limiting the operation to *removal* of a *toe* or several *toes* (fig. 9/1) is, of course, apparent. However, great care must be taken in the choice of patients for such an approach (p. 182). Otherwise, healing of the operative site will not occur and a second amputation site on the leg or thigh will have to be utilized, with all its attendant risks.

Surgical removal of all the toes and metatarsal heads (transmetatarsal amputation) (fig. 9/2a) has a great advantage in that rehabilitation of the patient can readily be accomplished. All that is required subsequently is the use of a foam rubber insert or a leather-covered steel shank placed in the toe of the shoe. An excellent functional lower limb still exists since removal of the metatarsal heads does not significantly affect the three-point bearing surface of the foot. However, there is loss of the normal 'push off' which is delivered by the movement of the toes. Transmetatarsal amputation is considered when there is gangrene of several toes and the necrotic process has begun to involve the distal portion of the dorsum of the foot. If the plantar surface is also affected, this practically contraindicates the use of such an approach since an adequate plantar flap to cover the operative site is no longer available under such conditions.

A supramalleolar amputation (Syme's procedure) [6] (fig. 9/2b) has the advantage that essentially the full length of the shank is retained and weight-bearing is practically similar to that existing with an intact heel. Also, this type of operation enables the amputee to walk or stand without support using a Syme's prosthesis. The procedure is applicable when the gangrenous process has extended over a good portion of the distal segment of the foot so that a transmetatarsal amputation is no longer feasible.

Evaluation of Local Circulation at Foot and Ankle Amputation Sites. In order to expect healing of the operative site to occur after toe or toes amputation, transmetatarsal amputation, or supramalleolar amputation, most of the following criteria must be satisfied: (1) At least one of the arteries of the ankle or foot (preferably the posterior tibial) must demonstrate a good pulsation. (2) Oscillometric readings at the lower segment of leg, just above the ankle, should be at least 1 unit or higher. (3) Blood pressure in the posterior tibial artery at the ankle or the dorsal pedal artery on the dorsum of the foot should be 70 mm Hg or higher [8], using the Doppler ultrasonic flowmeter (p. 67). (4) Any local inflammatory process must be controlled and signs of involvement of the foot proper must be minimal or absent at the time of operation. (5) Lines of demarcation between viable and necrotic tissue should have developed, a situation which is preferable but not essential. In the case of amputation of a toe or toes, an added condition is that the gangrenous process must be limited to the distal segment of the digit, with normal tissue intervening between it and the attachment of the toe or toes to the foot proper. If most of these criteria are not satisfied (especially pulsations in an artery in the foot and an adequate blood pressure at the ankle), the prognosis as to subsequent healing of the operative site is poor.

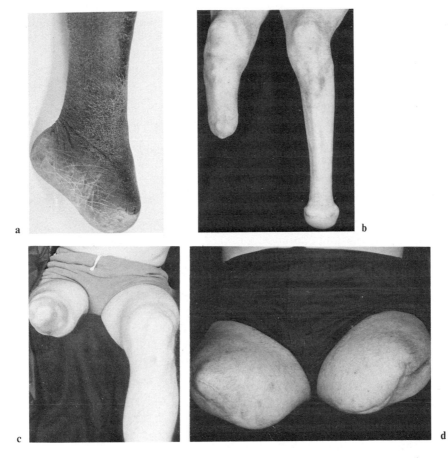

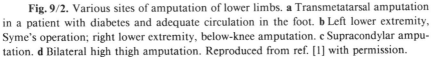

Fig. 9/2. Various sites of amputation of lower limbs. **a** Transmetatarsal amputation in a patient with diabetes and adequate circulation in the foot. **b** Left lower extremity, Syme's operation; right lower extremity, below-knee amputation. **c** Supracondylar amputation. **d** Bilateral high thigh amputation. Reproduced from ref. [1] with permission.

Results of Foot and Ankle Amputations in Different Types of Patients. The best candidate for a successful outcome following a foot or ankle amputation is the diabetic patient who suffers from occlusive disease of the terminal arteries to the digits but often has patent vessels in the thigh and leg, as reflected in good pulsations in the posterior tibial artery at the ankle and/or in the dorsal pedal artery. On the other hand, rarely can healing be expected to occur in the operative site if the patient is suffering from arteriosclerosis obliterans with stenosis or thrombosis of the main arteries in the thigh and leg and, of course, with no pulsations in the tibial arteries in the foot. In the case of the individual with thromboangiitis obliterans, who manifests signs of moderate or severe vasospasm as well as organic occlusion of arteries in the leg and foot, amputation of a toe or toes may have a successful outcome, provided a lumbar sympathectomy is performed at the time of operation and the patient has abstained completely from smoking for at least 2 months before the procedure. Such a good therapeutic response may be possible even if pulsations are absent in the tibial arteries in the foot.

Considerations of Leg and Thigh Amputations. There is no question that if a major amputation of a lower limb is being considered, all efforts should be made to preserve the knee joint and carry out a below-knee amputation (fig. 9/2b). In the case of the elderly patient, such a measure offers a greatly improved potential for the use of a prosthesis and hence for self-care. It also leaves him with better proprioceptive balance than does an above-knee amputation. Moreover, the available prostheses are much lighter than those applicable to the above-knee amputee, a very important consideration in the case of the individual who may also be suffering from chronic lung and/or heart disorders. Even if the patient is not a candidate for a prosthesis, the increased length of the remaining limb is of great advantage to him in moving about in bed and getting into a wheelchair. Another important point is that the below-knee amputation is associated with a lower mortality than is the above-knee level [4]. For all these reasons, removing the limb without sacrificing the knee joint should not be dismissed unless the physical findings indicate very little chance for a successful outcome. It is necessary to point out that to achieve the desired result with a below-knee amputation, meticulous surgical technique and careful control of wound complications are essential.

Despite all the advantages to a below-knee amputation, this procedure is also associated with certain difficulties which detract significantly from its overall usefulness. In many of the patients with ischemic gangrene due to atherosclerosis, the same process is present also in the larger vessels in the thigh and proximally, as well as in the leg arteries. Moreover, such a disorder is progressive, and for this reason, some surgeons prefer to operate at a higher level on the limb where a better blood supply can be expected to be found, as compared with the leg, thus facilitating healing of the stump.

Since elderly patients, as a group, are poor operative risks, of value in this regard is the fact that performing the surgery at the level of the thigh would significantly reduce the need for a second amputation, a possibility that would almost invariably be indicated in the case of lack of healing of a below-knee stump. Another point to consider is that generally a much longer period of bed confinement is required to obtain healing of a below-knee amputation than is necessary for an above-knee level, a situation conducive to postoperative complications, especially in the geriatric patient. Naturally, when there is a 15° or more permanent knee contracture (not uncommonly found in bedridden elderly patients), the possibility of a below-knee amputation is practically ruled out.

An above-knee amputation (fig. 9/2c, d) should therefore be considered only after the results of the various tests for determining the state of the circulation below the knee (see below) have revealed that a significantly compromised local blood flow exists in the leg and/or that there are associated medical conditions which make the patient a high risk for any operative procedures. The great advantage of a supracondylar or a mid-thigh amputation is that it can generally be anticipated that adequate stump healing will occur in a relatively short time.

Evaluation of Local Circulation at Below-Knee Amputation Site. Besides initial palpation of pulses in the limb, pertinent information regarding the state of the circulation in the leg below the knee can be derived from the results of several clinical and laboratory tests, one of the more valuable of which is oscillometry (p. 58). If the reading at the level of the calf is 3 units or more, this indicates that blood flow through the popliteal artery is adequate and that healing of a below-knee amputation will almost always occur without any difficulty. Even in the presence of a reading of 1 unit, there may still be a good possibility of a satisfactory result, since under such conditions the tissues are being nourished by circulation through both the main arterial tree (although to a significantly diminished degree) and the collateral channels. However, if the results are less than 1 unit or zero, the possibility of stump healing after a below-knee amputation is slim, since the skin and muscles will have to depend solely on blood flow through secondary collateral channels. If, at the same time, pulsations are absent in the common femoral artery in the groin, a below-knee amputation generally should not be considered.

A number of other tests may be helpful in determining the state of the circulation at the level of the proposed amputation. Among these are the reactive hyperemia test (p. 32), Doppler ultrasonic flowmeter (p. 65), contrast arteriography (p. 72), and xenon-133 [5].

The presence or absence of certain local symptoms and physical findings may also help evaluate the state of circulation existing at the level of contemplated amputation. For example, the presence of rest pain due to ischemic neuropathy (p. 14) indicates that the circulation to the entire limb is seriously compromised. The cutaneous temperature, skin color, degree of hair growth, quantity of subcutaneous fat, and pliability and elasticity of the skin all reflect the local nutritional status of the superficial tissues and the level of cutaneous blood flow. Specifically, if the segment of limb under consideration as a possible site for amputation demonstrates a low cutaneous temperature, slight cyanosis or pallor, pigmentation, atrophy of skin and subcutaneous tissue, absence of hair growth (with adequate hair growth on the opposite limb), and dryness and scaliness of the skin, attempts to utilize it for such a purpose may very well result in nonhealing of the subsequent stump. For all of these findings together signify the existence of a severely reduced local cutaneous circulation.

If the results of the various diagnostic tests are equivocal and insufficient on which to base a clear-cut conclusion, the decision regarding the proper level for amputation may have to be deferred until the patient is on the operating table. At this time, sites below and above the knee are surgically prepared and first a below-knee amputation is attempted. As the surgery proceeds, if brisk free bleeding and oozing from small vessels in the skin and subcutaneous tissue are encountered and if the muscles have a healthy red appearance and bleeders are found on making incisions into them, then such findings support the belief that the proper level for amputation has been selected. On the other hand, if free bleeding and oozing are minimal following incision through the skin and subcutaneous tissue and if the muscles are friable and brown or pale, demonstrating absence of adequate bleeders on section, under such conditions, it is probably expedient to change the operative site to above the knee and perform a supracondylar or mid-thigh amputation.

Results of Leg and Thigh Amputations in Different Types of Patients. In many individuals suffering from diabetes mellitus, the pathologic vascular changes are limited to the smaller arteries in the lower part of the leg and in the foot and, as a result, if a major amputation becomes necessary, one performed at a level below the knee has a good possibility of subsequent healing of the stump. The patient with thromboangiitis obliterans is frequently also a proper candidate for a below-knee amputation, since almost invariably the pathologic changes are found in the arteries of the leg and foot and not proximally. In the case of the individual with arteriosclerosis obliterans, with stenosis or thrombosis of proximal arteries in the thigh and even in the abdominal cavity, the decision to perform a below-knee amputation will depend heavily upon the results of the tests of circulatory efficiency, the state of the vascular tree at the time of operation, and the overall physical condition of the patient.

Generally, an above-knee amputation is performed on the elderly patient with arteriosclerosis obliterans, for the loss of the knee in such an individual does not present as much of a problem as it would in a younger person. Moreover, a prosthesis for an above-knee amputation is frequently adequate for the limited physical activity usually attempted. Also, it must be pointed out that a certain percentage of geriatric patients, because of the coexistence of mental or physical abnormalities, are not proper candidates for a prosthesis and must become reconciled to a wheelchair type of life. For most patients with diabetes unassociated with arteriosclerosis obliterans of large vessels and for those suffering from thromboangiitis obliterans, above-knee amputations are usually not indicated.

Complications of Major Amputations

Morbidity and Mortality

As already emphasized, major amputations of lower limbs for extensive ischemic gangrene are associated with high morbidity and mortality rates since most of the patients falling into this category are elderly and frequently poor candidates for any type of surgical procedure. The most frequent complications are pulmonary embolism and other thromboembolic phenomena, occurring most often after above-knee amputations. In the first month following operation, the morbidity rate has been reported to be as high as 37% and the mortality rate as high as 10% [7].

Postoperative Mental Depression

As discussed on page 179, the thought of having a lower limb amputated produces marked psychic trauma in the patient, a reaction which is considerably magnified when the procedure is actually carried out. As a result, particularly in some elderly patients, a state of depression may develop. This may not be immediately apparent, since some individuals may maintain an optimistic facade, but careful questioning will generally reveal that they consider themselves hopeless cripples who will remain in this state until they die. A supportive attitude and a realistic discussion with the patient of what to expect in the future may help decrease or even eliminate the depression.

Nonhealing Stump

One of the most serious complications of either a major or a minor amputation is nonhealing of the operative site. This may be due either to superimposed infection or to inadequate local circulation.

Infection. Despite the almost routine use of prophylactic antibacterial agents, wound infections are still common, although less than in the past. This is particularly true when the original lesion in the foot was associated with a severe infection, leading to lymphangitis and regional lymphadenitis. When such a situation exists preoperatively, it is advisable to delay the surgery for a week, if feasible, and intensively administer penicillin or other antibiotics in an attempt to destroy any bacteria which have penetrated tissues, lymphatics, and veins some distance proximal to the original lesion. Such a program should be continued for 10–14 days postoperatively. Also important in the prevention of infection of the stump are the use of meticulous care in tying off all bleeding points and attempts to reduce oozing and accumulation of serum in the operative site.

Once infection develops in the wound, the therapeutic approach will depend upon the degree of involvement. With only wound edges affected, antibacterial agents should be used locally, the stump should be given daily whirlpool treatments, and appropriate antibiotics should be administered orally or parenterally. In the presence of extensive signs of inflammation, it may be necessary to open the entire length of the incision and evacuate whatever pus or liquefaction products have accumulated. Necrotic material may have to be debrided. Secondary closure is attempted only after granulation tissue begins to cover the exposed surfaces. Until then, it is advisable to keep the wound open to prevent formation of pockets of pus, by means of daily whirlpool baths. At all times, care should be taken to prevent recontamination of the operative site.

Inadequate Local Circulation. Insufficient local blood supply is much more frequently the cause of nonhealing of the stump than is infection (see above). Such a situation may indicate that the site for the amputation was poorly selected or that the surgical procedure was unnecessarily traumatizing. There is also the possibility that the drop in blood pressure due to the general anesthesia was responsible for complete occlusion of a previously stenosed critical artery supplying the stump.

If the necrosis of the stump resulting from local ischemia is extensive, then reamputation is the best approach, the procedure being performed as soon as the physical state of the patient permits. Otherwise, there may be absorption of toxic materials from the involved site, as well as proximal spread of the thrombotic process into vessels supplying adjoining normal structures, with subsequent loss of viability and extension of the necrotic lesion.

If, on the other hand, the gangrenous process is limited to the skin edges of one of the flaps but without involvement of deeper structures, conservative therapy should be followed, particularly if the condition has become stationary. Attempts should be made to remove the necrotic material by debridement, and whirlpool baths are used to deal with noxious secretions and pus. As the area becomes covered by granulation tissue, skin grafting may be considered if the defect is large. Otherwise, the wound should receive daily meticulous aseptic care in the hope that epithelialization will take place spontaneously. All during the period of treatment, the patient should be receiving the proper oral or parenteral antibacterial therapy. Of course, if definite signs of improvement do not appear after an adequate period of conservative management, then reamputation may have to be performed.

Phantom Limb

Definition. Phantom limb refers to the illusion that the amputated limb or digits are still attached to the body, frequently with the patient experiencing the same pain that was triggered by the previous gangrenous process. In fact, often he is able to localize the symptom exactly to the original site of involvement.

Pathogenesis. The cause of phantom limb has not clearly been defined. Some workers believe that the symptom complex is of an organic origin, the painful sensations arising from an inflamed, compressed, or lacerated stump or from a neuroma developing at the end of the sectioned peripheral mixed nerve. On the basis of such a theory, afferent impulses originating in the involved nerve pass to the spinal cord where they initiate efferent impulses and, as a result, a reverberating current is set up in the internuncial pool of neurons which travels cephalad until it reaches the thalamus. As a consequence, a vicious cycle is set up between the thalamus and the cerebral cortex which is self-perpetuating and not affected by removal of the initial precipitating factors.

Others in the field have proposed that the symptoms of phanton limb have a psychogenic origin. This view, the 'body image' concept, assumes that, as a result of various sensations experienced over the years, the patient builds up in his own mind an image of himself in relation to the external world. Hence, loss of a lower limb or even digits has a marked psychologic effect, this being reflected in the development of symptoms referred to the amputated part.

Clinical Manifestations. At times, the phantom limb syndrome may be severe enough to incapacitate the patient. The complaint is usually described as a boring pain in the bone or a sense of tearing or pressing which is continuous or intermittent. It may be initiated by slight trauma to the stump, nervous tension, pain elsewhere, or changes in weather. There may also be signs of vasospasm in the stump, such as coldness, cyanosis of the skin, and hyperhidrosis.

Treatment. Management of phantom limb is varied, but no one approach has been found to be consistently effective. The surgical program consists of means to interrupt the pain pathways between the periphery and the pain centers in the thalamus and cerebral centers. The procedures include injection of alcohol into peripheral nerves, intradural incision of nerve roots, lumbar sympathectomy, and spinothalamic cordotomy. Generally, however, the late results from such measures are poor, although some improvement is usually noted initially. More conservative steps are repeated infiltration of the peripheral and sympathetic nervous system with procaine or longer-acting local anesthetics and extensive psychotherapy.

Other Abnormal Responses to Amputation
Symptomatic Neuroma Formation. This condition, a common complication of major amputation, is the result of some type of irritation of the cut end of the main nerve trunk. As a consequence, pain, tenderness, hyperesthesia, or hypesthesia of the overlying skin of the stump may be experienced, not infrequently to a degree which precludes the use of a prosthesis. The pathogenesis probably consists of compression of the distal part of the nerve by the forming scar tissue. Management includes local injection of

alcohol to cause nerve block, ultrasound application which probably has the same effect, and even excision of the involved structures.

Joint Abnormalities. The existence of contractures of joints proximal to the level of amputation may have a serious impact on prosthetic fitting and gait training. This applies particularly in the case of loss of hip and knee extension due to degenerative joint changes. Such findings are not uncommon in older amputees and when present definitely limit the ability to ambulate.

Bony Spurs. These sharp structures develop from the end of the stump, causing pain and even ulcerations of the overlying skin. In the case of a below-knee amputation, a sharp edge may form on the anterior surface of the distal segment of tibia which produces irritation and abrasion of the skin, at times to the point of requiring surgical revision of the stump.

Steps in a Rehabilitation Program

Management of the amputee is an interdisciplinary team function [3], involving the physiatrist, surgeon, prosthetist, physical therapist, podiatrist, social worker, and psychologist. The following measures are instituted as early postoperatively as feasible.

Early Bed Positioning
Proper bed positioning is begun when the patient is returned from the operating room. This involves placing a firm board between the mattress and springs to minimize the tendency toward hip and knee flexion, keeping the patient's pelvis straight to prevent abduction of the stump, and maintaining the latter flat on the bed, at the same time warning sympathetic hospital personnel against placing pillows under the stump to relieve local pain in the incision. At intervals during the day, the patient should be instructed to assume the prone position with a pillow under the anterior surface of the stump, so as to encourage hip extension.

Stump and General Conditioning Exercises
Supervised active and assistive stump exercises should be instituted as soon as the patient is fully recovered from the anesthesia. The purpose of this measure is to prevent abduction, external rotation, and flexion of the

hip (not infrequently noted after a conventional above-knee amputation) and flexion of the knee and hip (often present after a below-knee amputation). With diminution and then disappearance of postoperative pain, resistive exercises are initiated to strengthen all muscles involved in moving the stump.

At the same time that the above program is being carried out, exercises are also introduced to strengthen the muscles of the trunk and those of the remaining three limbs. As soon as feasible, the patient is encouraged to stand and balance between parallel bars. As improvement in performance appears, he then progresses to the pickup walker or crutch ambulation. The purpose of the program is to prepare the patient for the increased work load associated with gait training using a prosthesis.

Stump Bandaging

Proper shaping of the stump through stump bandaging is an essential preparatory step to the use of a prosthesis. The measure is begun several weeks after the operation, depending upon how rapidly the wound is healing. The purpose is to reduce the swelling of the stump, thus helping to shape it for insertion into the socket of a prosthesis and to facilitate wound healing. The greatest pressure in applying the elastic bandages in a diagonal pattern is exerted distally and then with gradually decreasing firmness as the proximal portion of the limb is approached. At no time should circular turns be taken around the limb, since they may be responsible for a buildup of local venous pressure and edema of the stump end. The bandage should be removed and reapplied 4–6 times during the day so as to maintain continuous pressure on the stump.

Criteria for Choice of Candidates for Prosthesis

Among the important factors contributing to the decision to prescribe a prosthesis for an elderly amputee is whether or not his knee joint has been preserved, the importance of which has already been discussed (p. 184). Others are the general physical and mental state of the prospective candidate, his socioeconomic status, the degree of involvement of the circulation in the remaining lower limb, and the manner in which he performs using a temporary prosthesis. Finally, his motivation and premorbid personality are both of great significance in the determination under consideration. Age per se does not appear to exert an important influence on the rehabilitative potential of the individual unless severe senility is also present.

Prosthetic Prescription

In prescribing a prosthesis for an elderly amputee, certain factors must be considered: fit, design, proper alignment, materials making up the artificial limb, and its weight. For an above-knee amputation, two types of prosthesis are commercially available: the standard and the suction socket. The suction socket is generally prescribed for younger patients who have normal cardiovascular-pulmonary systems and in whom the stump is well-shaped, cylindrical or conical, with little or no scarring. The standard prosthesis is the one generally applicable to the geriatric amputee suffering from arteriosclerosis obliterans. It can be used even if the stump is short, irregularly shaped, and scarred and if there are frequent changes in body weight and hence in size of the stump.

For a below-knee amputation, there are also two types of prosthesis: the patellar tendon-bearing laminated and the standard (with or without a pelvic band) with a leather lacer corset of varying height. The patellar tendon-bearing laminated prosthesis is light-weight and allows for complete freedom of the knee joint. Moreover, it takes less time to apply than does the standard type. However, even slight changes in body weight may affect the fit of the socket, leading to the need for frequent adjustments. The standard type, on the other hand, is quite durable and can be used on rough terrain. The leather thigh corset achieves considerable stability which is generally very helpful to the elderly amputee.

Gait Training

Once the patient has received the prosthesis and it has been tested and found satisfactory, the next step is training to achieve a gait which is as normal as possible under the circumstances. At all times, it must be kept in mind that the amount of energy being expended by the patient while ambulating must definitely be within the limits of capability of his cardiovascular-pulmonary systems. At first, training is given for short periods, so as to prevent abrasions of the skin of the stump, and then the duration is lengthened so as to develop a greater tolerance of the stump to weight bearing. The initial step is to achieve good standing balance by placing the patient between parallel bars and having him balance first on his own and the artificial limb and then on each leg separately. This step is followed by having him shift his weight from one side to the other, with little or no use of the upper limbs. Following the development of proficiency in these maneuvers, the patient begins to walk between parallel bars with steps of equal length and with the weight of his body distributed equally between both lower limbs. Once he is able to achieve these goals, the parallel bars are discarded and the ambulation program progresses to walking on level surfaces and to ascending and descending stairs and finally to walking on uneven terrain.

Local Care of Stump and Prosthesis

It is very important to maintain the skin of the stump in excellent condition by washing it daily using a mild soap, rinsing well, and thoroughly drying it, followed by application of talcum powder. The skin should be inspected frequently for the appearance of any type of dermatitis, particularly furunculosis due to sweating of the stump from long confinement in the stump sock and socket. Abrasions of the skin, which may develop from rough spots in the socket or poor fit or alignment, must immediately be treated. Otherwise, they may become severe enough to interfere with the use of the prosthesis. The stump sock should be washed frequently and the prosthetic socket should be cleansed often; all moving parts of the prosthesis should be properly lubricated and kept in good repair.

Role of the Podiatrist in Rehabilitation of the Amputee

The podiatrist should be included in the team approach to the rehabilitation of the amputee, as the status of the remaining foot is most important in the initiation and continuation of an ambulation program using a prosthesis, especially since a greater than normal stress will be placed on it. Hence, it should be carefully analyzed and prepared for weight bearing following a podiatric biomechanical examination. The severely subtalar pronated (calcaneal valgus) foot should be controlled with the use of the proper shoe and a fixed orthotic device. Those patients with plantar flexed metatarsals and/or hammer toes should be sufficiently treated to permit some semblance of normal weight distribution. However, since in most instances atherosclerosis is also present in the arterial vascular tree of the remaining lower limb, any type of therapeutic program involving a surgical approach is generally contraindicated.

References

1   Abramson, D.I.: Circulatory diseases of the limbs: a primer (Grune & Stratton, New York 1978).
2   Bradham, R.R.; Smoak, R.D.: Amputations of the lower extremity used for arteriosclerosis obliterans. Archs Surg., Chicago 90: 60 (1965).

3   Burgess, E.M.: Boston interhospital amputee study. Archs Surg., Chicago *107:* 830 (1973).
4   Lim, R.C.J.; Blaisdell, F.W.; Hall, A.D., et al.: Below-knee amputation for ischemic gangrene. Surgery Gynec. Obstet. *125:* 493 (1967).
5   Moore, W.S.: Determination of amputation level: measurement of skin blood flow with Xenon Xe 133. Archs Surg., Chicago *107:* 798 (1973).
6   Pinzur, M.S.; Jordan, C.; Rana, N.A.: Syme's two-stage amputation in diabetic dysvascular disease. Ill. med. J. *160:* 23 (1981).
7   Thompson, R.C.; Delbanco, T.L.; McAllister, F.F.: Complications following lower extremity amputation. Surgery Gynec. Obstet. *120:* 301 (1965).
8   Yao, J.S.T.; Bergan, J.J.: Application of ultrasound to arterial and venous diagnosis. Surg. Clins N. Am. *54:* 23 (1974).

10 Physiologic and Clinical Basis for Use of Physical Modalities as Therapy in Arterial Disorders

Some physical agents play a definite but limited role as therapy for arterial disorders of the lower limbs; others are unequivocally contraindicated for this purpose. Although these modalities do not permanently influence the pathologic process in the arteries, a number are effective in eliciting transient vasodilatation by their action on local arteriolar beds still capable of reacting in this manner and on collateral channels not affected by the occlusive process. The primary reason for devoting this chapter to a discussion of the physiologic and clinical evaluation of the common physical modalities is because of their rather extensive use in podiatric and medical practices, not infrequently without firm basis and, at times, with dire consequences. The fact that untoward responses may result emphasizes the need for caution in the application of the modalities, especially since skin suffering from a state of chronic ischemia is particularly vulnerable to mechanical, chemical, and thermal injuries.

Direct Topical Heating

Direct heating of a limb can be accomplished utilizing a number of different approaches: wet heat, hot dry air, Hydrocollator packs, melted paraffin, hot water bottle, electric heating pad, or a heat cradle. At no time should the maximum height of the temperature rise produced by the modality be permitted to exceed physiologic limits (level of 42 °C; 108 °F).

Physiologic Effects of the Procedure
Vascular and Metabolic Changes Elicited in the Limb with Normal Arterial Circulation. In the normal lower extremity, topical heat has a very potent vasodilating effect upon the arterial and arteriolar trees in the

exposed tissues, the change occurring almost immediately and continuing all during the treatment period and for a considerable time after removal of the physical agent (fig. 10/1a). The greatest increase in blood flow takes place in the skin, although vascular alterations are also noted in the underlying subcutaneous tissue and muscle, but to a lesser degree. At the same time, there is a considerable rise in tissue temperature, again the most marked change occurring in the skin (fig. 10/1b). As a consequence of such a response, there is a corresponding elevation of metabolic requirements of the heated structures (fig. 10/1a) [1, 4]. However, this can readily be satisfied by the marked augmentation in local blood flow that exists under such circumstances, and hence no untoward reactions follow the application of the heat, provided the intensity of the modality elicits a response which falls within physiologic limits. Another compensatory mechanism that comes into play is the cooling effect developed by the marked increase in local circulation. For, since the temperature of the blood passing through the heated tissues is much lower than that to which the skin is externally exposed, a means is at hand for the rapid removal of the deposited heat. As a result, the tissues never achieve a rise in temperature which approaches that supplied by the modality. Hence, the resulting elevation in metabolic needs is much less than would otherwise have occurred without the existence of the cooling mechanism.

Vascular and Metabolic Changes Elicited in the Limb with Compromised Arterial Circulation. In the presence of an impaired arterial circulation, the vascular responses to the direct application of heat are entirely different from those described above. Even this powerful vasodilating agent is unable to elicit much of a circulatory effect in blood vessels partially or completely occluded by clot or atheromatous plaques. As a result, the increase in local blood flow is minimal. At the same time, the cooling system inherent in a significant increase in circulation is not available or, if present, is very inefficient in removing the heat deposited in the tissues by the modality. Hence, a considerable rise in tissue temperature occurs, particularly in the the skin, followed by a correspondingly marked increase in metabolic needs of the exposed structures. In contrast to what occurs in the presence of a normal vascular tree, the magnitude of the resulting augmentation in local blood flow is far from capable of satisfying the elevated metabolic requirements of the tissues and hence viability of exposed structures is jeopardized and local necrosis can be expected to develop (see fig. 8/1e).

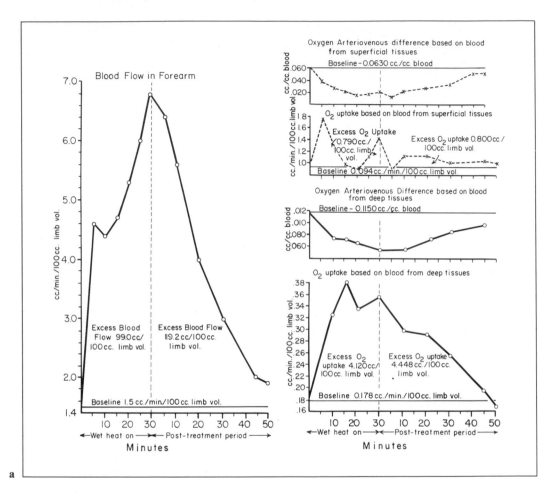

Clinical Application of, and Contraindications to, the Procedure

Organic Arterial Insufficiency. For reasons developed in the preceding section, direct heat in any form should *never* be prescribed for or administered to a lower limb of any adult patient before first determining whether he is suffering from local organic arterial disease. If he is, the procedure is unequivocally contraindicated. Such a precaution should significantly reduce the incidence of malpractice suits, as well as the grief and mental stresses triggered by the knowledge that an improper therapeutic measure was responsible for the loss of a lower limb.

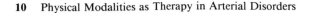

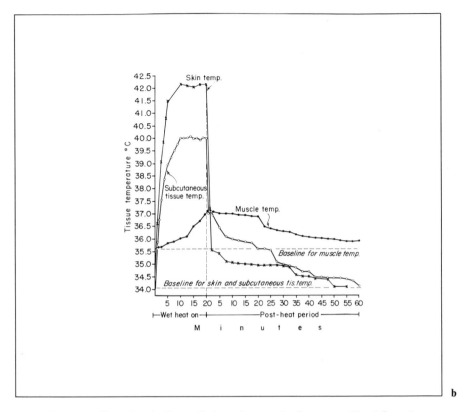

b

Fig. 10/1. Effect of topically applied wet heat to the forearm. **a** Blood flow changes produced by 30 min of direct heating. Alterations in oxygen uptake also noted. **b** Tissue temperature changes produced during and after 20 min of direct heating. Reproduced from ref. [4] with permission.

Arterial Vasospasm. The application of direct heat to a lower limb manifesting increased sympathetic tone generally results in disappearance of the symptoms and signs of vasospasm and an increase in local blood flow which approaches a normal level. Hence, the exposed structures are not placed in jeopardy by such a procedure, in contrast to what occurs in the presence of organic arterial disease (p. 198). However, it is frequently difficult to differentiate between the two states, which may introduce an element of risk unless it has previously been determined by means of temporarily blocking the pathway of vasoconstrictor impulses that the observed physical signs are due to vasospasm. Moreover, the vasodilating response elicited by heat is only transient, with the vascular tree reverting to the vasospastic state soon after the treatment is terminated. Therefore, in the presence of vasospasm, the use of direct heat to increase local blood flow has very little clinical application or usefulness. (For the use of direct heating in the treatment of venous stasis ulcers, see p. 299.)

Indirect Body Heating (Reflex Vasodilatation)

Physiologic Effects of the Procedure
Technique. Indirect vasodilatation in the lower limbs is achieved by applying heat in any form to distant portions of the body, such as the two upper limbs, the abdomen, and the chest, and covering the patient with blankets (except for the limbs under study) to prevent loss of heat. The heating procedures consist of either immersion of the upper limbs in buckets of hot water (up to 42 °C; 108 °F), hot water bottles or Hydrocollator packs to the chest or abdomen, or short-wave diathermy to the same areas. After about 15 min, the patient will begin to perspire and the temperature of the toes will begin to rise, associated with an increase in local circulation in the foot (fig. 10/2). There may also be a slight rise in body temperature. The vascular response will continue to increase and then level off during the latter part of the treatment period, which generally lasts for 30 min in all. At the termination of indirect heating, there is a fairly rapid decline in the magnitude of the blood flow response in the feet, the resting control level being reached in about 1 h in the posttreatment period (fig. 10/2) [5, 8].

Mechanisms Responsible for Vasodilatation. The increase in blood flow produced by body heating is limited to a great extent to the skin of the toes and feet proper, sites in which vasomotor control over the cutaneous arteries and arterioles is quite marked. The vessels in the skin elsewhere are very little affected and no change is noted in muscle blood flow.

In the lower limb with a normal circulation, the mechanism responsible for vasodilatation of cutaneous vessels is as follows: blood leaving the heated parts of the body initially has a higher temperature than the systemic level of temperature, but with prolonged application of heat, the latter will also eventually be raised. On passing through the temperature-regulating

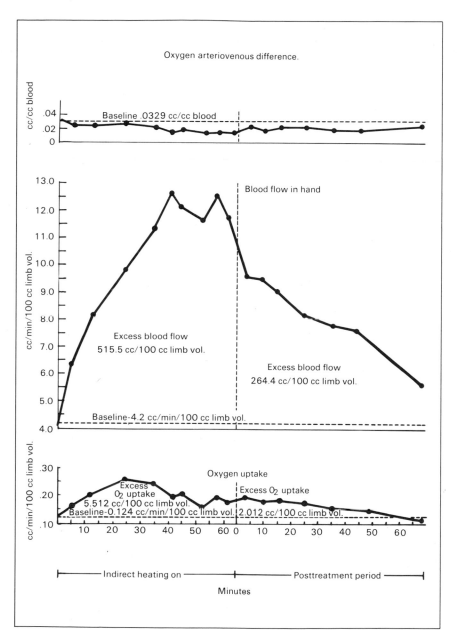

Fig. 10/2. Effect of indirect heating on blood flow in the hand. A marked increase in local circulation is noted, with very little associated rise in oxygen uptake (a similar type of change is produced in the foot). Reproduced from ref. [5] with permission.

center in the hypothalamus, the heated blood now acts to stimulate this structure, with the result that inhibiting impulses will be initiated which pass down to the vasomotor center in the medulla and depress its rate of formation of vasoconstricting impulses. Consequently, there will be a reduction in the number of such impulses which reach the cutaneous arterioles in the feet, and so these vessels will passively dilate, thus allowing a more rapid rate of blood flow through them. Normally, indirect heating may produce a doubling of the local cutaneous circulation, with the change persisting during the entire treatment period and for almost 1 h afterwards (fig. 10/2). It is obvious that in a foot in which the continuity of the sympathetic pathway has already been destroyed, as by lumbar sympathectomy, the local vascular bed will no longer respond to body heating by vasodilating.

Of importance is the finding that body heating produces only a small rise in oxygen uptake in the distal portions of the limb (fig. 10/2). The change appears to be related to the rise in local tissue temperature produced by the augmentation in blood flow.

Clinical Application of the Procedure

Organic Arterial Insufficiency. In the case of a lower limb suffering from occlusive arterial disease, indirect body heating initiates the same sequence of events as described above for the normal extremity. However, the magnitude of the increase in local blood flow will directly depend upon the number of arterioles that are unaffected by the pathologic process and hence are capable of dilating on removal or reduction of vasomotor control over them, the same applying to the compensatory collateral circulation which has developed in response to the state of ischemia existing in the tissues. If the magnitude of the vascular response approaches that observed in a limb with a normal circulation, then the accompanying minor increase in oxygen demands can readily be met by the marked augmentation in local circulation. On the other hand, if the vascular response is minimal because of extensive involvement of the arterial and arteriolar trees by the pathologic process, then the rise in tissue temperature and hence, in oxygen needs, will also be correspondingly low. In either situation, the tissues will not be in any jeopardy because a discrepancy between the oxygen requirements of the tissues and the capability of the vascular tree to satisfy them will never develop. Therefore, indirect body heating is a very useful procedure for increasing blood flow in the toes, unassociated with any harmful reactions or untoward responses other than the transient general sensation of discomfort and excessive perspiration which it initiates. Hence, it can be used with impunity as a therapeutic agent for organic occlusive arterial disorders of the feet.

Arterial Vasospasm. Indirect body heating is very effective in temporarily counteracting the low cutaneous blood flow observed in feet suffering from a vasospastic arterial disorder. It is also useful in removal of arterial vasospasm initiated by sudden occlusion of a main collecting vein in the lower limbs by a thrombus (p. 262). (For the use of indirect body heating as a means of determining the degree of existing vasospasm, see p. 69.)

Ion Transfer of Vasodilator Drugs

Orally or parenterally administered vasodilator drugs as therapy in arterial disorders of the lower limbs are, unfortunately, generally associated with an unwanted widespread relaxation of the cutaneous arteriolar bed, rather than the desired action – a circulatory response limited to the tissues requiring an increase in local blood flow (p. 147). Mainly for this reason, they have currently lost favor as therapeutic agents, and hence other means of administration of vasodilator drugs have been evaluated, one of which is ion transfer.

Technique of Ion Transfer

In an attempt to minimize or eliminate the adverse responses to vasodilator agents and still retain their therapeutic effects, ion transfer of agents having an inhibiting action on the circular muscle fibers in the blood vessel wall (myovascular relaxants) has been proposed. For this purpose, a number of medications have been studied, the one most commonly used at present being histamine diphosphate or dihydrochloride. This agent is capable of readily dissociating in solution into positive and negative ions; these are transferred through intact skin by passage of a galvanic electric current.

The procedure is performed in the following manner: a plastic basin, large enough to contain the foot and lower portion of the leg, is filled with a fresh solution of histamine diphosphate, 1:10,000 concentration, in water. The positive pole of a direct current generator is connected to an electrode which is attached to the inner surface of the container and so positioned that it is immersed in the solution but prevented from coming in contact with the skin of the limb under treatment. The negative pole of the galvanic machine is attached to a large dispersive electrode applied to the patient's back and held in place with elastic bandages.

The average current density used varies between 3 and 12 mA. Generally, the smaller dose is first applied and then the amount is increased until tolerance is reached, the dosage gradually rising with subsequent applications. The lesion being treated may be covered with a sterile gauze pad or directly exposed to the solution. The treatment schedule consists of 2 or 3 applications a week, each one being for 5–20 min. If originally the lesion is covered by an eschar, it is advisable to precede ion transfer by a 10-min period of whirlpool, followed by debridement of necrotic tissue [9].

Physiologic Response to Ion Transfer

Immediately with the onset of the procedure, the positively charged histamine ions are repelled away from the positive electrode immersed in the solution, to migrate in the direction of the negative electrode on the back. In the process, they are deposited locally in the skin and subcutaneous tissue. Most of the agent remains there to cause vasodilatation of exposed arterioles, the rest being absorbed into the blood stream. In the normal subject, the resulting increase in local cutaneous circulation is considerable, continuing during the entire period of exposure and for approximately 1 h afterwards (fig. 10/3) [7, 9]. In fact, the magnitude of the vascular change is greater for the post-treatment period than for the time the procedure is applied. Associated with the circulatory effect, there is either a small increase in oxygen needs locally or no change.

Clinical Application and Complications of the Procedure

Organic Arterial Insufficiency. Histamine by ion transfer has had limited clinical application in the treatment of complications of arterial insufficiency in the lower limbs, such as ischemic ulceration or gangrene. However, in view of the significant increase in cutaneous blood flow and minimal rise in oxygen needs of the exposed tissues observed in normal individuals, the procedure warrants further clinical trial, although it is realized that vessels occluded by a pathologic process cannot be expected to respond to any extent to the vasodilating agent. Nevertheless, healing of ulcerations of digits in scleroderma [9] and reduction in pain in thromboangiitis obliterans have been reported [10].

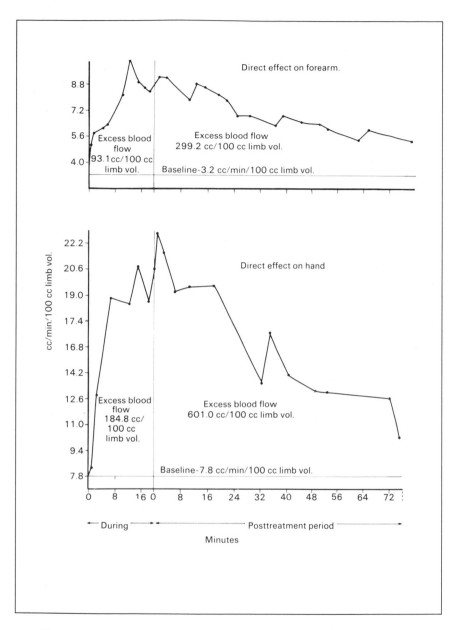

Fig. 10/3. Vascular response to histamine by ion transfer. A marked increase in blood flow is noted in the hand and a smaller response in the forearm (corresponding changes in local circulation are also produced in the foot and leg, respectively). Reproduced from ref. [7] with permission.

Arterial Vasospasm. Histamine by ion transfer has been used in patients with Raynaud's disease, with reported good results [10]. (For the use of histamine by ion transfer in the treatment of venous stasis ulcers, see p. 300.)

Possible Untoward Responses to the Procedure. The most common symptom produced by histamine by ion transfer is headache which generally responds to aspirin. Dizziness, lightheadedness, and local itching and swelling are also frequently experienced. Most of the complaints can be controlled by reducing the current density; rarely is it necessary to terminate the series of treatments because of such reactions. However, in the presence of a history of asthma, hay fever, or any type of sensitivity reaction, histamine by ion transfer should not be given. Especially in the case of the limb with an organic arterial disorder, great care must be taken to prevent skin contact with the electrode immersed in the solution, for otherwise, a third-degree burn may develop which can be expected not to heal.

Miscellaneous Procedures

Whirlpool Therapy

The whirlpool bath, a fairly common piece of apparatus in the conventional podiatric office, has only limited clinical applicability as therapy for occlusive arterial disorders of the lower limbs. Despite this, it has a history of being used quite frequently for a multitude of conditions.

Physiologic Effect of Procedure. There is very little evidence to support the view that the whirlpool bath has any significant lasting effect on the cutaneous circulation in the exposed leg and foot. The temperature of the water in the container is generally maintained at a level below body temperature (32 °C; 90 °F or less), and this may have a mild vasodilating action, but no more than would result from immersion in water that is stationary and at the same temperature. The only possible beneficial effect that can be attributed to the method is that the whirling water may have a massage-like action on the skin, which could psychologically cause a more relaxed state in the patient, with a resultant reduction in vasomotor tone and a temporary slight increase in cutaneous blood flow to the feet.

Clinical Application, Limitations, and Complications of the Procedure. Whirlpool baths are useful in the presence of some of the complications of arterial insufficiency, such as ischemic ulceration and gangrene of the legs and feet. For example, the procedure helps control the secretion and pus which frequently develop in such lesions. At the same time, it helps soften necrotic and callous tissue around and in the involved site, thus allowing the material to be more readily removed by debridement, especially if this step is performed immediately after the bath. The method is also of value in the management of sinus tracts leading from infected bone or abscesses, as may develop in an amputation site, for the moving water has a better possibility of entering and cleansing the lesion and keeping it open and free of pus than has a simple footbath. This is essential in the prevention of accumulation of infected secretion and its spread along tissue planes. As a consequence, formation of granulation tissue is hastened and healing is promoted.

In the case of the patient with chronic arterial insufficiency manifesting no cutaneous lesions of the legs and feet and demonstrating an intact skin, whirlpool baths are of no value and should not be used. Moreover, unless great care is taken to remove all moisture from between the toes following each treatment, repeated baths may be responsible for maceration of the skin in these sites and an increased vulnerability to dermatophytosis.

Manual Massage

Manual massage of the involved limb has a very limited use as a therapeutic procedure in arterial disorders of the lower limbs.

Physiologic Effects of the Procedure. There is no conclusive evidence that manual or mechanical massage of a limb increases local circulation. Nor is blood pressure or pulse rate affected by the procedure. However, kneading and stroking massage many cause accelerated lymph flow out of a limb. Depending on the type of movement employed, the procedure has either a sedative or a stimulating effect on the central nervous system. If the former, there may be some reduction in vasomotor tone and hence some slight passive increase in cutaneous circulation in the feet. The procedure does not appear to cause any change in oxygen consumption of the treated tissues or in the urinary output of acid or base.

Clinical Application of, and Contraindications to, the Procedure. Besides having little or no beneficial effect, manual massage may actually cause harm to the skin of a limb with compromised arterial circulation if the measure is applied with any force. For, under such circumstances, the procedure may lead to the appearance of ischemic ulceration or gangrene. In the presence of local infection superimposed on a vascular lesion, massage may be responsible for the dissemination of bacteria into the local lymphatic and venous systems and enlargement of the area of involvement.

Postural (Buerger's) Exercises

Currently, postural exercises are rarely utilized as therapy in chronic arterial occlusive disorders of the lower limbs. However, since the procedure is still occasionally mentioned in podiatric literature, it will be discussed briefly below.

Physiologic Effect of the Procedure. The method consists of successively placing the lower limbs in several positions, the changes being either actively carried out by the patient himself, or achieved passively by means of a Sanders' oscillating bed. First the patient lies on his back in bed for 2 min, maintaining his lower limbs elevated at an angle of 45°. Then he sits up with his limbs over the edge of the bed in dependency for 2–3 min. During this period the feet are moved inward and outward, the ankles are moved downward and upward, and the toes are alternately spread and closed. The next step is for the patient to lie back in bed with the whole body, including the lower limbs, in the horizontal position. After several minutes, the cycle is repeated. A treatment consists of 4 or 5 cycles in succession, and this is performed 2–4 times daily.

The beneficial effects attributed to postural exercises have been related to an increase in blood flow consequent to the emptying and filling of the vessels by gravity, a point which has never been satisfactorily proved. In fact, it has been shown that maintaining a limb in the elevated position (the first posture assumed by the patient performing the exercises) actually reduces arterial inflow [6], especially in the presence of stenotic or occluded main arteries.

Clinical Application of the Procedure. At one time postural exercises were used extensively as adjunctive therapy in arteriosclerosis obliterans and thromboangiitis obliterans. Although not having any beneficial effect on intermittent claudication, it was considered to cause temporary alleviation of rest pain associated with ulceration and gangrene. At present all that can be said in its favor is that it tends to occupy the time and mind of the patient and, to some extent, to distract his attention from the seriousness of his condition.

Short-Wave Diathermy

Although short-wave diathermy increases local blood flow, primarily in the muscles, at the same time it significantly elevates oxygen needs of tissues through its effect on raising tissue temperatures [2]. Therefore, as in the case of local use of heat in any form (p. 197), its direct application to a lower limb suffering from arterial impairment is definitely contraindicated.

Ultrasound

Ultrasound also increases local blood flow, but to a lesser degree than does short-wave diathermy, the greatest augmentation occurring in the subcutaneous tissue. Again, oxygen needs of the exposed tissues are significantly raised [3], and for this reason, the procedure should never be applied directly to a limb with an impaired arterial circulation. The basis for such a conclusion has already been discussed on page 197.

References

1 Abramson, D.I.; Kahn, A.; Tuck, S., Jr.; Turman, G.A.; Rejal, H.; Fleischer, C.J.: Relationship between a range of tissue temperature and local oxygen uptake in the human forearm. 1. Changes observed under resting conditions. J. clin. Invest. *37:* 1031 (1958).

2 Abramson, D.I.; Bell, Y.; Rejal, H.; Tuck, S., Jr.; Burnett, C.; Fleischer, C.J.: Changes in blood flow, oxygen uptake, and tissue temperatures produced by therapeutic physical agents. II. Effect of short-wave diathermy. Am. J. phys. Med. *39:* 87 (1960).

3 Abramson, D.I.; Burnett, C.; Bell, Y.; Tuck, S., Jr.; Rejal, H.; Fleischer, C.J.: Changes in blood flow, oxygen uptake, and tissue temperatures produced by therapeutic physical agents. I. Effect of ultrasound. Am. J. phys. Med. *39:* 51 (1960).

4 Abramson, D.I.; Mitchell, R.E.; Tuck, S., Jr.; Bell, Y.; Zayas, A.M.: Changes in blood flow, oxygen uptake, and tissue temperatures produced by the topical application of wet heat. Archs phys. Med. Rehabil. *42:* 305 (1961).

5 Abramson, D.I.; Bell, Y.; Tuck, S., Jr.; Mitchell, R.; Chandrasekharappa, G.: Changes in blood flow, oxygen uptake, and tissue temperatures produced by therapeutic physical agents. III. Effect of indirect or reflex vasodilatation. Am. J. phys. Med. *40:* 5 (1961).

6 Abramson, D.I.; Tuck, S., Jr.; Zayas, A.M.; Mitchell, R.E.: Effect of altering limb position on blood flow, O_2 uptake, and skin temperature. J. appl. Physiol. *17:* 191 (1962).

7   Abramson, D.L.; Tuck, S., Jr.; Zayas, A.M.; Donatello, T.M.; Chu, L.S.W.; Mitchell, R.E.: Vascular responses produced by histamine by ion transfer. J. appl. Physiol. *18:* 305 (1963).

8   Abramson, D.I.; Tuck, S., Jr.; Chu, L.S.W.; Lee, S.W.; Gibbons, C.; Richardson, G.: Indirect vasodilatation in thermotherapy. Archs phys. Med. Rehabil. *46:* 412 (1965).

9   Abramson, D.I.; Tuck, S., Jr.; Chu, L.S.W.; Buso, E.: Physiologic and clinical basis for histamine by ion transfer. Archs phys. Med. Rehabil. *48:* 583 (1967).

10 Kling, D.H.; Sashin, D.: Histamine iontophoresis in rheumatic conditions of deficiencies of peripheral circulation. Archs phys. Ther. *18:* 333 (1937).

II Venous Disorders of the Lower Limbs

11 Clinical and Laboratory Assessment of the Venous Circulation in the Lower Limbs

Vascular History (table 11/I)

In general, the outline to follow in eliciting a history from a patient presumably suffering from some types of venous involvement of the lower limb is similar to that utilized in determining whether arterial insufficiency exists (table 1/I), except that the direction taken by the examiner in his interrogation is different.

Elucidation of Pertinent Points in a Vascular History

Certain items enumerated in table 11/I require some elaboration. For example, a past history of episodes of thrombophlebitis, whether of the superficial or the deep venous system, places the patient in a category in which there is a greater vulnerability to subsequent attacks of intravascular clotting. This is particularly true if primary varicosities exist. Eliciting a history of iliofemoral thrombophlebitis may help explain the presence of marked signs of venous stasis in the limb previously affected, because of the presence of the postphlebitic syndrome. Unilateral swelling of a lower limb may be due to such a cause or, less frequently, it is associated with primary varicosities, congenital lymphatic disease, or destruction or obstruction of critical lymph channels. Pulmonary embolism may have its origin in thrombosis of deep venous plexuses of the calf muscles. A history of non-vascular operations may also have significance, since certain ones, like herniorrhaphy, gynecologic procedures, hip surgery, and cholecystectomy, are associated with a relatively high incidence of phlebothrombosis, iliofemoral thrombophlebitis, and pulmonary embolism.

Selective Physical Examination (table 11/II)

Through inspection and palpation of the skin of the lower limbs, considerable valuable information can be collected regarding the state of the superficial venous system and, to a lesser extent, that of the deep venous

Table 11/I. Pertinent points in the vascular history for venous disorders of the lower limbs

---

1   Chief complaint: list

2   Relevant family history: list those conditions which have a relationship to or result from venous disorders of the lower limbs, such as episodes of superficial or deep venous thrombophlebitis, primary varicosities, etc.

3   Past history of:
    (a)   Repeated attacks of superficial or deep thrombophlebitis
    (b)   Spontaneous ulcers of legs (cause, treatment, outcome)
    (c)   Spontaneous pitting or nonpitting edema of lower limbs
    (d)   Systemic conditions associated with venous manifestations in the lower limbs (hematologic disorders)
    (e)   Nonvascular surgical procedures

4   Habits and routine medications: tobacco smoking; use of contraceptive drugs; outpatient anticoagulants

5   Occupation: amount of standing and sitting required at work

6   Present complaints, including:
    (a)   Sense of tiredness, fatigue, and heaviness in the feet
    (b)   Presence of nocturnal cramps
    (c)   Responses of unilateral swelling to sitting, standing, and lying down with lower limbs elevated
    (d)   Pain due to stasis dermatitis, stasis ulceration, chronic indurated cellulitis

---

system. To make the superficial veins more visible, it is advisable, as an added routine measure, to have the patient stand on a stool and face the examiner so that the hydrostatic effect will distend the vessels with blood.

Differentiation of Prominent Superficial Veins

The appearance of prominent superficial veins may be due to a number of different and unrelated mechanisms.

Normal Manifestations. Dilated superficial veins may be found in normal individuals, particularly when there has been a rapid loss of body weight. Ordinarily subcutaneous tissue supplies an element of support for the superficial vessels, and if it is suddenly reduced in amount, the veins may become prominent on standing. A differential point from superficial thrombophlebitis (p. 235) is that elevation of the limb will result in

Table 11/II. Steps in the clinical and laboratory assessment of the venous and lymphatic circulations in the lower limbs

---

1   By inspection:
Venous system
(a)   Varicosities, superficial thrombophlebitis, dilated prominent veins which remain full on elevation of limb
(b)   Swelling (location, pitting, nonpitting)
(c)   Pigmentation, induration, and brawniness of skin of legs; presence of stasis dermatitis or ulceration
Lymphatic system
(a)   Lymphangitis
(b)   Lymphedema (location, severity, degree)
(c)   Elephantiasis

2   By palpation:
Venous system
(a)   Determination of presence of superficial thrombophlebitis
(b)   Determination of presence of a tender mass in calf muscles by deep palpation, as in phlebothrombosis
Lymphatic system
(a)   Determination of nonpitting quality of swelling

3   By clinical testing:
Venous system
(a)   Single (Trendelenburg) and multiple tourniquet tests for study of varicosities
(b)   Homans' test for study of phlebothrombosis
(c)   Perthes' test for study of state of deep venous circulation

4   By laboratory testing:
Venous system
(a)   Venous pressure determinations
(b)   Doppler ultrasonic flowmeter
(c)   Radioactive fibrinogen test
(d)   Impedance and mercury strain-gauge plethysmography
(e)   Contrast venography
(f)   Radionuclide venography
Lymphatic system
(a)   Lymphangiography

---

immediate collapse of the vessels which now become almost imperceptible, whereas the appearance of thrombosed superficial veins remains unchanged under such circumstances. No signs of a regurgitant flow are noted in normally dilated veins when studied by means of the Brodie-Trendelenburg or multiple tourniquet test (pp. 233, 234).

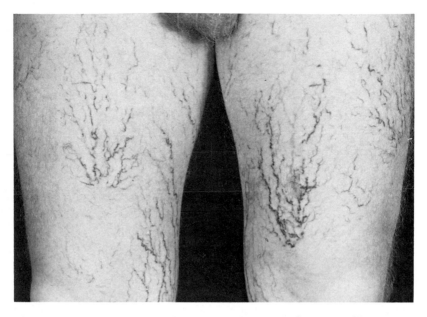

Fig. 11/1. 'Spider' veins on the thighs due to enlargement of the subpapillary venous plexus. Reproduced from ref. [2] with permission.

Spider Veins. These prominent, but small, thin-walled bursts of superficial vessels may likewise be a normal finding, especially in obese females (fig. 11/1), although also noted in association with primary varicosities. In contrast to the latter, however, the vessels feeding the spider veins never demonstrate regurgitant blood flow, since the valves in them are normal. The vascular lesions are usually located on the lateral aspect of the thighs, in the popliteal space, and in the region of the malleoli. They generally become more obvious during pregnancy, with no regression occurring following delivery. If primary varicosities coexist, their successful surgical treatment appears to prevent new batches of spider veins from developing. However, the operation has no effect on those already present, except that subsequently they will no longer enlarge or become more prominent. Aside from their unesthetic appearance, spider veins have no clinical implications. Nevertheless, some of the female patients with them will frequently try strong persuasion on their physician to utilize some medical means of obliterating the vessels, such as sclerosing technique. If such an approach is initiated, the end result, as judged from the appearance of the limb, may be worse (because of scarring) than before therapy. As a general rule, then, spider veins should not be treated, and instead, topical cosmetic creams should be applied to the lesions to make them less conspicuous. (For differentiation of spider veins from congenital diffuse dilatation of the subpapillary venous plexus and phlebectasia, see p. 363.)

Dilated Superficial Veins Developing during the Acute Stage of Collecting Vein Thrombosis. The sudden appearance of dilated veins on one or both lower limbs may be the first sign of the presence of inferior vena cava (fig. 11/2a), iliofemoral (fig. 11/2b), or popliteal thrombophlebitis (p. 260). The responsible mechanism is shunting of blood from the distal portion of the deep venous system into the superficial veins, in an attempt to bypass the blocked segment of main vessel. Under these circumstances, elevation of the lower limb has no effect on the distended appearance of the superficial vessels since the high venous pressure in their lumen prevents collapse, despite the counteracting effect of hydrostatic pressure facilitating venous drainage out of the limb. Unfortunately, this diagnostic sign is rarely available, because generally it is masked by the associated extensive local pitting edema invariably present.

It is necessary to point out that the sudden appearance of prominent dilated superficial veins due to occlusion of a main collecting vessel by a thrombus can be mimicked by extrinsic total compression of the inferior vena cava or its main tributaries by tumor in the pelvis or by a gravid uterus.

Dilated Superficial Veins Developing during the Later Stage of Collecting Vein Thrombosis. Later in the course of iliofemoral thrombophlebitis and subsequently in the stage of full recovery, a new superficial venous network becomes conspicuous on the lateral aspect of the thigh and the lateral and anterior portions of the abdominal wall. Such a response is a manifestation of the secondary collateral venous system which has become functional to permit blood to circumvent the obstruction in the deep venous system in its passage to the inferior vena cava.

Dilated Superficial Veins Developing in Postphlebitic Syndrome. As a sign of the existence of chronic venous hypertension, due either to persistence of the block in the iliofemoral vein or to recanalization of the clot with destruction of critical valves, large superficial dilated and incompetent veins (secondary varicosities) may appear on the involved lower limb or in

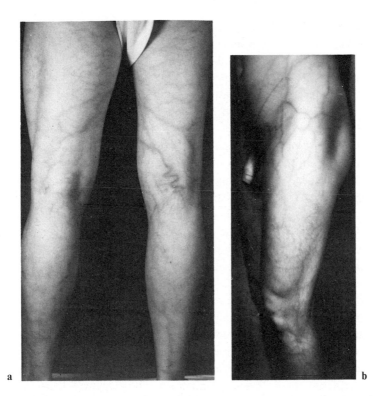

Fig. 11/2. Development of superficial venous collateral circulation following sudden occlusion of a collecting vein in the lower limbs. **a** Changes produced by total obstruction of the inferior vena cava. **b** Changes produced by total obstruction of the left iliofemoral vein.

the suprapubic region (see fig. 15/1b and c, respectively) months or even years after full recovery from iliofemoral thrombophlebitis. The development of these vessels is in response to prolonged overdistention of the superficial venous system by blood originating in the deep venous system and passing through incompetent communicating veins in a retrograde fashion. (For a detailed description of the physical findings in postphlebitic syndrome, see pp. 290–298.)

Phlebosclerosis (Venofibrosis). In this condition the superficial veins are prominent and appear dilated as a result of loss of normal elasticity, with replacement by fibrous, plaque-like thickening of the intima. Elevation of the limb has no effect on the appearance of the vessels, since they have also lost the ability to collapse. Such a change is found most often in older people. When noted in young individuals, it can be considered to be a distinct clinical entity, the cause of which is unknown. [For a discussion of primary varicosities (including tests for regurgitant flow) and superficial thrombophlebitis, see pp. 230 and 235.]

Clinical Testing of Deep Venous System

Depending upon the location of the thrombus in the deep venous system, the associated physical findings may either practically make the diagnosis, as in the case of popliteal or iliofemoral thrombophlebitis (p. 260), or contribute very little of value in this regard, as in the case of phlebothrombosis (p. 257). In the study of the latter condition, considerable reliance must therefore be placed on diagnostic laboratory testing (p. 220) to provide the essential information for this purpose.

Homans' Sign. A clinical test which may be helpful in the diagnosis of phlebothrombosis consists of forcibly dorsiflexing the foot while the lower limb is lifted off the bed. If pain or discomfort is produced in the calf, the test is considered to be positive for a clot in the deep venous plexus, but only after a variety of unrelated conditions causing a similar response can be eliminated from the differential diagnosis. These include local hemorrhage, acute or chronic cellulitis, myositis, dermatitis, laceration and contusion of muscle, and superficial thrombophlebitis, all located in the vicinity of the posterior surface of the leg, in its upper portion. A false-positive Homans' sign may also be elicited in the patient in whom the full weight of his leg had rested on his calf muscles for a protracted period while recovering from the effects of an anesthetic or in the one whose legs were in a stirrup during the entire course of an operation. However, it is necessary to point out that both of the latter individuals are potential candidates for thrombosis of venous plexuses located in the muscle mass, but the process does not occur immediately, and instead it requires 7–10 days to develop before it can be identified by clinical or laboratory means.

Other Tests for Phlebothrombosis. Neuhof's sign consists of carefully palpating the upper part of the calf while the patient rests his heels on the bed and bends his knees to relax the calf muscles. The presence of thickening and infiltration deep in the gastrocnemius and the elicitation of pain constitute a positive sign for thrombosis of the deep venous plexuses. An increase in cutaneous temperature in the region of the calf may also be present, as well as cutaneous dilated 'sentinel veins' in the upper part of the leg.

Study of Patency and Competency of Deep Venous System. In the patient who has recovered from an iliofemoral thrombophlebitis, it is important to determine whether the original thrombus still remains, resulting in an impatent deep venous system, or whether it has been recanalized, causing destruction of local valves and producing a patent but incompetent deep venous system. In the case of primary varicosities, it is also essential to obtain information regarding the state of the deep venous system before any serious consideration can be given to an operative approach to the management of the condition. A number of simple clinical procedures, available for the collection of such important data, are described below.

The *Perthes' test* consists of applying a tourniquet around the thigh while the patient is standing and then instructing him alternately to flex and extend his knee 10 times or to walk. If the deep veins are patent and competent, the blood in the distended superficial veins should be propelled into the deep venous system by the exercise and hence out of the limb, causing the superficial vessels to collapse and remain so after the exercise is terminated. If the deep veins are patent but incompetent, the superficial veins will empty during the physical effort but then refill as soon as the patient stands still. Finally, if the deep venous system is not patent, then the exercise will cause the superficial veins to become even more distended, remaining so in the postexercise period for some time.

A modification of the above procedure consists of applying a tourniquet to the upper part of the thigh with the patient standing, to prevent regurgitant flow and movement of blood out of the superficial venous system of the leg and thigh, and then having him lie down and elevate the limb under study. If the superficial veins remain distended under such circumstances, it can be assumed that a block exists in the deep venous system. In the absence of such a state, the superficial veins will collapse as blood drains from them into the deep veins by way of the communicating vessels and then out of the limb. To make certain that this has taken place, the patient stands again with the tourniquet still on. If the superficial veins now suddenly became distended, such a response negates the impression that patency of the deep veins exists.

The *elastic bandage test,* another means of studying the state of the deep venous system, consists of the following: The lower limb is elevated, and while in this position, careful measurements are made of the circumferences of the leg. Then, with the limb still elevated, a snug elastic bandage is applied to it, beginning with the toes and extending up to the knee. The next step is to have the patient walk at an average pace for approximately 30 min. At the end of this period, a second group of measurements of leg circumferences is made on the elevated uncovered limb. In the presence of a block in the deep venous circulation, definite discomfort is experienced during physical effort, and this increases in intensity as the exercise is continued. On removal of the elastic bandage, the symptoms are immediately relieved, due to the fact that the superficial veins, previously collapsed by the bandage, can again take over the task of removing blood from the lower limb. Together with the development and buildup of the pain, an increase in the size of the calf is generally noted at the end of the walk. If the deep venous system is patent and the valves in the communicating channels are competent, the test elicits no complaints.

Laboratory Testing of the Deep Venous System

Venous Pressure Measurements
Considerable pertinent information regarding the state of the deep veins in the lower limbs can be derived from measurement of the pressure in them.

Technique. A superficial vein on the dorsum of the foot or near the ankle is surgically exposed under local anesthesia and entered using a 14-gauge, thin-walled needle. Then a flexible polyethylene catheter, 30 cm (12 inches) long and with an internal diameter of 1 mm, is filled with sterile isotonic saline solution and threaded through the needle into the vein. The needle is now withdrawn and the skin is closed with one or two sutures previously placed. The free end of the polyethylene tubing is passed through an airtight cork of a reservoir bottle so as to extend below the level of sterile heparinized saline solution half filling the container. A water or mercury manometer is connected by a three-way stopcock to a blood pressure hand bulb and to a glass tube which also passes through the cork of the reservoir bottle but only reaches to above the level of the saline. A pressure reading is obtained by first raising the pressure in the system with the blood pressure bulb to above the anticipated venous pressure and then, when the cannula is cleared of blood, lowering it very slowly until blood is seen entering the translucent tubing arising from the vein. At this point, the venous pressure is read off the manometer. Data are obtained under three different conditions: first, with the patient lying on the examining table and the limb under study at heart level; secondly, with him standing quietly erect; and thirdly, while he walks briskly in place at a rate of one double step per second, each time lifting each of his feet 6 inches from the floor.

Interpretation of Results. In the normal person who is lying down, the venous pressure in the foot is 4.4–8.8 mm Hg (60–120 mm H_2O). On standing, it rises to 70–100 mm Hg, depending upon the height of the individual. With exercise, it falls to around 30–40 mm Hg, due to the pumping action of the muscles on the neighboring thin-walled veins, propelling the blood into the deep venous system and then out of the limb.

In the presence of primary varicosities, the venous pressure readings in the foot with the patient in the horizontal position are greater than normal, due to the increased circulating blood volume ordinarily present in this condition. In the standing position, the readings are the same as those found in the normal individual in this position. With exercise, the reduction in pressure normally observed does not occur because of the regurgitant blood flow from the deep into the superficial vessels that takes place due to incompetency of the valves primarily at the saphenofemoral junction. Previous application of a tourniquet high on the thigh will prevent such a response, and a normal fall in venous pressure with exercise will now take place.

When the postphlebitic syndrome (see chapter 15) exists, the readings in recumbency are normal, but on standing, they exceed the limits generally observed in normal individuals. With exercise there is no decrease in venous pressure, even when a tourniquet has previously been applied. Such abnormal responses result from a retrograde flow of blood into the superficial veins from the deep venous system, due either to a valvular incompetency or a block in the deep veins.

Evaluation of Procedure. Although venous pressure measurements are very helpful in determining the state of the deep venous system, they are of no value in distinguishing between extrinsic pressure on a collecting vein and a thrombus occluding its lumen. Nor do the results of the test differentiate between a rise in venous pressure resulting from local pathology and that produced by systemic disorders, such as congestive heart failure, pericarditis with effusion, or constrictive pericarditis. However, venous pressure determinations are very helpful in distinguishing postphlebitic syndrome from certain conditions which may mimic it, including lymphedema, cellulitis, and brawny induration of the leg; in all of the latter conditions, venous pressure measurements are normal in different positions and during exercise.

Transcutaneous Doppler Ultrasonic Flowmeter

The Doppler ultrasonic flowmeter, a noninvasive laboratory method, has a limited use in the identification of thrombi in the deep veins of the lower limbs. The principle involved in the use of this procedure and a description of the instrument required for the collection of data are discussed on page 65, dealing with the application of the method to the study of local arterial circulation.

Technique. The utilization of the Doppler ultrasonic flowmeter as a diagnostic tool in deep venous thrombosis rests on the fact that normally blood flow in the veins of the lower limbs displays spontaneous alterations related to respiration. For example, a deep inspiration, associated with depression of the diaphragm, causes transient obstruction of flow through the abdominal segment of the inferior vena cava and, hence, interference with movement of blood out of the lower limbs; expiration has the opposite effect as the diaphragm returns to its elevated position. Such cyclic changes in the velocity of the local venous circulation are identified by the ultrasonic flowmeter as corresponding alterations in the character of the sounds heard with the stethoscope.

For collection of data, the probe head is held lightly in contact with the skin overlying the vessels under study. Generally the common femoral, popliteal, and posterior tibial veins are examined, all of them running in proximity and parallel to the respective arteries. Since the angle between the incident sound beam and the vessel determines the pitch of the velocity signal, it is necessary to maintain this angle as constant as possible, one of 45 °C generally being satisfactory. The venous signal, a cyclic blowing high-pitched sound which resembles the noise produced by a strong wind or breaking surf, is altered in frequency by the phases of respiration. Of importance is to be able to distinguish and separate it from the arterial sounds arising from the movement of blood through the accompanying arterial channel. Besides obtaining data under resting conditions, another set of records is collected during a period when venous outflow is artificially increased by compression of the lower segment of limb, using an ordinary blood pressure cuff inflated to 40 mm Hg. In the presence of open collecting channels, such a step should momentarily alter the quality of the venous signal due to the resulting increase in velocity of the venous outflow from the limb. If normal cyclic respiratory sounds are not present over proximal veins and if an artificially produced increase in venous return has no effect in this regard, then it can be assumed that no blood is flowing through the vessel under study.

Evaluation of Procedure. A serious weakness of the Doppler ultrasonic flowmeter when used as a diagnostic tool in venous disorders is that the instrument is unable to detect clots in the small deep venous plexuses in the muscles of the calf [3], the site of origin of many of the pulmonary emboli. Nor is it effective in identifying the presence of thrombosis when only tributary vessels are involved or when patent collateral channels exist [6]. The reason is that under all these conditions, there is no significant interference with venous outflow through the main collecting veins. Naturally, when the thrombus is located in the latter vessels, especially the popliteal and common femoral veins, venous return is markedly reduced, with the result that this situation is readily identified by the absence of the cyclic respiratory sounds, even when attempts are made to facilitate venous outflow by compression applied to the lower part of the limb. However, as already mentioned, occlusion of the popliteal or iliofemoral veins produces such a characteristic clinical picture (p. 260) that laboratory tests are not necessary for its recognition. Also of great importance is the fact that clots which do not totally obstruct main venous channels may likewise go undetected by the ultrasonic flowmeter [3]. This constitutes a serious disadvantage of the test since such thrombi are generally extensive and friable and may be responsible for occlusion of large pulmonary arteries once dislodged. Finally, it is necessary to point out that there is an almost 27% occurrence of false-negative responses with the procedure [4].

Strain-Gauge Plethysmography and Impedance Rheography (Plethysmography)

Both strain-gauge plethysmography and impedance rheography are noninvasive procedures which measure variations in either limb volume or in tissue electrical resistance (also dependent upon limb volume), respectively, during a deep inspiration or a Valsalva maneuver and after compression of the lower segment of leg to increase venous outflow. Since blood is a better conductor of electricity than solid structures, interference with venous return from the lower limb produced by a deep inspiration or a

Valsalva maneuver will result in a momentary reduction in limb resistance and then a return to the previous baseline as expiration is carried out. As in the case of the Doppler ultrasonic flowmeter (p. 222), the two methods primarily collect information regarding the presence of clots which totally occlude main collecting veins. Those in deep venous plexuses of the calf are not identified because the involved vessels are not important in removal of blood from the limb and hence thrombi in them do not materially affect venous outflow. Therefore, there is little change in the respiratory alterations in venous outflow produced by a deep breath or by carrying out a Valsalva maneuver. Another weakness of the two tests is that they require the active cooperation of the patient in performing the above steps, which may be difficult to obtain if he is acutely ill. For all these reasons, strain-gauge plethysmography and impedance rheography have only limited use as diagnostic aids in deep venous thrombosis. (For the technique involved in the application of the two procedures to the limb, see p. 70.)

Radioactive Fibrinogen Test

The radioactive fibrinogen test plays a very important but limited role as a sensitive diagnostic tool in deep venous thrombosis of the lower limbs, especially as a means of screening high risk populations.

Technique. The test is carried out by injecting 100 µCi of ^{125}I-fibrinogen intravenously, followed by surface counting over selected regions of each leg, using a shielded external probe and a single-channel analyzer spectrometer. To protect the thyroid gland from the effects of radioactivity, an oral dose of Lugol's solution or of sodium iodide (100 mg) is given 24 h before the test.

The basis for the procedure is that the radioactive fibrinogen will be adsorbed to the surface of any fresh clot with which it comes in contact. It does not accumulate on a thrombus early in its inception (for the first 3–4 days), nor does it have any effect on a clot which is already organized (after the 11th day of formation). Moreover, it becomes attached to any freshly clotted blood, regardless of the location, as for example, a hematoma, such a response reducing and limiting the value of the method.

Evaluation of Procedure. The radioactive fibrinogen test is particularly helpful when thrombi are confined to the sinusoids in the soleus muscle, since these are almost impossible to visualize completely by radiologic means (p. 228). Also of great importance is that with the method, nonocclusive thrombi in a large collecting vein which are floating in the lumen of the vessel and hence can readily be dislodged to form pulmonary emboli, are identifiable. On the other hand, complete occlusion of such vessels, preventing the blood containing the radioactive fibrinogen from passing over the clot, cannot be diagnosed. But, as already indicated, in this type of situation, the clinical pattern is readily recognized. A potential complication of the test is a slight risk of hepatitis transmission with the fibrinogen.

Contrast Venography

Roentgenographic visualization of the deep venous system through the use of radiopaque material (fig. 11/3) is a procedure which reveals in detail the anatomy of the vessels and at the same time accurately locates blocks in venous plexuses in the calf (see fig. 14/2a), as well as partial and complete occlusions of main venous channels (see fig. 14/2b). There is no question that it is the most effective and precise means for establishing or eliminating the possibility of a disease process in the deep venous tree in the lower limbs. However, besides being an expensive test to carry out, it is an invasive procedure, responsible for certain mild and also serious adverse responses and complications, including postinjection and radiation venous thrombosis.

Technique. Although a number of approaches are available, the one most commonly used is the percutaneous injection of the radiopaque material into a superficial vein on the dorsum of the foot, using a tourniquet applied to the lower portion of the leg to direct the material into the deep venous circulation. The films are exposed at intervals, the contrast medium is washed out of the vein with saline solution, and the needle is removed. When there is need to determine venous valve competency, descending venography is indicated. This involves the slow injection of the contrast medium into the common femoral vein under fluoroscopic control with the patient in the semi-erect position. The principle of contrast venography is similar to that utilized in contrast arteriography (p. 72). (For adverse reactions to the contrast medium, see p. 76.)

Interpretation of the Venogram. Thrombi in the deep venous plexuses in the calf muscle are identified as constant, elongated filling defects which persist in shape and location in well-opacified vessels in at least two films. A thrombus which is floating in the lumen and partly occluding the vessel appears as a well-defined translucent area surrounded by a rim or narrow border of contrast medium (see fig. 14/2b). Generally, the ends of the clot have rounded tips. Partial obstruction of a collecting vein may be identified as a reduction in size and irregularities in contour of segments of the vessel. In the presence of complete occlusion, the portion of the vein proximal to the obstruction shows no opacification (see fig. 14/1b). Collateral vessels may be visualized through filling with contrast medium.

Certain artifacts may be found in the records. For example, venospasm, initiated by the injection of the radiopaque material, may cause almost complete occlusion of a segment of vein, with tapering distally and normally appearing vessel on either side of the apparent block. Another situation which may cause incorrect interpretation of the film is produced by a greater velocity of blood flow in the center of the vessel, causing translucency in the area which resembles a partial block. Additional films can readily demonstrate the artifact because it will no longer be present on the second examination. Contraction of voluntary muscle toward the end of the procedure may be responsible for changes which are misinterpreted as filling defects of varying length.

In the case of descending venography, fluoroscopic visualization demonstrates the movement of the contrast medium injected in a retrograde fashion into the common femoral vein. In the normal individual with competent valves in the main venous channels, the column of radiopaque material is seen fluctuating up and down in synchrony with every heart beat and with respiration, but still steadily passing upward in the direction of the inferior vena cava. In the patient with moderate incompetence of the valves in the common femoral vein, the contrast medium moves both in a retrograde fashion and proximally. When extreme incompetence exists, the column of contrast medium falls precipitously straight down the vessel in the thigh from the point of injection. The difference can be exaggerated by having the patient perform a Valsalva maneuver. In the normal individual, the radiopaque medium will accumulate just above the location of compe-

---

Fig. 11/3. Normal venous tree in lower limb visualized by contrast venography. **a** EIV = External iliac vein; FV = common femoral vein. **b** FV = Superficial femoral vein; PV = popliteal vein; PT = venae comites of posterior tibial artery; P = venae comites of peroneal artery; AT = venae comites of anterior tibial artery. **c** Diagrammatic representation of the venous tree in the lower limb. Designations are similar to those in **b**. Reproduced from ref. [1] with permission.

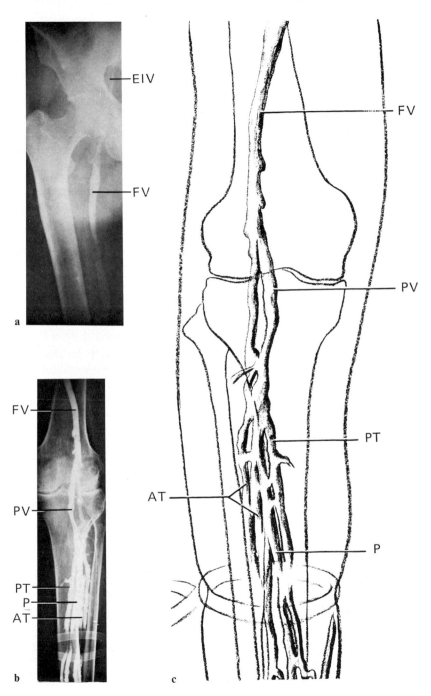

tent valves, whereas in the patient in whom these structures are destroyed, the material will rapidly fall to a low level of the venous tree.

Evaluation of Procedure. As already mentioned, contrast venography is most helpful as a diagnostic procedure when a clot is located in the deep venous plexuses in the calf. However, with the method, there is a possibility of inadequate visualization of the soleal venous sinuses, the anterior tibial veins, and the profunda femoris system, all of which may be sites of origin of pulmonary emboli. Perhaps with modifications of the conventional technique of venography, such weaknesses in the procedure may be eliminated.

Among other situations in which the method is applicable and useful is one in which there is a problem in determining why surgical removal of primary varicosities was not successful. In this regard, it may be able to identify the presence of Klippel-Trenaunay syndrome (p. 364), in which the dilated superficial veins are associated with congenital abnormalities of the deep venous system. It also calls attention to the presence, location, and extent of incompetent perforating vessels responsible for maintaining a state of venous stasis in the vicinity of a chronic nonhealing ulcer and thus contributing to the lack of improvement despite appropriate therapy. Finally, contrast venography may clarify the cause of persistent edema of a lower limb by either demonstrating an old block in the main venous channel or eliminating such a possibility.

Radionuclide (Radioisotopic) Venography
Radionuclide venography is a noninvasive relatively simple and rapid procedure for the visualization of the venous tree in the lower limbs, unassociated with significant morbidity or much pain. It has been used as a substitute for contrast venography under certain circumstances, for it can be repeated many times if necessary without harm to the patient. However, the method is not as accurate as contrast venography in presenting a detailed study of the anatomy of the venous tree and in identifying the exact location of a thrombus. Nor is the full length of the thrombotic process visualized with the method. Furthermore, a completely blocked vessel cannot be identified since the clot cannot pick up the radioisotopic tracer in the blood stream because of lack of flow. An advantage of the method is that lung scanning (p. 267) can be performed at the same time, thus supplying pertinent information regarding the presence of pulmonary emboli. Or the findings can be used as a baseline scan for future reference [6].

Technique. A suspension of human serum albumin microspheres incorporating ^{99m}Tc-sulfur colloid is injected into a superficial vein on the dorsum of the foot with a small-calibered plastic needle, after double ankle tourniquets have been applied to direct the material into the deep venous system. Before administration of the suspension, the patient is carefully positioned under an Anger-type scintillation camera. Using a Gamma camera, rapid sequence scintiphotography is made of blood flow through the veins of the calf, thigh, and groin. At the same time, the image is recorded by Polaroid camera photography. After the peripheral vein scan of the limb is completed, scintiphotographs of the lungs are taken in four views with the patient in the supine position, using the same Gamma camera.

Interpretation of Results. Radioisotopic venography may reveal the following abnormalities: absent flow in the deep venous system, with normal visualization of the superficial veins; obstruction in the deep veins with collateral vessels bridging it; irregular deep veins, with collateral and superficial venous system also visualized; 'hot spots' representing entrapment of the microspheres in the thrombus, and filling defects in large veins [5].

References

1   Abramson, D.I.: Vascular disorders of the extremities (Harper & Row, Hagerstown 1974).

2   Abramson, D.I.; Miller, D.S.: Vascular problems in musculoskeletal disorders of the limbs (Springer, Berlin 1981).

3   Sigel, B.; Popky, G.L.; Wagner, D.K; et al.: A Doppler ultrasound method for diagnosing lower extremity venous disease. Surgery Gynec. Obstet. *127:* 339 (1968).

4   Sigel, B.; Felix, W.B., Jr.; Popky, G.L.; et al.: Diagnosis of lower limb venous thrombosis by Doppler ultrasound technique. Archs Surg., Chicago *104:* 174 (1972).

5   Yao, J.S.T.; Henkin, R.E.; Conn, J., Jr.; et al.: Combined isotope venography and lung scanning: a new diagnostic approach to thromboembolism. Archs Surg., Chicago *107:* 146 (1973).

6   Young, J.R.: Thrombophlebitis and chronic venous insufficiency. Geriatrics *28:* 63 (1973).

12 Physical Signs of Venous Disorders

This chapter is devoted to those abnormal physical findings which indicate the presence of incompetency, impatency, or both in the superficial or deep venous system in the lower limbs. The discussion supplements the material found on page 212, dealing with the clinical steps involved in a study of the venous circulation. In each of the physical signs or states considered below, the pathogenesis, clinical description, and differential diagnosis are presented.

Varicosities

Besides those conditions enumerated on page 213, both primary and secondary varicosities also fall into the category of prominent superficial veins of the lower limbs.

Primary Varicosities

Primary varicosities are probably the most common vascular disorder affecting the lower limbs. Although generally found in women, men may also demonstrate signs of the disorder, especially if they are over 6 feet (183 cm) tall and have a mother or father with the same condition.

Pathogenesis. Primary varicosities consist of superficial dilated, tortuous, and distended venous channels on the lower limbs, in which there is a regurgitant flow of blood due to incompetent or absent valves at sites where the superficial veins enter the deep venous system. Since the pressure in the latter is greater than that in the superficial vessels, the abnormality permits blood from the deep veins to pass in a retrograde fashion into the superficial veins, overdistending them and causing their valves to become functionally incompetent. The leaks into the superficial venous system may occur in three locations: where the great saphenous vein enters the common femoral vein at the level of the fossa ovalis (fig. 12/1a); where the small saphenous vein enters the popliteal vein in the popliteal fossa (fig. 12/1b),

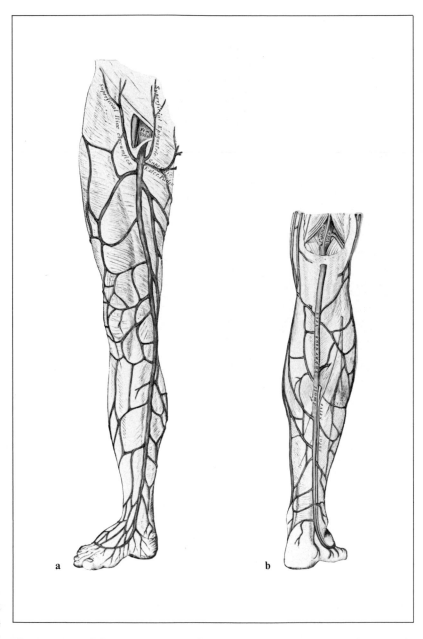

Fig. 12/1. Superficial venous system of the lower extremity. **a** Great saphenous vein and its tributaries. **b** Small saphenous vein and its tributaries. Reproduced from ref. [3] with permission.

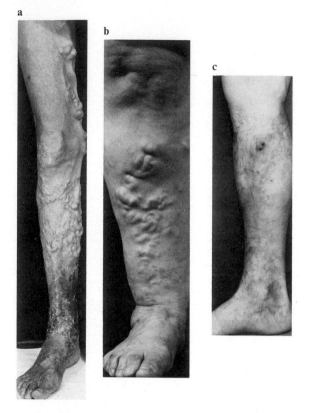

Fig. 12/2. Primary varicosities in the lower limbs. **a** Marked involvement of the entire length of great saphenous vein. Pigmentation (sign of venous stasis) also noted. **b** Involvement of the great saphenous vein in the leg. **c** Erosion of a varicose vein on right leg leading to hemorrhage. Reproduced from ref. [2] with permission.

and anywhere on the leg and thigh where superficial veins empty blood into communicating channels which penetrate the muscle mass to join the deep venous system.

Clinical Manifestations. Generally the uncomplicated case of primary varicosities is associated with only minor complaints, such as tiredness and heaviness of the lower limbs at the end of the day and night cramps, together with slight swelling of the ankles, and the appearance of dilated and tortuous superficial veins on the thigh and leg (fig. 12/2a, b). However, complications of a much more serious nature may develop, including

a   b

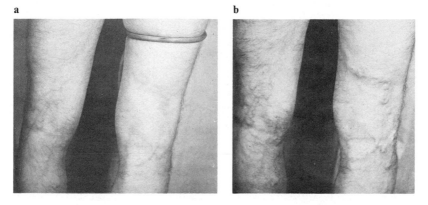

Fig. 12/3. Demonstration of incompetency in the great saphenous vein on the left thigh at the level of the saphenofemoral junction, using the Trendelenburg test. **a** Tourniquet applied high on the thigh with the patient lying down and the extremity elevated. On standing, no varicosities are noted. **b** Tourniquet removed, with immediate appearance of varicosities on posterior aspect of thigh and leg. Reproduced from ref. [1] with permission.

repeated attacks of superficial benign thrombophlebitis (p. 235), external hemorrhage (fig. 12/2c), chronic indurated cellulitis, stasis dermatitis, and stasis ulceration. (For discussion of the latter three states, see pp. 294–296.)

Diagnosis. A regurgitant flow must be demonstrated in a superficial dilated vein before a diagnosis of primary varicosities can be made, and for this purpose, several clinical procedures are available. One of these, the *Brodie-Trendelenburg test* (better known by the latter name) (fig. 12/3), is performed as follows: The patient lies down, the lower limb being studied is elevated to drain blood out of the superficial vessels, and while in this position, a tourniquet is applied around the thigh just below the level of the fossa ovalis. The amount of compression utilized is approximately 30–40 mm Hg, much less than that which would obstruct arterial inflow or deep vein outflow, but great enough to collapse the superficially located great saphenous vein. Then the patient stands facing the examiner who observes the sites previously demonstrating clusters of varicose veins. After 10 s the tourniquet is released. Immediate filling and distention of the great saphenous system indicates that the valves in the proximal segment of the main vein are incompetent, generally at the level of the fossa ovalis, and that blood is leaking backward into the superficial venous system from the deep veins through the saphenofemoral junction. Slow filling of the vessels after removal of the tourniquet (30 s or more) is a normal response, due to the upward movement of blood from the capillary system.

The *multiple tourniquet test* is helpful in determining whether more than one leak is present and the location of the abnormalities on the limb. It is performed as follows: Three tourniquets are placed around the elevated extremity: one high upon the thigh, one above the knee, and one just above the upper limits of the calf; then the patient stands. The immediate appearance of varicosities on the leg below the level of the most distal tourniquet indicates that incompetent communicating veins are present in the lower part of the limb above the ankle. If removal of the tourniquet on the leg results in the appearance of varicose veins distally, this means that the small saphenous vein is incompetent. If the varicosities return only after removal of the tourniquet just above the knee, then it can be assumed that the difficulty is in a main tributary of the great saphenous system. Finally, a leak in the great saphenous vein will manifest itself when the last tourniquet is removed and the entire superficial venous system is flooded with blood.

Secondary Varicosities

Etiologic Factors. Secondary varicosities generally develop in response to significant rises in pressure in the deep venous system, either as a result of impatency of a main collecting vein or incompetency of the valves in the latter. Either state may develop following occlusion of the popliteal or iliofemoral vein by a thrombus, whether due to initial intrinsic pathology or to prolonged, persistent extrinsic pressure. (For a discussion of the signs and pathogenesis of secondary varicosities resulting from iliofemoral or popliteal thrombophlebitis, see p. 292.)

Another cause of secondary varicosities is flooding of the proximal superficial veins with blood at a high venous pressure, a situation found in congenital arteriovenous fistula (p. 362) and in acquired arteriovenous fistula (p. 310). In both conditions, the high venous pressure is imparted to the blood by the arterial blood pressure, very little of which is dissipated by the passage of blood from the arterial side of the circulation, through the fistulous tract or tracts, into the large superficial veins located proximal to the lesion. The resulting venous hypertension and the large quantity of blood entering and distending these vessels contribute to functional incompetency of their valves and the development of secondary varicosities.

Superficial Thrombophlebitis

Superficial thrombophlebitis must also be differentiated from the various states characterized by prominent superficial veins of the lower limbs (pp. 213, 230). However, in most instances, clear-cut clinical signs observed in this condition make its presence readily identifiable.

General Considerations
Pathogenesis and Etiologic Factors. The occlusion of a superficial vein by a thrombus is almost invariably associated with a severe local phlebitic reaction but no constitutional responses. The precipitating cause is some type of injury to the intimal lining produced either by extrinsic trauma or by intrinsic factors, such as sclerosing or hypertonic solutions injected into the vessel. Hematologic changes may also contribute to the formation of the intravenous thrombus. Under some circumstances, no apparent etiologic agent can be identified.

Clinical Manifestations. A thrombus in a superficial vein located in the subcutaneous tissue of the lower limbs is readily diagnosed by its characteristic physical findings: the presence of one or more linear-shaped areas of erythema of varying lengths, representing the alterations in the skin overlying and outlining the thrombosed vein (fig. 12/4); local swelling, elevated cutaneous temperature, and tenderness, contributed to by the phlebitic reaction; and a cordlike mass beneath the skin, determined by palpation – the occluded and inflamed vein. Elevation of the limb has no effect on the physical findings. At no time is superficial thrombophlebitis associated with edema of the leg and foot. Rarely, if at all, is it followed by pulmonary embolism. When there appears to be an apparent relationship, not infrequently a similar thrombotic process is also found in the deep veins of the calf or elsewhere.

Types of Superficial Thrombophlebitis
Several categories of superficial thrombophlebitis are identifiable clinically, each demonstrating some differences in clinical manifestations, treatment, or prognosis from the others.

Superficial Benign Thrombophlebitis. This entity is by far the most common type of thrombotic involvement of superficial veins. The pathologic process is generally found in the course of the great or small saphenous vein. Usual sites on the limbs for the lesions are the medial aspect of the leg and thigh and the lateral and posterolateral aspect of the leg up to the level of the knee. Each thrombosed segment of vein is about 1 cm (less than 0.5 inches) in width and 3–15 cm (1–6 inches) or longer in length. The clinical picture is similar to that already described, the involved portion of vessel usually remaining palpable for several days or even weeks after all signs of inflammation have disappeared.

Recurrent episodes of superficial benign thrombophlebitis on the lower limbs is a relatively common complication of primary varicosities (p. 232), due to the persistent venous stasis and venous hypertension that exist in such vessels when the patient assumes the upright position. The precipitating mechanism is usually some minor trauma to the skin and subcutaneous tissue overlying the vessel. When the condition appears in the absence of any apparent etiologic factor, it may or may not have serious implications. For example, it may be found in obese people, in the elderly, in patients who have been subjected to a slow return to ambulation after prolonged bedrest, and in people recovering from a major operation or from a delivery. In all such individuals, venous stasis plays a role in the development of the thrombotic process in the superficial veins. Other etiologic factors are hypercoagulability of the blood and injury to the venous endothelium. Among the much more serious conditions associated with benign thrombophlebitis are congestive heart failure, neoplastic disease of visceral organs, blood dyscrasias, occult ulcerative bowel difficulties, and connective tissue disorders (especially systemic lupus erythematosus). Iatrogenic superficial benign thrombophlebitis may follow intravenous injection of hypertonic medications, sclerosing or irritant solutions, and drugs causing marked vasoconstriction, such as norepinephrine (Levophed), and the use of indwelling catheters.

Superficial Migratory Thrombophlebitis. This type of superficial thrombophlebitis has some clinical manifestations which help differentiate it from superficial benign thrombophlebitis. The lesions are generally much smaller, their length being only about 2–3 cm (1.5 inches or less), and they are found anywhere on the leg and thigh (fig. 12/4) (as well as on the upper limbs), in no relationship to the location of the major superficial venous systems. Moreover, they may be present on a number of separate sites on one or both lower limbs at the same time, developing in the form of crops in one location and receding in another. This gives the impression that the small discrete nodules are migratory and fleeting in character, each one

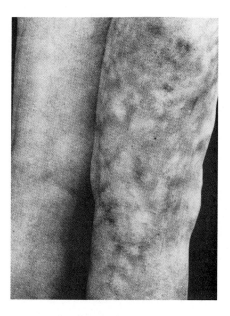

Fig. 12/4. Numerous lesions of thrombophlebitis migrains (similar to those observed in thromboangiitis obliterans) on the thigh. A number of different segments of superficial veins are involved. Reproduced from ref. [2] with permission.

persisting for only 7 or 8 days. The skin over them is red and hot, and the lesions themselves are felt as tender, firm indurated cords. As the process subsides, the hard masses resolve, eventually to disappear, except for the residual of deposits of brown pigment in the overlying skin in some areas (fig. 12/4).

Superficial migratory thrombophlebitis has been noted in association with thromboangiitis obliterans (Buerger's disease) in about 40% of cases (p. 106). In fact, it may be the earliest finding in the disease before signs of arterial involvement are noted. If the patient persists in smoking, the crops of superficial migratory thrombophlebitis will continue to appear at intervals, together with progression of the occlusive process in the arterial tree.

Superficial migratory thrombophlebitis may also be followed for many years without the appearance of any etiology and without signs of occlusion of arteries in the limbs, despite the fact that the patient continues his smoking habit. This condition, termed thrombophlebitis migrans (idiopathic recurrent superficial migratory thrombophlebitis), has been reported to be associated on occasion with thrombosis of abdominal and intracranial veins which, of course, results in a very poor prognosis. If limited to the superficial veins on the limbs, it will cause very little difficulty except local pain on walking when active lesions are present.

Finally, superficial migratory thrombophlebitis may be found in patients suffering from severe congestive heart failure and from visceral carcinoma, particularly of the body and tail of the pancreas and, less often, the liver, stomach, gallbladder, and lungs.

Differential Diagnosis of Superficial Thrombophlebitis

Superficial Benign Thrombophlebitis. There should be little difficulty in differentiating this condition from other entities because of the clear-cut physical findings invariably present. At times dilated distended superficial veins may pose a problem, but this can quickly be clarified (p. 213). Acute lymphangitis may bear some resemblance to superficial benign thrombophlebitis except that the linear red streaks are much narrower and no mass can be palpated beneath them. Furthermore, the condition is always associated with a systemic reaction, in the form of a high fever, leukocytosis, and malaise, whereas superficial benign thrombophlebitis displays none of these findings. Nor is there any tenderness in the popliteal space or in the groin (locations of lymph glands), a finding almost invariably present in connection with lymphangitis.

Superficial Migratory Thrombophlebitis. Because this condition is characterized by small discrete lesions under the skin, it must be distinguished from a number of different disorders which are associated with various types of subcutaneous nodules. Among these are neoplastic infiltrations (neurofibroma, lymphosarcoma, myosarcoma) and benign masses (neuromas). In some instances, only a biopsy study reveals the true nature of the nodules.

Venous Edema

Swelling of the lower limbs is a fairly common finding in local venous disorders. Initially it is of the pitting type, except on occasion when the quantity of fluid that has accumulated in the tissue spaces is so marked that, as a result, the skin is tightly stretched. Generally, if the edema persists uncontrolled for a protracted period of time, eventually it loses its pitting quality, thus making it indistinguishable from lymphedema (p. 242).

This section is devoted to the pathogenesis of the type of edema found in such venous disorders as iliofemoral or popliteal thrombophlebitis, the postphlebitic syndrome, and primary varicosities. Also discussed is the differentiation of venous edema from swelling due to nonvenous disorders.

Edema of Popliteal and Iliofemoral Thrombophlebitis

When a main collecting vein in a lower limb is suddenly occluded by a thrombus, one of the first manifestations of such a situation is the rapid appearance of pitting edema affecting the foot, leg, and thigh if the clot is in the iliofemoral vein (see fig. 14/3), or the foot and leg, if the popliteal vein is occluded. The swelling frequently develops within 6–8 h following the onset of the pathologic process in the vessel.

Pathogenesis. The mechanism responsible for the edema is primarily interference with the movement of venous blood out of the involved lower limb, due to occlusion of the main vein. As a consequence, there is a rapid buildup of venous hypertension and stasis in the small venules and capillaries, followed by a rise of pressure within their lumens – sometimes to a level five times greater than normal. Such a response acts to raise capillary filtration pressure markedly, thus causing the expression of fluid from the blood stream into the extravascular spaces. At the same time, the normal movement of fluid from the tissue spaces into the venular end of the capillaries is prevented by the existing high capillary and venular pressure. The venous stasis also contributes to the development of some anoxia of the capillary wall, thus increasing its permeability. All of these factors facilitate transudation of fluid from the lumen of the capillaries and venules into the tissue spaces, with the production of pitting edema.

Several other mechanisms are involved, but to a lesser degree, in the development of edema following occlusion of a main collecting vein. One of these is interference with lymphatic drainage from the limb due, in part, to inflammation of the large lymphatic trunks, resulting from their proximity to the periphlebitic reaction of the thrombosed vein. Further lymphatic stasis follows the increased burden placed on the lymphatic system through the loss of the normal mechanism of removal of blood via venous channels. Another factor which exaggerates lymph stasis is spasm of medium- and small-sized arteries due to a vasomotor reflex triggered by the occluded segment of vein. The resulting reduction in pulsations in the arterial tree causes a decrease in the pumping action with each heart beat that this mechanism normally has on neighboring lymphatic channels. Hence, stagnation of tissue fluids and accumulation of proteins in the perivascular spaces occur. Such a situation is also conducive to edema formation since the osmotic pressure exerted by the large molecules remaining in the tissue spaces prevents resorption of tissue fluid into the vascular bed. Finally, the existing vasospasm produces anoxia of the capillary endothelium, which causes greater capillary permeability and thus facilitates transudation of fluid from the lumen of the vessels into the tissue spaces.

Edema of Postphlebitic Syndrome
Following the disappearance of the edema developed during the acute stage of iliofemoral or popliteal thrombophlebitis, there may be a recurrence of swelling weeks or months later. This may be the first manifestation of the existence of the postphlebitic syndrome (p. 290).

Pathogenesis. The edema of the postphlebitic syndrome reflects an inefficient and inadequate local venous system, unable to cope with the problem of venous return from the affected extremity when the patient assumes the upright position. The mechanism responsible for the swelling is a state of venous hypertension transmitted back into the capillary bed as an elevated capillary filtration pressure, the latter causing a rapid transudation of fluid from the blood into the tissue spaces. The venous stasis and the elevated local venous pressure are the result of either a persisting incompetency of the deep venous system, due to destruction of valves in the process of recanalization of the old clot in the collecting vein, or retention of the thrombus, producing an impatent system. Under either condition, there is interference with venous outflow and hence the development of venous hypertension.

Edema of Primary Varicosities
In patients with primary varicosities of the lower limbs (p. 232), swelling of a minor degree generally accumulates around the ankles and the lower portion of the legs at the end of the day. This does not readily pit, and the amount is generally related to the length of time the patient is on his feet. After a night's rest, it is usually minimal or absent.

Pathogenesis. The edema is related to the state of venous hypertension which exists in superficial varicose veins when the upright position is assumed. Such a situation arises because the incompetent valves in these vessels permit retrograde flow into the distal segment of limb and the development of venous stasis and a rise in venous pressure. As a consequence, capillary filtration pressure in the capillary bed becomes elevated, causing a greater transudation of fluid into the tissue spaces and hence mild edema.

Differentiation of Venous Edema from Edema of Nonvenous Origin
Swelling of the lower extremities can be produced by a large number of unrelated conditions or states.

Dependency Edema. Prolonged standing or sitting with the feet in dependency can produce swelling, at times of a marked degree, in the lower limbs of normal people. The lack of contraction of voluntary muscles of the legs and thighs and the significant rise in hydrostatic pressure in the veins of the lower limbs, both contribute to a buildup of venous pressure, followed by a similar change in capillary filtration pressure, producing a greater than normal movement of fluid from the blood into the tissue spaces. The response is more apparent in women than in men and is particularly evident in a warm or hot environment. A night's rest with the lower limbs elevated generally results in complete disppearance of the edema. There is no significance attributed to its development. (For information on dependency edema in the patient with severe arterial insufficiency of a lower limb associated with ischemic neuropathy, see p. 144).

Arterial Vasospasm. In certain vasospastic disorders, like major causalgia and post-traumatic vasomotor disorders (pp. 327, 330) and in the acute stage of frostbite (p. 320), swelling is not infrequently present (see fig. 16/5a). The mechanisms responsible for this finding are ischemia of capillaries, due to impaired arterial inflow, which causes increased permeability of the capillary wall; reduced pumping action of the constricted arteries on neighboring lymphatic channels, resulting in lymphatic stasis; and voluntarily maintained immobility and dependency of the limb for fear of precipitating more pain. The latter factor raises hydrostatic and hence venous pressures due to loss of pumping action on thin-walled veins and lymphatics ordinarily supplied by contracting muscles.

Drug Edema. Administration of such hormones as corticosteroids, adrenocorticotropins, estrogen, progesterone (including birth control agents), aldosterone-like substances, and testosterone may cause swelling of the lower limbs, as well as elsewhere. Antihypertensive agents, including guanethedine sulfate (Ismelin), hydralazine hydrochloride (Apresoline Hydrochloride), methyldopa (Aldomet), the rauwolfia preparations, and diazides, have the same effect. Certain anti-inflammatory drugs, such as phenylbutazone (Butazolidin) may also cause edema. In most instances, the swelling subsides soon after withdrawal of the responsible agent.

Systemic Disorders. Naturally, before attributing the edema to abnormal local mechanisms, it is necessary to eliminate those systemic conditions which are associated with bilateral swelling of the lower limbs. Among these are congestive heart failure, cirrhosis of the liver, nephrosis, vitamin and nutritional deficiency diseases, and hypothyroidism.

Lymphatic Disorders. Interference with lymphatic outflow from a lower limb is characterized by mild to severe swelling, which at the beginning may be pitting in character but invariably becomes nonpitting and firm. Two etiologic types of lymphedema are observed clinically: the congenital or primary and the acquired, or secondary.

Congenital abnormalities of the lymphatic system consist of an absence of formed lymph trunks (aplasia); unconnected lymph spaces; reduced number or size of lymph channels (hypoplasia); and widening and tortuosity of the lymphatics (hyperplasia) producing incompetency of the vessels. All of these changes fall into the category of primary lymphedema, causing such clinical entities as simple congenital lymphedema (fig. 12/5a), congenital familial lymphedema (Milroy's disease), and lymphedema praecox (observed almost exclusively in girls around the time of puberty or in young women).

Lymphedema may also be secondary to a number of different conditions in which there is interference with movement of lymph out of a lower limb, resulting in lymph stasis. This latter state may follow malignant occlusion of lymph nodes (fig. 12/5b, c), destruction of local lymphatic channels by trauma (fig. 12/5d), and repeated lymphangitic episodes, eventually causing fibrosis and obliteration of the affected lymph vessels.

Soft-Tissue Dystrophic Calcification on a Venous Stasis Basis

Soft-tissue dystrophic calcification, an abnormal accumulation of lime salts in an injured tissue, is found in a number of unrelated conditions, among which is protracted venous stasis of the lower limbs [5, 6]. The

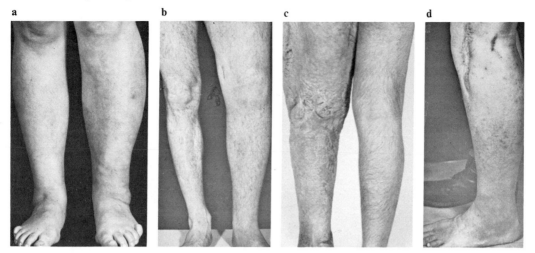

Fig. 12/5. Lymphedema resulting from various etiologic agents. **a** Simple congenital lymphedema of left lower extremity. **b** Lymphedema of left lower extremity following metastasis of fibrosarcoma of fifth toe to inguinal lymph nodes. **c** Secondary lymphedema due to repeated attacks of cellulitis followed by lymphangitis and lymphadenitis. **d** Secondary lymphedema following extensive destruction of lymphatic channels by shell fragment wound in the leg. Reproduced from ref. [2] with permission.

change can be demonstrated on soft-tissue roentgenograms and microscopically, as well as by clinical observation and palpation, as in chronic indurated cellulitis.

General Considerations of Calcium Deposits in Venous Stasis

Pathogenesis. The exact mechanism which alters the invisible calcium carbonate and phosphate in the blood stream so that aggregates of these salts are deposited in the tissues as gross collections is not known. Normally there is a dynamic equilibrium between the circulating calcium and phosphorus which, in turn, is dependent upon the absorption of these ions from the gastrointestinal tract, their resorption from or deposition in the bony storehouse, and their excretion by the kidneys and bowel. If there is an increase of calcium without a compensatory decrease in phosphorus, or if the reverse exists, precipitation of insoluble calcium phosphate occurs.

Injured tissue is especially prone to deposition of calcium salts, due to an associated lowered carbon dioxide tension which allows fewer calcium and posphate ions to be held in solution. It may very well be that this is the etiologic agent which is responsible for the deposition of calcium in an area of persistent venous stasis in the lower part of the leg, as occurs in chronic indurated cellulitis (p. 294), one of the facets of the postphlebitic syndrome. A contributing factor is a low-grade infection.

Clinical Manifestations. The plaques of subcutaneous ossification are found almost exclusively in postmenopausal obese women suffering from chronic venous insufficiency of the lower limbs, as well as epidermophytosis of the feet and, in some instances, recurrent stasis ulcers in the involved area (p. 296). Serum calcium, phosphorus, and alkaline phosphatase values are generally all normal in such individuals. There appears to be little question that in the case of local ulceration, the calcium deposits interfere with healing of the lesion, removal of the ossified mass with excision of the overlying ulcer having a therapeutic effect in some instances [4].

Other Types of Calcium Deposits in Soft Tissues
Metastatic Calcification. This response is due to an altered calcium and/or phosphorus regulation distant from the site of deposit of the salt. Associated findings are elevated levels of ionized calcium and phosphorus in the serum, the local process being initiated by precipitation of calcium phosphate, usually in an alkaline medium. Although the tissues in which the deposits develop are normal, some type of underlying systemic difficulty always coexists. Such disorders as hyperparathyroidism, vitamin D intoxication, pseudohypoparathyroidism, destructive bone diseases, and renal insufficiency have all been implicated in the local response.

Calcinosis. This type of change has been noted most often in the connective tissue disorders (p. 370), in the form of *calcinosis circumscripta.* The process is generally found in older female patients, being confined to the extensor surface of the knees, as well as to the elbows and fingers. The avidity of calcium for degenerated tissue is clearly demonstrated in this category.

Vascular Calcification. In blood vessels, calcium deposits may take place on ulcerated atheromas in the intima, or the change may be noted in the media, as occurs in Mönckeberg's sclerosis (p. 109). The vascular alterations are intensified in conditions in which there are elevated serum calcium levels, as in hyperparathyroidism and vitamin D intoxication.

Heterotopic Bone Formation. This type is associated with normal serum calcium, phosphorus, and pH values. The process is noted in many sites, including insertions of tendons, soft tissues in paraplegics, and postoperative abdominal scars. *Myositis ossificans progressiva* is typical for heterotopic bone formation. This condition is usually characterized by progressive ossification of the connective tissue of muscles. It may result from injury to deep muscle tissue, with the production of edema and cellular proliferation, followed by ingrowth of masses of collagen. The latter generally accepts the deposition of calcium salts, then osteoid, cartilage, and finally bone. The quadriceps of the thigh is most frequently involved in the process.

References

1 Abramson, D.I.: Practical procedures in bedside diagnosis of peripheral vascular disorders. Am. Practnr Dig. Treat. *6:* 546 (1955).

2 Abramson, D.I.: Diagnosis and treatment of peripheral vascular disorders (Hoeber-Harper, New York 1956).

3 Abramson, D.I.: Vascular disorders of the extremities (Harper & Row, Hagerstown 1974).

4 Condon, R.E.; Harkins, H.N.: Subcutaneous bone formation in chronic venous insufficiency of the legs. Ann. Surg. *157:* 27 (1963).

5 Lippmann, H.I.: Subcutaneous ossification in chronic venous insufficiency: presentation of 23 cases. Preliminary report. Angiology *8:* 378 (1957).

6 Lippmann, H.I.; Goldin, R.R.: Subcutaneous ossification of legs in chronic venous insufficiency. Radiology *74:* 279 (1960).

13 Factors Contributing to Deep Venous Thrombosis and Their Control

Acute occlusion of segments of the deep venous system of the lower limbs is a very serious condition which has the potential for drastically and dramatically altering the entire outlook of a relatively benign illness or a surgical procedure, primarily because of its close alliance with pulmonary embolism and infarction (p. 263). For this reason, the present chapter is devoted to a discussion of (1) those factors, either extrinsic or intrinsic, which predispose to intravascular coagulation, and (2) clinical measures to combat, eliminate, or minimize their deleterious effects.

Factors Responsible for or Predisposing to Venous Thrombosis (Virchow's Triad)

Intravascular clotting occurs when the efficiency of the various mechanisms involved in maintaining the fluidity of circulating blood is impaired. The fact that the rate of blood flow is much slower in venous than in arterial channels contributes to some extent to a greater incidence of clot formation in veins, particularly of the lower limbs. Although retarded circulation, by itself, cannot initiate intravascular coagulation, this factor tends to facilitate the process when one or several of the mechanisms discussed below coexist [6].

Venous Stasis

Slowed venous blood flow (venous stasis) plays a very important role in the formation of thrombi in the deep veins of the lower limbs. It may result from physical inactivity associated with protracted bedrest, from immobilization of a lower limb in a cast, and from various situations producing interference with venous outflow, as in the case of an enlarging uterus due to pregnancy compressing the pelvic veins. It may be present in congestive heart failure and in quadriplegia, paraplegia, and hemiplegia in which the lower limb or limbs are held in dependency and local muscles are incapable of voluntary contraction. Old age is associated with a high incidence of deep venous thrombosis probably because elderly patients are frequently subjected to prostatectomy, herniorrhaphy, surgical treatment of hip fractures, and gynecologic procedures, all associated with protracted periods of bedrest and an attendant state of venous stasis.

Damage to Venous Endothelium

Pathogenesis. Trauma to a deep vein, resulting in exposure of the subendothelial collagen, is followed by adhesion of platelets to the injured site and damage to the platelets, with release of biologically active compounds, such as adenosine diphosphate and biphosphate, serotonin, and pyrophate. All of these substances, in turn, produce an increase in 'stickiness' of the platelets already deposited locally and hence growth of the aggregation until a thrombus develops.

It is necessary to point out, however, that injury to venous endothelium resulting from trauma is assumed to occur rather than being positively proved. For, by the time a histologic examination of the affected vessel is possible, it is rarely clear as to whether this type of abnormality preceded or followed the development of a clot.

Etiologic Factors. A number of different types of agents may be responsible for damage to the endothelium of deep veins. These consist of direct surgical trauma, endotoxins, antibody complexes, crush injuries, dislocations, fractures, and deep wounds in a lower limb producing bruising, contusion, or laceration of the vessel wall. Endothelial trauma may also result from prolonged pressure of the weight of the leg on the calf muscles, as during an operative procedure with the limb supported on a metal stirrup, or immediately postoperatively when the patient is content to lie on his back in bed without moving his limbs. Intermittent compression of a vein by a nearby bony projection will have a similar effect. Sitting in one position on long bus, train, or plane trips may lead to endothelial trauma in the leg veins due to protracted pressure of the edge of the seat against calf muscles. Direct malignant invasion of deep veins will cause injury to the intima, as well as involvement of the other layers of the venous wall. In pregnancy, trauma to pelvic veins during delivery may predispose to intravascular clotting. Contributary factors include physical inactivity and improper gait, among others.

Besides the above factors, physical effort or strain may also be responsible for endothelial damage to the deep veins of the leg. For example, lifting heavy objects, twising a knee, setting up exercises, squatting, running, landing on the feet after a fall, jumping, and climbing stairs may all be associated with such a change, especially in the nonathletic individual. Another mechanism which may be responsible for endothelial damage is muscular contraction in the limb. In most instances, with physical effort the large flat muscles of the leg and the quadriceps group of the thigh contract simultaneously, with the result that the deep veins of the calf are sharply compressed against the posterior surface of the tibia, this causing venous blood to be forcibly pumped into the collecting channels traversing Hunter's (adductor) canal (which is surrounded by relaxed muscular compartments). Violent or repeated muscular contractions when combined with the high venous pressure existing during physical exertion may exert a bursting force great enough to contuse the thin-walled veins or bruise their vasa vasorum.

Alterations in Coagulability of Blood

A number of states and disorders favor blood coagulation. Among the latter are such hematologic conditions as polycythemia vera and severe anemia. Marked dehydration, by producing a significant concentration of the blood, has a comparable effect to that existing in polycythemia vera. Neoplastic infiltrations, particularly those located in the head and tail of the pancreas, are also associated with changes in the blood that are conducive to intravascular clotting. Such a response may result from destruction of tissue by the tumor, followed by liberation into the blood stream of substances which raise the clotting tendency of the blood. Infectious diseases of bacterial origin, such as typhoid fever, rheumatic fever, and pneumonia, are also associated with changes in the blood which contribute to the formation of intravascular clotting. In the periods of gestation and puerperium, the increased incidence of venous thrombosis noted under such circumstances may be due to a number of factors, including changes in the coagulability of the blood.

Whether oral contraceptive drugs alter the coagulability of blood and thus predispose to venous thrombosis has not been definitely settled. Experimental studies have shown that antithrombin III activity, which normally constitutes a natural protective barrier against intravascular clotting, is reduced when contraceptive drugs are administered. Moreover, it has been found that women on such medications require a greater than usual dose of oral anticoagulants to maintain prothrombin activity at a therapeutic level. However, there is also evidence which supports the view that contraceptives do not affect coagulation mechanisms in a manner which facilitates intravascular clotting. Therefore, all that can be stated at present is that although these medications are not by themselves thrombogenic, they do aggravate the severity of a thrombotic stimulus and thereby enhance the possibility of the development of a venous thrombus.

Clinical Measures for Prevention of Venous Thrombosis

Ideally, the management of deep venous thrombosis is its prevention, particularly in people who are prone to this state: the elderly requiring complete bedrest for protracted periods; patients of any age undergoing a major surgical procedure; and individuals who have already suffered an episode of intravascular clotting and are therefore very prone to a second one. The goal of a prophylactic treatment program is to eliminate or minimize the influence of those factors which contribute to intravascular clotting, discussed on page 246. The same approach is also applicable to the prevention of pulmonary embolism.

Measures to Control Venous Stasis
A very important prophylactic step in the case of bedridden patients and in those who have been subjected to major surgery is to counteract pooling of blood in the deep venous system of the lower limbs inevitably present under such circumstances. This can be achieved through a number of different therapeutic means, as described below.

Physical Measures. For the bedridden geriatric patient, frequent planned and supervised exercises of the lower limbs, including active flexion and extension of the feet, legs, and thighs and movement of the feet against a bed board, are very useful in propelling blood out the deep venous tree; at the same time such steps help prevent deconditioning (p. 332). The program should be continued during the entire period of bed confinement in the hospital, generally under the supervision of a physical therapist. At home, a relative who has been instructed in the procedure can see to it that the patient carries out the same exercises properly.

In the case of the surgical patient, the lower limbs should be passively moved as soon as he has been returned to his bed and while he is still under the general anesthesia. The program consists of repeatedly dorsiflexing and plantar flexing the feet. Such an approach is not affected by any muscle relaxants given previously or by the depth of anesthesia.

All attempts should be made to facilitate venous return from the lower limbs. To be avoided in this regard are the Fowler's position and application of tight abdominal binders. Immediately on reaching a conscious state, the patient should be encouraged to take 12–15 deep breaths every hour during the day, since the associated movements of the diaphragm with respiration will move blood out of the lower limbs and into the inferior vena cava. This regimen is facilitated by restriction of sedatives, for otherwise, there may be some depression of respiration.

To remove the mild to moderate degree of vasospasm which generally accompanies a surgical procedure and persists during the early stage of the postoperative period, dry heat is applied to the lower limbs, provided the local arterial circulation is intact. If not, then indirect vasodilatation (p. 200) should be initiated by applying heating pads or short-wave diathermy to the abdomen or pelvic region posteriorly. As a result of either procedure, there will be an increase in local cutaneous arterial blood flow, followed by a similar response in the venous bed, thus facilitating venous return from the limb.

If the patient does not suffer from congestive heart failure, threshold cardiac function, or severe chronic obstructive lung disease, the lower limbs should be elevated approximately 15° by raising the foot of the bed about 18 cm (6 inches), at the same time preventing a hump in the mattress to develop at the level of the break in the bed. In the case of the surgical patient, if feasible, this measure should be instituted at the beginning of the operation and continued in the recovery room. Such a step has been found to be very effective in reducing the incidence of venous thrombosis, even in patients treated for fracture of the hip, a group in whom this complication is fairly common [3].

To prevent venous stasis in a lower limb held immobile in a rigid cast, the patient should be instructed to make a practice of attempting to contract the muscles in the involved extremity. Although he will not notice any obvious movement (isometric contraction), the tensing of the muscles locally will help the movement of blood and lymph out of the limb and thus relieve venous and lymph stasis. Besides this maneuver, the opposite normal limb should be exercised so as to maintain muscle tone reflexly in the extremity in the cast. At the same time, cardiac output will be increased as a result of the physical effort, and this should have the beneficial effect of greater perfusion of the involved limb.

Early ambulation appears to decrease the risk of deep venous thrombosis. At the same time, deconditioning (p. 332) is reduced in severity and recovery from this state is facilitated.

Elastic Compression of Limbs. Various types of elastic supports have been utilized to control venous stasis during bedrest, among the most common of which are elastic bandages and antiembolism elastic stockings. A serious objection to the latter is that in most hospitals, little attempt is made by nursing personnel to supply the patient with proper fitting ones. As a result, the stockings may apply too much pressure to some sites and too little to others, and consequently, control of venous stasis is not achieved. Moreover, the discomfort that develops from poorly fitting stockings may cause the patient to discard them, frequently without the hospital staff being aware of this, especially if there is no close nursing supervision of his activities. It would appear, therefore, that the use of standard stockings as a prophylactic procedure in the control of venous pooling is of very little value [5]. Of course, if stockings fabricated to the size of the patient's lower limbs are available, wearing such garments would be very helpful in this regard. However, this approach is generally not practicable since at least a week is required to manufacture properly fitting elastic stockings possessing a built-in gradient of pressure. A definite disadvantage of all types of elastic stockings when applied continuously on bedridden patients is that they predispose to heel ulcers and prevent proper care of the skin of the feet, both of which may cause serious complications if the individual is elderly and has some degree of arterial insufficiency of the lower limbs.

When elastic bandages are substituted in the case of the surgical patient, they should be placed around his lower limbs immediately after the operation, beginning with the foot and extending upward to the groin. In this manner, the superficial veins are maintained in a collapsed state and the blood is shunted into the deep venous system, with an acceleration of flow, and then out of the limb. However, there are also disadvantages to this procedure, one of which is the inability to apply the bandages so that they continuously exert the proper amount of tension on the skin and deeper tissues. To accomplish this correctly, the bandages have to be repeatedly rewrapped during the day, a measure which is generally not carried out by inadequate and busy nursing personnel. Moreover, there is no definite evidence to support the view that the application of elastic bandages prevents postoperative venous thrombosis.

Intermittent Calf Compression. Another means of controlling venous pooling in the lower limbs of surgical patients is to apply inflatable pressurized plastic boots to them before, during, and for some time after an operation. The apparatus is fitted over the foot and reaches up to the knee. It inflates for 12 s of each minute to an air pressure of 40 mm Hg, supplied by a pneumatic pump. Whether the boot is effective in reducing postoperative venous thrombosis and pulmonary embolism has not definitely been determined. It is contraindicated for the limb with a severely impaired local arterial circulation.

A modification of the pressurized boot consists of pneumatic leg sleeves or leggings connected to a power source that uses compressed gases and ambient air at a pressure up to 45 mm Hg. With it both calves and thighs are sequentially squeezed every 2 min. It has the advantage of increasing pulsatility of venous outflow rather than mean blood flow.

Electric Stimulation of Calf Muscles. This procedure is useful primarily during the operation when venous thrombosis may have its inception. It consists of applying a galvanic current to the calf muscles to produce intermittent contraction, reversal of polarity being carried out with each pulse to prevent tissue ionization. Two electrodes, enclosed in pads soaked in saline, are applied to the back of each leg, one at the ankle and the other at the knee. The voltage is adjusted to produce brisk calf-muscle contraction throughout the operation. Once the patient has regained consciousness, the procedure is terminated, since now the electric stimulation may produce discomfort.

Measures to Reduce or Eliminate Damage to Venous Endothelium

In the course of an operative procedure on the lower limbs, care must be taken to prevent damage to vascular elements, particularly deep veins, that are in the surgical field. Also important is to protect the venous tree from forced stretching and manipulation. Knee crutches and leg holders should be well padded and restraining straps should not be too tight. If a cast is to be applied, minimal pressure should be used in the vicinity of main collecting veins.

General Principles in Reducing Blood Coagulability

Precautions during Operative Procedure. Care to minimize trauma to neighboring nonvascular structures is also important, for destruction of tissues may cause changes in blood plasma which contribute to intravascular clotting. Since dehydration results in increased viscosity of the blood, this state should be prevented by intravenous infusion of 5% glucose solution or isotonic saline solution.

Low-Dose Heparin Administration. Currently this prophylactic program is having extensive clinical trial. Small doses of heparin are injected subcutaneously on the following schedule: 5,000 U 2 h before operation and 5,000 U every 12 h for 7 days thereafter or until the patient is fully ambulatory. Another regimen consists of 5,000 U subcutaneously every 8 h postoperatively. Although more effective, in preventing venous thrombosis than the one utilizing longerspaced intervals, this program is also associated with bleeding episodes, a response rarely noted with the use of less frequent doses.

Although the amounts of heparin utilized are too small to have a direct antithrombin action, still the procedure has a definite effect on reducing venous thrombosis. The rationale for its use is based on the fact that small doses of heparin help prevent platelet aggregation and act to form a complex with a naturally occurring plasma inhibitor (antithrombin III; antifactor X^2; heparin cofactor), the resultant product greatly enhancing the ability of antithrombin III to inactivate factors IX^a, X^a, XI^a, and thrombin. As a consequence, the conversion of prothrombin to thrombin is inhibited. At the same time, the small doses of heparin generally do not seriously impair normal hemostasis.

Prophylactic Oral Anticoagulant Therapy. The use of warfarin sodium (Coumadin) and dicumarol as prophylactic agents has never been given extensive clinical trial, primarily because of the possibility of bleeding into the surgical site during and after the operation. However, there is some experimental evidence indicating that the derived benefits, in the form of a significant reduction in postoperative thromboembolism, more than compensates for the possible development of local hemorrhage.

Dextran Therapy. The use of the glucose polymer, dextran, as a prophylactic agent against intravascular clotting has been advocated, especially in the case of patients who are unable to take heparin or oral anticoagulants because of associated bleeding tendencies. The therapeutic effect is due to the fact that the drug inhibits vascular stasis and platelet adhesiveness without blocking fibrinogen-fibrin conversion (as occurs with anticoagulants). The dextrans also expand plasma volume and decrease blood viscosity, enhance the microcirculation, and coat erythrocytes and endothelial walls, all desirable responses in the attack on thromboembolism.

The medication, in the form of 10% dextran 40 (Rheomacrodex; low molecular weight dextran), is given as follows: 200–500 ml in either normal saline solution or 5% glucose during the operation; 500 ml in the next 6–8 h; 500 ml daily for the first 3 days postoperatively, and 500 ml every other day thereafter until the patient becomes fully ambulatory.

Certain complications may follow administration of low molecular weight dextrans. Among these are anaphylactic reactions, hypotension, and pulmonary edema (in patients with reduced cardiac reserve). When administered to individuals with reduced kidney function, the medications may precipitate renal failure.

Discontinuation of Contraceptive Medication. In patients with a hereditary predisposition to intravascular clotting or who give a history of venous or arterial thrombosis, contraceptive drugs are contraindicated since they may raise the incidence of these difficulties if given to such a group of individuals. Such medications should also be discontinued if catheterization of veins, angiography, or elective surgery is contemplated. As a general rule, abstinence from smoking should be followed by the patient on contraceptives, for it has been shown that when this habit is continued while the individual is on such drugs, there is an increase in the indicence of death from thromboembolism [1].

Other Medical Approaches. In recent years it has been shown that aspirin inhibits the liberation of adenosine diphosphate from platelets, thus preventing platelet aggregation and adherence to sites of damaged endothelium. Because of such a property, the drug is being given extensive clinical trials as a means of combatting venous thrombosis in patients who are potential candidates for this state. Of interest is the clinical finding that in the case of total hip replacement, aspirin has the desired therapeutic effect only in male patients [2].

Another antiplatelet drug, dipyridamole (Persantin), has also been studied for its prophylactic effect in thromboembolism. When it is given in conjunction with 1 g of aspirin daily, less of the drug is necessary to achieve the desired effect. As a result, the maintenance dose can be reduced from 400 to 100 mg daily [4]. Sulfinpyrazone (Anturane) has likewise been used as an antiplatelet drug on the basis that it may be a competitive inhibitor of cyclooxygenase in platelets, thus preventing synthesis of prostaglandin endoperoxides and thromboxane A_2.

References

1   Frederiksen, H.; Ravenholt, R.T.: Thromboembolism, oral contraceptives, and cigarettes. Publ. Hlth Rep. *85:* 197 (1970).

2   Harris, W.H.; Salzman, E.W.; Athanasoulis, C.A.; et al.: Aspirin prophylaxis of venous thromboembolism after total hip replacement. New Engl. J. Med. *297:* 1246 (1977).

3   Hartman, J.T.; Altner, P.C.; Freeark, R.J.: The effect of limb elevation in preventing venous thrombosis. J. Bone Jt Surg. *52A:* 1618 (1970).

4   Renney, T.J.G.; O'Sullivan, E.F.; Burke, P.F.: Prevention of postoperative deep vein thrombosis with dipyridamole and aspirin. Br. med. J. *i:* 992 (1976).

5   Rosengarten, D.S.; Laird, J.; Jeyasingh, K.; et al.: The failure of compression stockings (Tubigrip) to prevent deep venous thrombosis after operation. Br. J. Surg. *57:* 296 (1970).

6   Wessler, S.: The role of stasis in thrombosis; in Sherry, Brinkhous, Genton, Stengle, Thrombosis, p. 461 (National Academy of Sciences, Washington 1969).

14 Venous Thrombosis and Pulmonary Embolism and Infarction

Deep Venous Thrombosis in Lower Limbs

Because of its close association with pulmonary embolism and infarction (p. 269), deep venous thrombosis or thrombophlebitis of the lower limbs may entirely alter prognosis when it develops during the course of a relatively benign illness or a minor operative procedure. Even if the condition is not followed by liberation of emboli into the venous circulation, it may still considerably prolong the convalescent period of the original illness or operative procedure. Moreover, it may be responsible for the development of the postphlebitic syndrome (see chapter 15), a disorder which is frequently disabling because of the high incidence of stasis dermatitis and stasis ulceration of the lower limbs found in this condition.

Types

On the basis of significant differences in clinical manifestations, deep venous thrombophlebitis of the lower limbs has been arbitrarily divided into two categories: *phlebothrombosis,* in which there is a partial or complete obstruction by a thrombus or thrombi of deep venous plexuses in the muscles of the calf (fig. 14/1a), and *popliteal* or *iliofemoral thrombophlebitis,* in which there is a total occlusion by a thrombus of the popliteal or iliofemoral vein (fig. 14/1b), respectively. Although such a classification does not have universal acceptance, there are certain advantages to its adoption, since it permits more accurate localization of the thrombus in the venous tree and the development of more appropriate treatment programs in each instance. However, it must be recognized that the pathologic process is the same in both conditions, but merely located in different portions of the deep venous system. Moreover, propagation of a thrombus initially located in the deep venous plexuses in the calf (and responsible for the appearance of the clinical signs of phlebothrombosis) may eventually result in total occlusion of the popliteal or iliofemoral vein (and in the development of the clinical picture of popliteal or iliofemoral thrombophlebitis). On the other hand, the primary initial site may have been a segment of

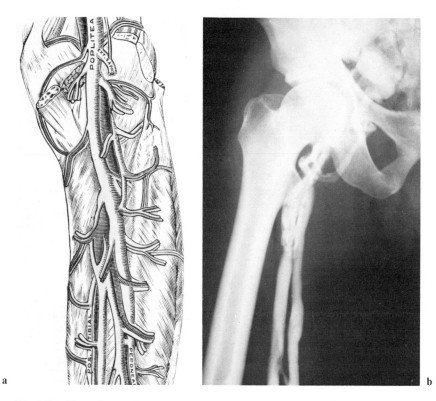

a   b

Fig. 14/1. Sites of occlusion of deep venous system in the lower limbs. **a** Diagrammatic representation of the deep venous plexus draining blood from the muscles into the venae comites of the posterior tibial and peroneal arteries. These plexuses are potential sites for phlebothrombosis. **b** Contrast venogram demonstrating complete occlusion of the iliofemoral vein (iliofemoral thrombophlebitis). Reproduced from ref. [3] with permission.

either of the two collecting veins, due to some local pathologic change, without any previous involvement of the deep venous plexuses in the calf. (For a discussion of the various factors responsible for intravenous clotting, see p. 246.)

Manifestations of Phlebothrombosis

Symptoms and Signs. The clinical picture of phlebothrombosis may be ambiguous, meager, and nonspecific and, as a result, when such a diagnosis is made, it is frequently considered provisional. In fact, the condition may be overlooked and only identified in retrospect, after a pulmonary embolism has developed and is clinically apparent (p. 265). The reason for such difficulty in accurately interpreting the clinical findings is because initially the thrombus is located in venous plexuses of small caliber in the muscles of the calf and hence there is little, if any, interference with venous return from the limb. As a consequence, no significant rise occurs in local venous pressure, so that the clinical changes, which are primarily a reflection of the degree of existing venous hypertension, are minimal or even absent.

The symptoms and signs generally found in phlebothrombosis are as follows: aching or a cramp-like pain in the calf and occasionally in the foot, experienced at rest and exaggerated by walking; pain in the calf on dorsiflexing the foot (positive Homans' sign); tense or spastic muscles due to the local inflammatory process; slight enlargement of the circumference of the upper segment of leg, frequently discernible only after careful measurement; an indefinite mass between the bellies of the gastrocnemius muscle; a slight rise in cutaneous temperature in the vicinity of the calf as determined clinically; some duskiness of the skin of the limb when placed in dependency; and nonspecific systemic signs (minor rises in body temperature, heart rate, and respiration). There may also be a general sense of apprehension, restlessness, a feeling of impending disaster, or an ill-defined sensation of something being wrong.

Of further importance with regard to differential diagnosis are the absence of edema of the foot and the lower part of the leg and a normal venous pressure in the superficial vessels on the dorsum of the foot as determined by their collapse on elevation of the limb. Such findings are in contrast to the signs invariably noted when the thrombus is in a main collecting channel, such as the popliteal or iliofemoral vein (p. 260).

Laboratory Aids. Because of the generally minimal and nonspecific symptoms and signs in phlebothrombosis, it is frequently necessary to rely heavily upon the results of laboratory testing. Of the various procedures available for this purpose, contrast venography is the most dependable (fig. 14/2). Radioactive fibrinogen test is also very helpful, provided the thrombus is not in a very early or a rather late stage of development. Radionuclide venography is useful, but the data are not as definitive as the results obtained with contrast venography. Recently, thermographic techniques have been used with reported good diagnostic results [5, 18]. It is necessary to call attention to the fact that impedance plethysmography, Doppler ultrasonic flowmeter, and strain-gauge plethysmography contrib-

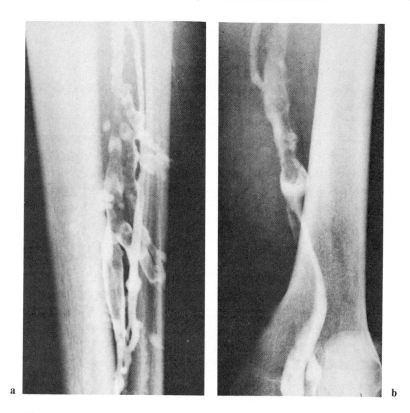

Fig. 14/2. Changes in the venogram due to thrombi in the deep venous tree of the lower limb. **a** Thrombi in the tibial veins seen as filling defects in an otherwise well-opacified vessel in two successive films, without any alteration in shape and location. **b** Partially occluding thrombi in the popliteal and superficial femoral veins, seen as well-defined translucent areas surrounded by a rim of contrast medium. Reproduced from ref. [11] with permission (Butterworth & Co., Surrey, England).

ute little of significance in the diagnosis of thrombi located below the knee in the deep venous plexuses. (For a description of all of these techniques, except thermography, see pp. 221–229.)

Differential Diagnosis. There are a number of conditions in which symptoms and signs are located in the vicinity of the calf and hence they must be distinguished from phlebothrombosis. Among these are a ruptured popliteal (Baker's) cyst, tennis leg (p. 10), muscle strain due to a hematoma, and muscle hernia (myocele) [21]. Other entities which may mimic the condition are sudden occlusion of the popliteal artery at its bifurcation, a superficial thrombophlebitis (p. 235) located subcutaneously in the vicinity of the calf, dermatitis or acute cellulitis in the same site, myositis of calf muscles, and rupture of the plantaris tendon.

Manifestations of Popliteal and Iliofemoral Thrombophlebitis

Because a main collecting vein is occluded in popliteal or iliofemoral thrombophlebitis, there is marked interference with venous outflow from the limb, followed by a very significant rise in venous pressure (venous hypertension). As a consequence, the local changes are very evident, in contradistinction to those present in phlebothrombosis (p. 257). Accordingly, the diagnosis is readily made on the basis of the clinical manifestations.

Symptoms and Signs of Nonsuppurative Thrombophlebitis of a Main Collecting Vein. The clinical picture of uncomplicated iliofemoral or popliteal thrombophlebitis consists of the following: the sudden appearance of variable amounts of pitting edema of a lower limb, generally developing in the course of 8–10 h (fig. 14/3a); pain along the course of the involved vessel; distention of the superficial veins on the foot and leg, partially masked by the swelling; signs of arterial vasospasm (coldness and cyanosis or pallor of the skin of the limb); and systemic responses – fever up to 38.9°C (102°F), tachycardia, an increase in white blood count and sedimentation rate, malaise, loss of appetite, and chilly sensation. The findings in popliteal thrombophlebitis and in iliofemoral thrombophlebitis are similar except for the following: In the case of the former, the swelling extends from the dorsum of the foot to the level of the knee and the pain is located primarily in the popliteal space and below, whereas in iliofemoral thrombophlebitis, the edema is found as high as the groin (fig. 14/3b) and the complaints are experienced in this area and on the inner aspect of the thigh, along the course of the superficial femoral vein. (For a discussion of the pathogenesis of the edema of iliofemoral and popliteal thrombophlebitis, see p. 239.)

Symptoms and Signs of Phlegmasia Cerulea Dolens. In some instances of iliofemoral thrombophlebitis, there is extensive thrombosis not only of the iliofemoral vein but also of the tributaries entering the involved vessel proximal and distal to the occluded segment. Such a state is responsible for

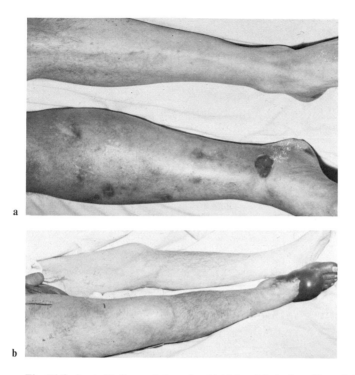

Fig. 14/3. Acute iliofemoral thrombophlebitis. **a** Marked swelling of right lower limb, with some superficial ulceration. **b** Phlegmasia cerulea dolens of the right lower limb with bullae and venous gangrene of the foot. Reproduced from ref. [1] with permission.

severe circulatory disturbances in the affected limb, with the local venous pressure rising to a level which may actually interfere with arteriolar inflow. As a consequence, the skin of the entire extremity assumes a deeply violaceous or cyanotic hue, with purpuric areas or petechial lesions scattered over the limb. Because of the significant interference with venous outflow, edema of the extremity is generally marked, associated with the appearance of cutaneous blebs or bullae filled with serum or blood (fig. 14/3b). The peripheral pulses are usually found to be reduced or even absent. At times there may be actual gangrene of the distal portion of the limb (venous gangrene) (fig. 14/3b) which may even require an amputation. Excruciating pain in the limb is a common complaint. This clinical entity is termed phlegmasis cerulea (purple) dolens, as compared with the usual type of iliofemoral thrombophlebitis, phlegmasia alba (white) dolens, in which the skin of the involved limb is generally pale. The release of serotonin (a vasoconstrictor agent) through the breakdown of platelets has been implicated as an etiologic factor in phlegmasia cerulea dolens [4].

Symptoms and Signs of Suppurative Iliofemoral Thrombophlebitis. Although in the great majority of cases of iliofemoral thrombophlebitis bacterial invasion plays no role, in the occasional patient, a suppurative process exists [17]. The cause of such a very serious condition is generally some type of pelvic manipulation (intrauterine insertion of radium), post-abortal or postpartum infection, a difficult delivery, or a pelvic abscess. As a consequence of one of these etiologic agents, a thrombus develops in a pelvic or iliofemoral vein which is infected, resulting in liquefaction of the clot and liberation of emboli containing the bacterial agent. These then lodge in the pulmonary vascular bed to form multiple abscesses.

The clinical manifestations of suppurative iliofemoral thrombophlebitis consist first of a marked systemic response in the form of high, spiking, relapsing fever, associated with chills and other signs of a serious blood-borne infection, including tachycardia and a rapid respiratory rate. In the lungs are found physical signs of abscess formation. The changes in the involved lower limb are similar to those described for the nonsuppurative type of iliofemoral thrombophlebitis (p. 260).

Laboratory Findings. Because of the dramatic clinical manifestations generally observed with iliofemoral or popliteal thrombophlebitis, rarely are laboratory procedures necessary to confirm the diagnosis. In the occasional case, if there is some question, then contrast venography can be employed, since this test readily identifies the site of block in the main collecting venous channel. Also useful in this regard, but less definitive in localizing the lesion, are transcutaneous Doppler ultrasonic flowmeter, strain-gauge plethysmography, impedance rheography, and radionuclide venography. All of these procedures are described on pp. 222–229.

Differential Diagnosis. Popliteal thrombophlebitis may have to be differentiated from acute cellulitis of the leg because of the local swelling and systemic responses found in the latter. Not infrequently, thrombosis of a collecting vein is associated with superimposed vasospasm, and for this reason, the clinical picture may demonstrate some findings in common with post-traumatic painful vascular disorders (pp. 326, 329). There should be no difficulty differentiating popliteal and iliofemoral thrombo-phlebitis from superficial benign thrombophlebitis (p. 235) and from the postphlebitic syndrome (p. 287).

Pulmonary Embolism and Infarction

Incidence

Although great strides have been made in the diagnosis and treatment of pulmonary embolism, this condition still continues to be a major and potentially fatal complication of a great number of states and disorders, some even of minor importance by themselves. Hence, it is necessary at all times to be alert to the development of such a possibility so as to be able to identify its presence early in its inception and institute proper therapeutic measures. Such vigilance is particularly important in the case of elderly patients, especially when injured, all types of individuals undergoing pod-iatric or orthopedic elective surgical procedures, and those people suffering from cardiac difficulties or malignant neoplasm. For example, it has been estimated that more than a third of the patients with cerebrovascular acci-dents, almost a third of general surgery cases, and more than a third of those with acute myocardial infarction are potential candidates for pulmonary embolism. The incidence of this condition is also relatively high in patients who have sustained fracture of the pelvis, spine, femur, and tibia [22] and extensive body burns [6]. As a consequence of all these factors, pulmonary embolism has become one of the most frequent problems encountered in an adult hospital population, unfortunately, often misdiagnosed and hence mistreated.

Source of Emboli

As already implied, many of the emboli which lodge in the pulmonary vascular bed originate as thrombi in the deep venous plexuses in the calves of the legs and in the small muscles of the feet. The early process in the venous tree becomes clinically important only when the clots propagate into the vena comites of the anterior and posterior tibial arteries and finally into the popliteal and superficial femoral veins but not necessarily occlud-ing the latter vessels. Other sites from which emboli arise are the common femoral, pelvic, and prostatic veins, and occasionally the axillary and sub-clavian veins, as well as the right atrium and right ventricle.

Dislodgment of the clots from any of the above locations results in their liberation into the systemic venous system, passage to the pulmonary arterial system, and occlusion of vessels in this vascular bed which have a smaller diameter than the thrombi themselves.

Pathogenesis

Since the pulmonary arterial system is located at the termination of the venous circulation, it acts as a filter for particulate matter circulating in the blood stream. There is a very good possibility that during a normal lifetime, small clots develop repeatedly which, however, produce no clinical signs of their presence since they are immediately dissolved by the efficient fibrinolytic system of the lungs. Only when thrombi obstruct one or two large vessels or a great number of smaller ones are they recognized in the form of clinical manifestations of pulmonary embolism. Even then, in many instances, underlying compromised pulmonary and bronchial circulations must coexist in order to be able to recognize the difficulty clinically. The explanation for such a situation lies in the fact that an efficient vascular mechanism and a reserve are found in the normal pulmonary circulation, particularly in the form of ready distensibility of the small vessels and the presence of large number of bronchial-pulmonary arterial anastomoses. Although not functioning under ordinary circumstances, when the need arises, the latter structures can permit blood to pass from gradually enlarging bronchial arteries into the pulmonary vascular bed. Opposed to such compensatory mechanisms, however, is reflex vasoconstriction of unaffected pulmonary arteries, which commonly develops when a thrombus occludes even small vessels. Because of this possibility, minor pulmonary artery obstruction may be responsible for a patient's death if the superimposed vasospasm is extensive and severe in the pulmonary vascular bed.

Pathology

The degree of the anatomic changes in the lungs following pulmonary embolism depends upon the size of the vessel or vessels occluded and upon the state and efficiency of the bronchial vascular tree. In the case of involvement of the main pulmonary artery or its principal branches, the marked alterations in hemodynamics that follow may be of such magnitude as to cause immediate death, without time for the development of pulmonary infarction. The latter pathologic change may also be absent when showers of minute emboli are released into the venous circulation, the result being occlusion of terminal pulmonary vessels, associated with very few significant anatomic alterations in the lung parenchyma. Even in the presence of obstruction of major arteries, pulmonary infarction is noted in only about 10% of cases [24, 25]. When the condition occurs, there is generally occlusion of the smaller muscular branches, particulary in sites where two or more pleural surfaces are in contact. Also of significance in the production of pulmonary infarction is the previous existence of some pathologic changes in lung parenchyma and bronchial blood supply, resulting in a high bronchial venous pressure.

Pulmonary infarcts may vary in size from 0.3 to 10.0 cm in diameter. They may be single but usually are multiple, most of them being located in the lower lobes. In the early stage, histologic examination of involved lung parenchyma demonstrates marked congestion of the capillary bed, with the alveolar spaces being filled with red blood cells and debris. Within about 3 days, the alveolar wall becomes necrotic and there are signs of red blood cell breakdown. Organization of the affected area begins within the second week following pulmonary infarction. However, in the presence of minimal involvement, the process may be completed by resolution within several days.

Clinical Manifestations of Pulmonary Embolism
General Considerations. The diagnosis of pulmonary embolism is frequently difficult to make with certainty because the clinical symptoms and signs are usually not specific enough. As already alluded to, this is due to the great reserve capacity that normal lung possesses. In fact, in the presence of obstruction of less than half of the pulmonary bed, the clinical manifestations may still be minimal provided the vascular tree, particularly the bronchial arterial system, was not previously compromised. With occlusion of large pulmonary arterial branches or of numerous small ones, causing greater interference with pulmonary blood flow and oxygenation of blood, symptoms and signs will develop. Contributing significantly to the paucity of clinical manifestations frequently observed is the efficient fibrinolytic system in the lungs which is able to lyse small pulmonary emboli and thus reestablish local circulation. For all these reasons, it is possible for pulmonary embolism to go unrecognized when the diagnostic study is based solely on clinical manifestations. Hence, in many instances, heavy reliance on laboratory aids is necessary for its detection (p. 267).

Nonmassive Pulmonary Embolism. Initial signs when moderately large pulmonary arteries are suddenly obstructed are dyspnea (in the great majority of cases), tachypnea, a dry nonproductive cough, and rales at the base of the lungs. Less commonly observed are pleural pain (in about half the cases), sweating, tachycardia, apprehension, dizziness, and syncope. Hemoptysis, which was previously considered to be a prominent finding, is actually noted in about a quarter or less of the patients. Audible wheezing may be heard over the affected site due to the associated bronchospasm. The systemic responses consist of a low-grade fever, leukocytosis, and an increase in sedimentation rate.

Massive Pulmonary Embolism. Occlusion of a main branch of the pulmonary artery or of this vessel itself causes a dramatic clinical picture. Although initially the findings may be minimal, they soon become very marked, with the patient manifesting anxious facies and apprehension of a severe degree and demonstrating labored breathing and air hunger, associated with severe substernal pain, tachycardia, a rapidly falling blood pressure to a shock level, and the appearance of pulmonary edema. Two auscultatory signs which have been considered almost pathognomonic for pulmonary embolism are a wide, fixed split second heart sound and an acquired nonprecordial peripheral pulmonary murmur [19].

Unless the condition can immediately be managed medically or surgically, it usually leads to the death of the patient. If this does not occur, then the early symptoms or signs gradually disappear, with hemoptysis generally developing in about 20% of the cases and persisting for 2 or 3 weeks. There may be signs of right heart failure, such as epigastric discomfort due to liver enlargement and distention of jugular veins in the neck.

Pulmonary Infarction. When this condition appears, due to insufficient local blood supply to alveolar tissue, the manifestations consist of knifelike pleuritic chest pain, splinting of the chest in an attempt to minimize the symptom, restriction of breathing, and hemoptysis.

Multiple Small Pulmonary Emboli. The identification of this condition, which may recur repeatedly over months and years, is very difficult. Because clear-cut symptoms and signs of pulmonary embolism are rarely apparent, the disorder may go unrecognized until right ventricular overload and pulmonary hypertension intervene, thus calling attention to such a possibility.

Diagnostic Laboratory Aids

Since pulmonary embolism may mimic a number of other conditions (p. 272) and since the clinical manifestations may in some instances not be definite enough on which to base the diagnosis (p. 265), it is frequently necessary to resort to diagnostic laboratory procedures in order to obtain confirmatory evidence of its presence. Some of the tests routinely used for this purpose are briefly evaluated below.

Chest Roentgenography. This approach is helpful but not necessarily diagnostic in pulmonary embolism. In fact, at times the X-ray may be normal, or radiolucency rather than opacity may be noted in the presence of an occlusion of a branch of the pulmonary artery. Of importance is the absence of vascular markings in the area of involvement, an abnormality which, unfortunately, is only infrequently encountered. If pulmonary infarction exists, the involved site may be identified by the presence of a truncated cone whose base is located on a pleural surface.

Electrocardiography. This procedure rarely supplies pertinent information on which a diagnosis of pulmonary embolism can be made. Actually, at times the record may be normal, or there may be nonspecific changes and a tachycardia. In the presence of extensive involvement of the pulmonary circulation, changes suggesting the presence of right heart strain may appear.

Radioisotopic Pulmonary Perfusion Scanning. The lung scan is a widely used and sensitive method for the identification of pulmonary embolism (fig. 14/4). Rarely, if ever, is it negative when the condition exists, a well-performed normal perfusion scan therefore virtually eliminating the diagnosis of clinically significant pulmonary embolism [13]. In this regard, however, it is necessary to point out that small emboli could be present without producing any change on the lung scan because they would not be large enough to cause a perfusion defect. Fortunately, such a situation usually also presents no major clinical problems.

False-positive lung scans can result from a number of other conditions besides pulmonary embolism, notably chronic obstructive pulmonary disorders, since avascular areas (as represented by sites of absent perfusion) may be present in both types of conditions. Hence, differentiation must be made between them by resorting either to simultaneous lung scanning and ventilation scanning (p. 270) or to repeated lung scanning alone at intervals of a week (p. 270).

Lung scanning gives information regarding the state of terminal arteries, arterioles, and capillaries of the pulmonary vascular bed. The technique provides no direct data on the exact location of an embolus in the arterial tree, information which can only be obtained from pulmonary angiography (p. 271).

Lung scanning is carried out by injecting macroaggregated human albumin particles (10–15 μm in diameter), tagged with either ^{131}I or ^{99m}Tc, into a peripheral vein and using an external scintillation counter applied immediately after administration. The rationale for the test is that the radioactive particulate matter is temporarily trapped in the pulmonary capillary bed, thus reflecting the distribution in the pulmonary parenchyma of blood coming from the right side of the heart. The resulting perfusion pattern, detected with the external scintillation counter, is recorded (fig. 14/4). The procedure is completed within about 15 min, and after approximately 90–120 min, the particles of albumin in the lungs are broken down to molecules capable of passing through the pulmonary capillary bed into the systemic circulation and then metabolized by the reticuloendothelial system in the liver and spleen, as well as elsewhere. The previously attached isotope is excreted by the kidneys. If ^{131}I has been used, the thyroid gland must be protected by a preliminary dose of iodides, for otherwise the material will accumulate in this site and cause damage to the glandular tissue.

In areas of involvement, the interference with blood flow in the lung parenchyma will manifest itself as regions in which there is no accumulation of radioactive material on the scan (areas of absent perfusion)

Fig. 14/4. Lung scans. A Perfusion patterns in normal subjects. 1 = Anterior view. Area of reduced perfusion in lower portion of lung field is normally noted due to compression by the heart. 2 = Posterior view. 3 = Right lateral view. 4 = Left lateral view. B Patient with multiple pulmonary emboli. 1 = Anterior view. Areas of reduced perfusion noted in right lung, upper portion, and in left lung, upper portion. 2 = Posterior view. Areas of reduced or absent perfusion present in both lungs. 3 = Right lateral view. Areas of absent or reduced perfusion noted along posterior border. C Lung scan performed 2 weeks later on same patient as in B. 1 = Anterior view. Area of reduced perfusion in right lung is no longer present. 2 = Posterior view. Areas of reduced perfusion in both lungs have disappeared. 3 = Right lateral view. Area of reduced perfusion along posterior border is no longer present. 4 = Left lateral view. Area of reduced perfusion along posterior border has disappeared. In each instance in B, areas of involvement are indicated by arrows. Reproduced from ref. [2] with permission.

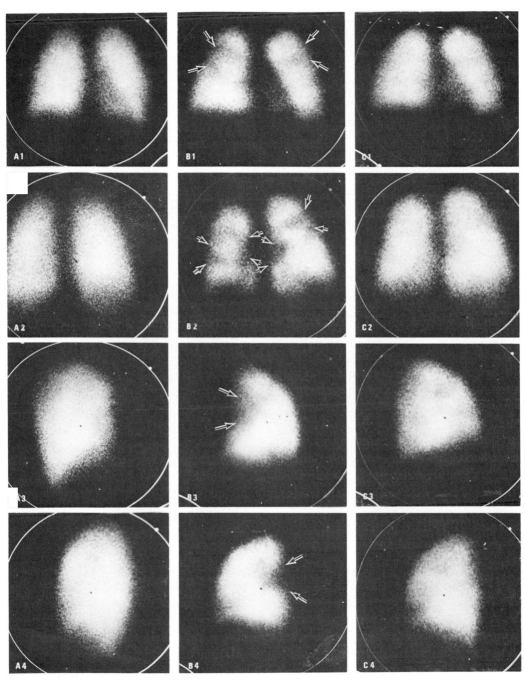

(fig. 14/4B). The abnormal changes are generally located along the lateral and basal portions of the lung fields, appearing as crescent-shaped defects (fig. 14/4B).

The test has the advantage of being safe to carry out and hence can be frequently repeated. Hence, it is possible to distinguish a perfusion defect produced by pulmonary embolism from one resulting from chronic lung disease, since in the case of the former, dramatic reductions in the size of the areas of decreased or absent perfusion or even the development of a normal pattern can be expected in a matter of a week or so (fig. 14/4C). On the other hand, in the presence of emphysema, chronic bronchitis, pneumothorax, asthma, atelectasis, and lung tumors, the areas of reduced perfusion due to such conditions will remain unchanged in this short period of time.

Lung Ventilation Scanning. This procedure, unfortunately available in very few hospitals, is very helpful in differentiating lung perfusion scanning defects caused by pulmonary embolism from those produced by chronic types of lung disease. It consists of the inhalation of a radioactive gas (xenon-133 or xenon-127), introduced through a closed system. An area of reduced or absent perfusion on the lung scan due to pulmonary embolism generally shows a normal response to the ventilation scan, whereas in the case of chronic lung pathology, results of both tests correlate with each other to identify an abnormal response in the same portion of pulmonary tissue. If a pulmonary infiltrate is being considered in the differential diagnosis of pulmonary embolism, the gallium-67 lung scan is very helpful in the elucidation of the problem. This substance concentrates in areas of an inflammatory process but not in sites of pulmonary embolization. Another approach is to use isoproterenol, since this drug reverses the vasoconstriction that causes the perfusion defect in the lung scan in the case of pneumonitis but has no effect on the changes produced by pulmonary embolism.

Arterial Oxygen Tension. It frequently is necessary to determine the oxygen tension of the arterial blood, since a reading below 80 mm Hg (normal range of 90–120 mm Hg) is a common finding in pulmonary embolism. The hypoxemia results from the interference with oxygenation of the blood in the pulmonary alveolar spaces. However, a reduced reading is not necessarily diagnostic for pulmonary embolism since it may also exist in a large number of other conditions in which the same abnormal situation is present in the pulmonary bed. Another point to consider is that normal oxygen tension may still be found in patients with occlusion of moderate-sized pulmonary arteries. In the presence of extensive involvement of the pulmonary bed, of course, PO_2 values are invariably depressed, associated with a similar change in PCO_2 (to below 40 mm Hg) due to hyperventilation that is frequently present in pulmonary embolism. Such changes may persist for about a week after the onset of the clinical manifestations despite appropriate treatment. It would appear, therefore, that alterations in arterial blood gas levels cannot be considered as highly sensitive or specific for the diagnosis of pulmonary embolism.

Enzymes. In the presence of pulmonary infarction, changes may be found in the levels of enzymes in the blood. In the uncomplicated case of pulmonary embolism, serum lactic dehydrogenase (LDH) activity is generally increased, whereas serum glutamic oxaloacetic transaminase (SGOT) remains unchanged. In about half the cases, there may be a rise in serum bilirubin during the first few days of pulmonary embolism. The triad of increased LDH, normal SGOT, and elevated serum bilirubin as diagnostic for pulmonary embolism was given considerable weight at one time in identifying the presence of this condition. However, it has fallen into disrepute because of a demonstrated lack of sensitivity and specificity.

Pulmonary Angiography. This procedure is a precise method for diagnosing pulmonary embolism. However, it is used in relatively few centers because it is an expensive invasive test requiring specialized equipment and personnel; moreover, it may be associated with serious complications (to the extent of 4–5% of cases), such as pulmonary artery rupture.

The conventional technique consists of catheterizing an antecubital vein after a cut-down and, under fluoroscopic control, passing the catheter up into the right ventricle; then the contrast material is injected, followed by exposure of films at appropriate intervals. Modifications of the method involve the use of a percutaneous injection of radiopaque material into a peripheral vein and insertion of a catheter into the femoral vein.

Recently, the data obtained with intravenous digital subtraction pulmonary angiography have been compared with those derived from contrast pulmonary angiography and the conclusion was reached that the former technique could be substituted for routine pulmonary angiography in most patients without loss of pertinent information [20]. Intravenous digital subtraction pulmonary angiography has the advantages of being less expensive, safer, faster, and easier to perform than conventional pulmonary angiography. However, there are some common technical and clinical problems which prevent adequate diagnostic studies with the procedure, such as transmitted cardiac motion, low cardiac output, respiratory motion, and a combination of these three factors.

Pulmonary angiography gives accurate information of the site of location of the occluded vessel or vessels in the pulmonary vascular tree (fig. 14/5). The lesion is identified either by an intraluminal filling defect in the pulmonary artery or its branches, an abrupt cutoff of the radiopaque stream, or absence of visualized vessels in a segment of the lung field (fig. 14/5).

The procedure is essential as a preliminary to pulmonary embolectomy, since it precisely identifies the presence, site, and extent of the lesion, information essential for the surgical removal of the thrombus. It has also been used when the clinical evidence for a pulmonary embolism is clearcut, but the perfusion scan is interpreted as normal, or a definite differential diagnosis from chronic lung disease cannot be made.

However, pulmonary angiography is not to be used as a diagnostic procedure in the great majority of cases of pulmonary embolism, for less invasive methods (see above) are available for this purpose. Besides the possibility of adverse reactions, the technique is difficult to perform properly and it is associated with a definite element of risk to the patient. In the presence of multiple small emboli or microemboli, the test may give a false-negative result since it does not visualize the smaller vessels in the pulmonary bed, information on this score being derived through pulmonary perfusion scanning (p. 267).

Differential Diagnosis of Pulmonary Embolism

As already emphasized, the clinical manifestations of pulmonary embolism are often nondiagnostic because they may mimic those observed in a large number of other disorders. Some of the more important of these are discussed below.

Myocardial Infarction. Since symptoms in this condition are generally located in the chest, they may be confused with the pleuritic pain found in massive pulmonary embolism and in pulmonary infarction. However, the evolution of the ST segment and T wave changes in the electrocardiogram typical for myocardial infarction is not seen in pulmonary embolism. Moreover, the enzyme studies are helpful as a differential point. In myocardial

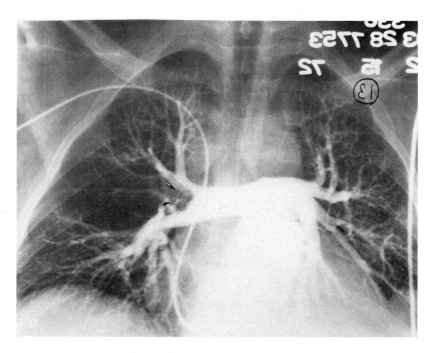

Fig. 14/5. Pulmonary angiography demonstrating an occlusion of a main branch of the right pulmonary artery by an embolus. Film shows normal extensive vascularization of the left lung field and only a few visualized vessels in the midportion of the right lung field. There is a partial filling defect in the right branch of the pulmonary artery (as indicated by arrows) which is the location of the embolus. Reproduced from ref. [2] with permission.

infarction, both the LDH and SGOT are raised, as contrasted to pulmonary embolism in which only the former is increased. Certain other enzymes, like the MB isoenzyme of serum creatine phosphokinase (CPK), are also elevated in myocardial infarction, while being unaffected in uncomplicated pulmonary embolism.

With regard to clinical manifestations, in pulmonary embolism there may be a sudden onset of severe substernal pain, whereas in myocardial infarction the complaints appear more gradually, with definite premonitory symptoms frequently preceding the acute pain by several days or hours. Furthermore, the characteristics of the pain are different in the two conditions. In pulmonary embolism, it is sharp and pleuritic in type and not located in any one area, whereas in myocardial infarction, it is pressing and constricting and is generally present substernally with radiation to the shoulders, arms, or neck. Such symptoms as dyspnea and tachypnea are prominent complaints in pulmonary embolism and may be mild or even absent in myocardial infarction. Systemic responses, including fever and increased white blood count and sedimentation rate, are found early in the inception of pulmonary embolism and appears later in myocardial infarction.

Lobar Pneumonia. When pulmonary embolism is associated with pulmonary infarction, the clinical picture may be confused with lobar pneumonia. For in both, there may be pleural pain, fever, and physical and X-ray signs of consolidation of a segment of lung. Ascertaining that the patient has had previous attacks of deep venous thrombosis and/or embolism supports the possibility of one of the latter conditions being present again. The early appearance of hemoptysis with blood clots in the sputum is in accord with a diagnosis of pulmonary infarction, whereas in lobar pneumonia the sputum generally becomes rusty in color and blood-tinged later in the clinical picture and blood clots are not observed. Of importance, also, is the fact that LDH is rarely elevated in lobar pneumonia; in contrast, a significant rise is frequently noted in pulmonary embolism and infarction. Finally, using the pulmonary perfusion scan, the lung ventilation scan, and the gallium-67 lung scan, it is possible to make the distinction between an area of infiltrate and inflammation and one of pulmonary embolism and infarction. To complicate the problem of making a differentiation, however, is the relatively frequent finding of a pneumonic process superimposed upon an area of pulmonary infarction.

Atypical Pneumonia. This condition may be confused with the clinical picture produced by repeated episodes of occlusion of small branches of the pulmonary artery. The symptoms and signs are so similar that difficulty exists in making the differential diagnosis on a clinical basis. However, a history of previous attacks of pulmonary embolism or the history or presence of deep venous thrombosis may help in determining which condition exists.

Miscellaneous Conditions Mimicking Pulmonary Embolism. Among these are pulmonary artery thrombosis (rarely diagnosed clinically), spontaneous pneumothorax, chronic lung disease, and pulmonary atelectasis. The use of pulmonary perfusion scans and lung ventilation studies should generally be very helpful in making the differential diagnosis (p. 267). Asthma may be confused with the clinical manifestations of episodes of small pulmonary emboli. Besides myocardial infarction (p. 272), certain other cardiac conditions may be confused with pulmonary embolism, including paroxysmal tachycardia, dissecting aortic aneurysm, and congestive heart failure. Idiopathic pleuritis and costochondritis must likewise be considered in the differential diagnosis of pain in the chest.

Principles of Therapy for Deep Venous Thrombosis and Pulmonary Embolism and Infarction

The material presented in this section is not intended to prepare the podiatrist for the responsibilities of medical management of the patient with deep venous thrombosis and venous thromboembolism, for obviously such a function belongs in the province of the internist or, on occasion, the vascular surgeon. Nevertheless, the podiatrist should be in a position of understanding in general terms the rationale for the various therapeutic steps being carried out on his patient, so that he or she is able to discuss them intelligently with the consultants on the case.

General Medical Adjunctive Measures
In conjunction with the specific program described below, all patients suffering from deep venous thrombosis of the lower limbs and/or pulmonary embolism should immediately be hospitalized, placed at bedrest with the foot of the bed elevated 15 cm (6 inches), allowed no bathroom privileges, and started on anticoagulant therapy at once. In the case of deep venous thrombosis, it is generally useful also to apply wet heat to the involved limb, provided local arterial circulation is intact. The procedure consists of wrapping the thigh, leg, and foot in hot, wet Turkish towels and then covering the limb with an electric cradle; the heat is maintained for periods of 3 h during the day, in each instance, with 1 h intervening without heat between applications. Such a measure is helpful in controlling the local pain due to the periphlebitis and in counteracting any superimposed arterial vasospasm, a not uncommon response to occlusion of a main collecting vein.

In the case of pulmonary embolism, local heating is eliminated, unless there are associated signs of activity in the deep veins of the lower limbs. Oxygen is given by nasal catheter if there are signs of hypoxemia, so as to maintain the PO_2 between 60 and 120 mm Hg. For severe pleuritic pain or marked apprehension, morphine sulfate may have to be given slowly intravenously 1 mg at a time. For lesser symptoms, codeine sulfate may be adequate.

Medical Therapy for Phlebothrombosis

In the case of phlebothrombosis, anticoagulation involves the intravenous administration of heparin, either by intermittent injection or, preferably, by continuous infusion, the goal of therapy being a rise of the activated partial thromboplastin time (APTT) to 1.5–2 times the control level (average normal range of 40–43 s). This state is then continuously maintained until all signs of activity in the calf muscles have disappeared and full recovery has occurred.

The question of whether the patient with phlebothrombosis should be prepared for outpatient oral anticoagulant therapy has not been fully resolved. As a general rule, if suggestive activity still persists in the calf muscles close to the end of the hospital stay or if the individual has a past history of chronic pulmonary disease or congestive heart failure, it is prudent to prepare him for this type of program. However, before such a course is initiated, it is necessary to weigh very carefully the need for the treatment against the possible risks from hemorrhage.

If the decision is in the affirmative, warfarin sodium (Coumadin) administration is started during the anticipated last week of hospitalization, in conjunction with the previously instituted intravenous injected heparin. With such a plan, usually a depression of prothrombin activity by Coumadin to a therapeutic level (a prothrombin time that is double the control figure) is achieved when the patient is ready to leave the hospital. On the date of discharge, heparin therapy is terminated, whereas the oral anticoagulant is continued, but now on an outpatient basis (p. 282).

At about a week before the patient leaves the hospital, he is measured for an elastic stocking which will contain a built-in gradient of pressure, with the greatest force being exerted at the ankle (40 mm Hg). Then he is placed on an ambulation program, temporarily applying an elastic bandage to the involved limb. Generally by the time of discharge, the fitted elastic stocking should be available for him to take home, substituting it for the compression bandage.

In those instances in which complete recovery from phlebothrombosis appears to have occurred and the patient's cardiopulmonary system is normal in all regards, heparin is also stopped with the end of hospitalization, but without previously initiating an oral anticoagulant program.

Conservative Management of Occlusion of a Main Collecting Vein

Medical Measures. If a nonsuppurative popliteal or iliofemoral thrombophlebitis exists, both intravenously administered heparin and oral Coumadin are given simultaneously early in the inception of the disorder and, following 6 or 7 days of combined therapy, heparin is then stopped. The oral anticoagulant is continued until full recovery has been achieved and the patient has completed a week of an ambulation program (see below). At this point, the oral anticoagulant is also terminated since the patient is now ready for discharge from the hospital.

While the patient is in the hospital, complete bedrest is maintained until all signs of systemic responses to the condition have completely subsided, as recognized by a fall to normal levels of the body temperature, pulse rate, respiration, sedimentation rate, and white blood count, accompanied by disappearance of manifestations of local involvement, such as tenderness in the groin and along the medial aspect of the thigh. Most importantly, the edema of the affected limb must be completely controlled, with the local venous pressure showing signs of approaching approximately normal levels, as reflected in collapse of superficial veins on elevation of the extremity.

With the appearance of all of the above findings, indicating subsidence of the inflammatory process and the development of an effective secondary venous circulation in the involved limb, the patient is now prepared for an ambulation program. First, with all the swelling gone, he is measured for an elastic stocking containing a gradient of pressure. In the interval required for fabrication of the support, he is instructed to walk for 15-min periods using an elastic bandage applied up to the knee. At the beginning, before each session of physical activity, the leg is measured at several levels and again after walking is terminated. If no enlargement has occurred following the initial periods of ambulation, their number during the course of the day are gradually increased, so that by the end of a week (at which time the fabricated elastic stocking is generally available), the patient is ready for discharge from the hospital. He is advised to do as little standing or sitting with his legs in dependency as possible.

If the edema returns during the early periods of ambulation, this indicates that the collateral venous circulation, developed in response to occlusion of a main collecting vein, is not adequate to cope with the great strain placed on the venous system in the involved lower limb when the patient assumes the upright position and begins to walk. Hence, he is again placed at complete bedrest, in the hope that a longer period under such conditions would help in the formation of a more efficient secondary venous circulation.

Normal ambulation is again initiated only after a program of repeated short periods of walking is no longer responsible for the appearance of edema.

Very recently a new medical approach to the treatment of deep venous thrombosis has been proposed, namely the use of such thrombolytic drugs as streptokinase and urokinase in order to preserve venous valve function and thus prevent the onset of the postphlebitic syndrome. However, this expensive and potentially dangerous form of therapy has had only limited application in this regard and hence its evaluation must await much more extensive clinical trials [15]. (For a discussion of fibrinolytic drugs as treatment in pulmonary embolism, see p. 280.)

Therapy for Phlegmasia Cerulea Dolens. In the presence of extensive thrombosis of a main collecting vein and its principal tributaries, the medical approach is generally the same as for the usual type of iliofemoral thrombophlebitis except that even more intensive anticoagulation is instituted. Early administration of fibrinolytic drugs has been proposed in order to lyse the clots in critical vessels and thus reduce the level of raised venous pressure. (For use of thrombectomy in phlegmasia cerulea dolens, see p. 279.)

Therapy for Suppurative Iliofemoral Thrombophlebitis. If an infected thrombus develops in a main collecting vein, measures must be taken immediately to prevent liberation of septic material into the blood stream and the formation of abscesses in the lungs. Of importance is to obtain cultures of blood immediately and then at 10-min intervals for sensitivity studies on bacterial growth so as to be able to administer appropriate antibacterial agents in massive dosage. Until the reports are available, the patient is given large amounts of a wide-spectrum antibiotic. After 24 h of intensive medical therapy, the patient's condition is reevaluated and if improvement is present, the same regimen is continued. If no significant changes are observed, some type of surgical approach should be introduced to arrest blood flow through the inferior vena cava and thus prevent further infected material from reaching the pulmonary vascular bed; at the same time, antibiotic therapy should be continued. (For the surgical methods applicable to such a situation, see p. 281.)

Surgical Management of Occlusion of a Main Collecting Vein
Although the treatment of choice of deep venous thrombosis is chiefly medical, for certain limited conditions, a surgical approach may be applicable.

Venous Thrombectomy. One of the measures proposed as treatment for iliofemoral thrombophlebitis is surgical removal of the thrombus from the lumen of the vessel (thrombectomy). For the most part, the recent clinical data on the assessment of this operation have led to considerable question concerning its utility [13, 14]. Thrombectomy has been primarily attempted in phlegmasia cerulea dolens (p. 260) to prevent venous gangrene. An objective evaluation of the results obtained with the procedure in this type of condition is not available.

Segmental Venous Replacement. Venous surgery has been hampered by the lack of a suitable venous substitute in the form of a graft, only autogenous veins having demonstrated a satisfactory long-term success rate. Experimental studies on dogs using lyophilized venous homografts have been found to be moderately successful as venous substitutes [23]. However, the results with such an approach on patients with iliofemoral thrombophlebitis are still not available and hence its application as a therapeutic procedure must await clinical proof.

Therapy for Pulmonary Embolism with or without Infarction
Treatment of pulmonary embolism and infarction varies depending primarily upon the severity of involvement of the pulmonary bed.

Medical Management of Nonmassive Occlusion. If the pathologic process affects only from 20 to 50% of the pulmonary vascular system and if blood pressure soon returns to a stable fairly normal level, then the therapeutic program is solely medical. This consists of intravenous administration of heparin in much larger doses than those used for deep venous thrombosis, at least for the first 24-hour period. The rationale for such a step is the ability of the drug in high concentrations to counteract the direct bronchoconstrictive action of the serotoninlike factors released from platelets during the early stage of pulmonary embolism. Subsequently the dosage of heparin is regulated so as to maintain the APTT of the blood at a level about twice that of the patient's control readings. This program is continued until there is no further clinical or laboratory evidence of activity in the deep venous plexuses in the legs and in the pulmonary vascular bed. As soon as such a situation is reached, the patient is placed on an ambulation program, and several days before discharge from the hospital is contemplated, Coumadin is added to the anticoagulant regimen. When he leaves the hospital, heparin administration is terminated, but Coumadin is continued on an outpatient basis (p. 282).

Medical Management of Massive Occlusion. When more than 50% of the pulmonary vascular bed is involved or when there is significant cardiopulmonary decompensation, heroic measures are indicated in order to combat the inevitable appearance of the shock state. If the condition is not too severe, initially medical therapy is attempted, in the form of large doses of heparin, treatment of cardiac failure with digitalis, and attempts to raise blood pressure, first with intravenous administration of isoproterenol hydrochloride (Isuprel) and, if this is not effective, by levarterenol bitartrate (Levophed).

If the hypotension cannot be controlled by the above measures, then fibrinolytic drugs (streptokinase or urokinase) should be substituted in an attempt to lyse the thrombus. Urokinase, which is collected from human urine or fetal kidney cell culture, enhances endogenous fibrinolysis by directly activating circulating plasminogen in the blood stream to plasmin; the latter, in turn, degrades fibrin in thrombi and fibrinogen in plasma and releases fibrinogen-fibrin degradation products. The end result is dissolution of clots in the blood vessels. Streptokinase, derived from streptococcal bacterial cell culture, also enhances fibrinolysis, but it accomplishes this by binding to plasminogen to form an activator complex (SK plasminogen) which then converts plasminogen to plasmin.

Both fibrinolytic drugs have been found to be effective in dealing with large emboli in the pulmonary bed and hence have been used with excellent results as a substitute for pulmonary embolectomy. However, their use may be associated with serious adverse reactions, especially hemorrhagic episodes, and therefore they should only be administered by physicians who have had extensive experience in the field of fibrinolytic drugs. It is necessary to point out that when the thrombolysis has been accomplished, as determined by the improvement in the clinical picture, the medication is discontinued and intravenous heparin is substituted in order to prevent rethrombosis.

Surgical Management of Massive Occlusion. In the presence of a medically uncontrollable shock state, it may be necessary to perform a pulmonary embolectomy to reestablish pulmonary blood flow, although such a measure is associated with a very high mortality rate (as great as 57%) [8]. The first step in the procedure consists of performing a pulmonary angiogram to determine the exact location of the thrombus (provided there is time to carry out this procedure) and then doing a pulmonary embolectomy utilizing cardiopulmonary bypass. Also proposed is the use of an intraluminal catheter technique (transvenous catheter embolectomy), which eliminates the need for cardiopulmonary bypass [9, 10].

Surgical Approach to the Prevention of Subsequent Pulmonary Emboli. A number of operative procedures have been proposed which have for their goal partial or complete interruption of blood flow through the inferior vena cava, in an attempt to prevent thrombi originating in the venous tree of the lower limbs or the pelvis from reaching the pulmonary vascular bed. The measures which have had clinical trials are ligation, plication, and clipping of the vessel or insertion of an intracaval device (Mobin-Uddin umbrella filter [16]; Greenfield vena caval filter [10]). In the case of partial obstruction of the vessel (as by a filter), there is a better possibility that edema of both lower limbs and other signs of venous hypertension will not subsequently develop.

Besides the relatively frequent appearance of a clinical entity which resembles the postphlebitic syndrome (p. 287), it is also necessary to point out that surgical partial or complete interruption of blood flow through the inferior vena cava may not always accomplish the desired goal of preventing venous emboli from reaching the lungs [7], for pieces of clot originating proximal to the site of partial or complete occlusion of the vessel may still be responsible for pulmonary emboli. Moreover, with the formation of collateral channels and enlargement of existing vessels (such as the ovarian veins) which rapidly follow surgical interruption of blood flow through the inferior vena cava, alternate pathways are available for the passage of emboli from the lower limbs to the pulmonary vascular bed. Also of great importance in the evaluation of this surgical approach is the report that the combined early operative and embolic mortality after caval ligation is severalfold higher than that for embolic and hemorrhagic deaths during anticoagulant treatment of pulmonary embolism [7]. (For a discussion of an outpatient anticoagulant program, see p. 282.)

Post-Hospital Therapeutic Measures
Physical Steps. At home, the patient who has just recovered from an episode of deep venous thrombosis or pulmonary embolism must continue to sleep with the foot of the bed elevated about 15 cm (6 inches), in order to facilitate venous drainage and prevent accumulation of edema. This can be accomplished by placing blocks of wood, bricks, or books of proper height

under each of the two distal legs of the bed. Pillows should never be used for this purpose since they are generally flattened out by the weight of the limb or are displaced upward into the patient's popliteal fossa, where they act to obstruct venous outflow. Or, as the patient turns in bed, the involved limb rolls off them onto the mattress. With all such responses, venous stasis, rather than venous drainage, results.

The patient's elastic stocking must be readily available in the morning so that he can put it on while still lying in bed with the legs elevated. This will necessitate taking a shower or bath on retiring rather than in the morning. The stocking is worn all day and is only removed when the patient prepares for sleep. It is advisable to have two stockings so that one can be used alternately with the other, thus permitting the one worn during the day to be washed. Even with great care, generally effective elasticity is lost in several months, at which time new stockings should be fabricated.

In the case of both pulmonary embolism and phlebothrombosis, since edema of the lower limb is usually not present, the elastic stockings are worn in order to prevent venous stasis, a situation conducive to intravascular clotting. Hence, several months after the acute episode, they are discarded, provided, of course, that all signs of activity in the calf muscles have disappeared.

Following popliteal or iliofemoral thrombophlebitis, the elastic stockings are permanently discarded only when trials of daily activity without them cause no edema formation. Such a situation may develop weeks, months, or even years after the acute episode, depending upon how many of the critical collateral veins were also occluded during the original attack and upon the rate of formation of new channels and communications in the venous tree of the involved limb. On occasion, the patient may be compelled to wear the stockings for the rest of his life in order to prevent the buildup of edema. Careful attention of the patient to all of the measures outlined in table 14/I will help prevent the appearance of the postphlebitic syndrome (p. 287).

Anticoagulant Regimen. If an oral anticoagulant program has been initiated in the last week of hospitalization, certain facilities and conditions must exist in order to continue it on an outpatient basis. Among these is a laboratory where prothrombin time determinations can be accurately and readily performed. Moreover, the patient must be willing to accept his role in the treatment program and be able to take care of the financial costs resulting therefrom. Also, the program must at all times be under the super-

Table 14/I. Directions for the prevention of postphlebitic syndrome in patients recovered from acute iliofemoral thrombophlebitis

---

Having been discharged from the hospital, it is now advisable for you gradually to assume normal physical activity, including swimming if feasible. In order to prevent any further difficulty with your affected leg, you must meticulously follow the schedule described below.

1. Sleep with the foot of the bed elevated about 6 inches. To accomplish this, raise both feet of the bed by placing the appropriate thickness of books, blocks, or bricks under them. Do not use pillows on the bed or place them under the mattress to elevate it.

2. In the morning, put the fitted elastic stocking with a built-in gradient of pressure on the lower limb *while still lying in bed.* For this purpose, it will be necessary for you to take your shower or bath the night before. You will also have to keep the stocking near at hand. You should continue wearing the stocking all during the day, only removing it in preparation for sleep. A new stocking should be ordered when the old one becomes loose or worn (generally in a matter of several months). It is advisable to have two stockings available so that the one you have worn can be washed each evening.

3. During the course of the day, elevate your legs as frequently as possible. Try not to sit for any period of time with the legs hanging down. Limit your periods of standing. Brisk walking is useful in returning the blood in your legs to the heart. On long train or plane trips, you must take short walks every hour or less.

4. Do not wear any tight or constricting garment or circular elastic garters; remove all elastic tops from socks. Do nothing which would interfere with the movement of blood out of your legs.

5. Take special care of the skin of the affected leg (especially around the ankle) and the foot. Do not expose the limb to strong sunlight (avoid sunburn). Be careful not to injure the leg in any way, as by scratching the skin. If the skin of the leg is dry and scaly, apply a lotion containing lanolin to it. Avoid athlete's foot by always wearing shoes or slippers in the house, carefully drying and powdering between toes after a bath or shower, and changing socks or stockings daily. If you use a public shower, immediately afterward apply one of the common fungicidal powders between the toes.

6. If a minor buildup of swelling develops in the leg around the ankle at the end of the day, do not be alarmed, provided that it is gone on arising the next morning. However, if this does not take place or if the amount of swelling increases with each successive day, seek medical attention. This approach also applies if you have injured your leg or broken the skin around the ankle.

7. Consider discarding your elastic stocking only after trial periods without it do not cause the swelling to return.

8. Avoid constipation and try not to gain weight.

---

vision of a physician knowledgeable in the use of anticoagulants. Close contact must always be maintained between him or her and the patient so that the dosage of the anticoagulant can readily be altered if the need arises. Tests should be performed at least every 2 weeks and the readings should be kept at double the control or within a small range of that figure. As a general rule, a 6-month period of outpatient anticoagulant therapy is sufficient to prevent recurrences of phlebothrombosis, whereas in the case of pulmonary embolism, the period should be extended to at least 1 or even 1.5 years. The patient who has suffered a popliteal or iliofemoral thrombophlebitis is generally not placed on a post-hospital anticoagulant regimen.

References

1 Abramson, D.I.: Diagnosis and treatment of peripheral vascular disorders (Hoeber-Harper, New York 1954).
2 Abramson, D.I.: Vascular disorders of the extremities (Harper & Row, Hagerstown 1974).
3 Abramson, D.I.: Circulatory diseases of the limbs: a primer (Grune & Stratton, New York 1978).
4 Anlyan, W.G.; Hart, G.: Special problems in venous thromboembolism. Ann. Surg. 146: 499 (1957).
5 Bergqvist, D.; Efsing, H.O.; Hallböök, T.: Thermography. A noninvasive method for diagnosis of deep venous thrombosis. Arch. Surg. 112: 600 (1977).
6 Coleman, J.B.; Chang, F.C.: Pulmonary embolism: an unrecognized event in severely burnt patients. Am. J. Surg. 130: 697 (1975).
7 Coon, W.W.: Operative therapy of venous thromboembolism. Modern Concepts cardiovasc. Dis. 43: 71 (1974).
8 Cross, F.S.; Mowlem, A.: A survey of the current status of pulmonary embolectomy for massive pulmonary embolism; in Kittle, Cardiovascular surgery, American Heart Association Monograph 16. Circulation 35: suppl. 1, p. 86 (1967).
9 Greenfield, L.J.: Transvenous pulmonary embolectomy; in Najarian, Delaney, Vascular surgery, p. 545 (Symposia Specialists, Miami 1978).
10 Greenfield, L.J.; Peyton, R.; Crute, S.: Greenfield technique for catheter pulmonary embolectomy and vena caval filter insertion. Vasc. Diag. Ther. 3: 45 (1982).
11 Kakkar, V.V.; Flanc, C.; O'Shea, M.J.; et al.: Treatment of deep-vein thrombosis with streptokinase. Br. J. Surg. 56: 178 (1969).
12 Karp, R.B.; Wylie, E.J.: Recurrent thrombosis after iliofemoral venous thrombectomy. Surg. Forum 17: 147 (1966).
13 Kipper, M.S.; Moser, K.M.; Kortman, K.E.; et al.: Longterm follow-up of patients with suspected pulmonary embolism and a normal lung scan: perfusion scans in embolic suspects. Chest 82: 411 (1982).
14 Lansing, A.M.; Davis, W.M.: Five-year follow-up study of iliofemoral venous thrombectomy. Ann. Surg. 168: 620 (1968).

15 Mich, R.J.; Bell, W.R.: Thrombolytic therapy of deep-vein thrombosis. Pract. Cardiol. *8:* 43 (1982).

16 Mobin-Uddin, K.; Trinkle, J.K.; Bryant, L.R.: Present status of the inferior vena cava umbrella filter. Surgery, St. Louis *70:* 914 (1971).

17 Munster, A.M.: Septic thrombophlebitis. A surgical disorder. J. Am. med. Ass. *230:* 1010 (1974).

18 Nilsson, R.; Sundén, P.; Zetterquist, S.: Leg temperature profiles with a simplified thermographic technique in the diagnosis of acute venous thromboses. Scand. J. clin. Lab. Invest. *39:* 171 (1979).

19 Okada, R.D.; Ewy, G.A.: The acquired nonprecordial murmur of pulmonary embolism. Chest *83:* 762 (1983).

20 Pond, G.D.; Ovitt, T.W.; Capp, M.P.: Comparison of conventional pulmonary angiography with intravenous digital subtraction angiography for pulmonary embolic disease. Radiology *147:* 345 (1983).

21 Schechter, D.C.; Waddell, W.R.; Coppinger, W.R.: Diagnosis and therapy of muscle hernia. Am. Surg. *29:* 483 (1963).

22 Sevitt, S.: Diagnosis and management of massive pulmonary embolism (abridged). Proc. R. Soc. Med. *61:* 143 (1968).

23 Smith, D.E.; Hammon, J.; Anane-Sefah, J.; et al.: Segmental venous replacement. A comparison of biological and synthetic substitutes. J. thorac. cardiovasc. Surg. *69:* 589 (1975).

24 Smith, G.T.; Damin, G.J.; Dexter, L.: Postmortem arteriographic studies of the human lung in pulmonary embolization. J. Am. med. Ass. *188:* 143 (1964).

25 Smith, G.T.; Hayland, J.W.; Piemme, T.; et al.: Human systemic-pulmonary-arterial collateral circulation after pulmonary thrombo-embolism. J. Am. med. Ass. *188:* 452 (1964).

15 Postphlebitic Syndrome

One of the most serious sequelae of acute iliofemoral thrombophlebitis (p. 260) is the subsequent development of venous hypertension in the involved limb due to interference with venous outflow from the extremity, resulting in local venous pooling. If venous hypertension is left unchecked for several years, almost inevitably such a state will be responsible for the production of the postphlebitic syndrome, a condition associated with a serious, frequently disabling, clinical pattern. This chapter is devoted to a discussion of the factors responsible for its appearance, the symptoms and signs indicating its presence, and the treatment of its various manifestations.

General Measures for Prevention of Postphlebitic Syndrome

In many instances the type of management initiated for the acute stage of iliofemoral thrombophlebitis determines whether the postphlebitic syndrome will subsequently develop. If properly instituted early in the inception of the condition and continued during the entire period of hospitalization, as described on page 277, the possibility of later complications is markedly diminished. On occasion, however, despite attempts to reduce the thrombotic tendency by the use of anticoagulants, extensive involvement occurs in the existing collateral channels, as well as in the main collecting vein, and under such circumstances, very little else can be done to prevent the almost inevitable development of the postphlebitic syndrome. The same outlook exists if the patient delays seeking medical aid for 7–10 days after the onset of swelling of the limb or if the condition is misdiagnosed during such a period and hence anticoagulants and complete bedrest are not prescribed until later.

Another factor which significantly influences the subsequent course of the patient who has suffered an episode of acute iliofemoral thrombophlebitis is how faithfully he carries out the instructions for his post-hospital treatment program, as discussed on page 281. Not infrequently, after a while he becomes lax in controlling the edema of the involved limb and discards the elastic hose before he should. If elevation of the limb during the night only minimally reduces the swelling, so there is still some when the patient awakens, and if this significantly increases in amount during the day, eventually irreversible local changes will develop which also make the patient a good candidate for the postphlebitic syndrome.

Clinical Manifestations and Treatment of Postphlebitic Syndrome

The clinical picture observed in the postphlebitic syndrome resembles that produced by prolonged pooling of blood in the superficial veins of the lower limbs due to primary varicosities (p. 232) except that the symptoms and signs are much more severe.

Nocturnal Leg Cramps

Symptoms. Night cramps are commonly present in patients suffering from venous hypertension. They are painful, paroxysmal, involuntary, and transiently sustained, contractions of muscle groups, most often located in the calf, but also involving the small muscles of the feet and the large muscles of the thigh. The cramps occur at night, while the patient is lying in bed and generally awaken him. To obtain relief, he massages the contracted muscles or gets out of bed and walks around the room. Each episode may last from several to 20 min or more, and the cramps may recur a number of times in the same night. They are frequently associated with discomfort or actual pain if the contraction of the muscles is strong. Infrequently, this may be intense enough to cause rupture of thin-walled veins in the involved site. Unless the latter occurs, relief is experienced soon after the spasm of the muscles is released, although a sense of aching and muscle soreness may remain for several hours.

It is necessary to point out that nocturnal leg cramps are by no means specific for venous hypertension. In fact, they may be present in normal people, as well as in a variety of different abnormal conditions, including chronic occlusive arterial disorders, static foot deformities, and peripheral neuropathy, among others. They are also found in such states as hypocalcemia, hyperphosphatemia, hypochloremia, and pregnancy.

Etiologic Factors and Pathogenesis. In the case of night cramps located in the calf muscles, the initiating stimulus is involuntary or voluntary stretching of the Achilles tendon. This acts as a trigger mechanism to cause simultaneous contraction of agonists and antagonists, the position assumed by the leg depending upon which group of muscles is the stronger. The explanation for such a response is not clear, although it is believed that there is a piling up of products of metabolism in the vicinity of the neuro-muscular junctions, causing these structures to become hyperresponsive to even minor stimuli or impulses. The underlying factor responsible for such a situation is either the slow movement of blood out of the limb or a local metabolic alteration.

Therapy. There is no specific treatment program for the control of night cramps. However, certain measures are very helpful in this regard. The patient should be advised to decrease the amount of standing and sitting, he should be warned against extending his legs while in bed, steps must be taken to decrease venous stasis, and oral quinine sulfate, 320 mg, should be given before retiring and, at times, also before the last meal in the evening. Ordinarily such a regimen will cause a reduction or even elimination of the attacks; however, the beneficial effect of quinine sulfate will only be present during the period the medication is given. One explanation for its thera-peutic action is that it hastens the removal, destruction, or conversion of the waste products that have accumulated in the muscles or at the neuromus-cular junction. Another is that it acts to block neuromuscular transmission by prolonging the refractory period of the peripheral nerves. Patients may develop sensitivity to quinine sulfate, a point which must always be kept in mind if it is being administered. Also it may initiate or aggravate tinnitus. If contraindications to its use exist, then oral diphenhydramine (Benadryl), 50 mg, should be given before retiring. Other drugs which have been advo-cated for the control of night cramps are large doses of calcium lactate or gluconate and dilute hydrochloric acid (only in the absence of signs of a peptic ulcer).

Postphlebitic Neurosis

Symptoms. Some patients who have apparently recovered from an acute iliofemoral thrombophlebitis and are back at home may become anxious, tense, apprehensive, and fearful of developing some serious disor-der, such as myocardial infarction, pulmonary embolism, or deformity or gangrene of the involved limb. To reinforce these worries, there may be pain in the extremity on weight-bearing and local coldness, hypersensitivity to cold, diffuse tenderness, or paresthesias, frequently without any organic basis. Each time swelling recurs in the limb following prolonged standing, the patient is convinced that he is suffering from another acute episode of iliofemoral thrombophlebitis or that he has 'chronic thrombophlebitis'. This collection of symptoms has been termed postphlebitic neurosis.

Etiologic Factors. The basis for the difficulty generally stems from the fact that the patient was improperly treated psychologically during the episode of acute iliofemoral thrombophlebitis and was left in complete ignorance of the condition which was causing his hospitalization. Thus, his imagination was permitted to go far afield. Such a situation arises because of poor communication between him and his physician, for which the latter is fully responsible. The previous existence of certain mental stigmata also makes the patient a more probable candidate for postphlebitic neurosis. Unnecessarily long periods of physical inactivity during the acute state of the underlying disease may likewise contribute to such a situation.

Therapy. The management of postphlebitic neurosis properly begins with prophylactic measures instituted during the early stage of acute iliofemoral thrombophlebitis. It takes the form of a clear and simple explanation to the patient of his difficulty, stressing the possibility that certain of his clinical findings may persist for some time although amenable to control. Reassuring him and his relatives on this score will frequently relieve their fears and reduce the severity of the patient's response to his condition. If there are some underlying psychiatric traits, then postphlebitic neurosis may prove to be a much greater problem to treat.

Venous Claudication

Symptoms and Signs. A small number of people who have a history of acute iliofemoral thrombophlebitis will begin to suffer from severe, ill-defined calf pain, experienced while walking. In a sense, this symptom, which may at times be almost disabling, resembles arterial intermittent claudication (p. 5). But since it is not associated with signs of impaired muscle circulation, it cannot be attributed to local ischemia during physical exertion. Another important differential point is that the patient does not always experience relief on standing for several minutes (as occurs in the case of intermittent claudication) and the pain will disappear much sooner if he assumes a seated or reclining position. Usually the symptom is less severe than intermittent claudication and it does not increase in severity to any extent if walking is continued after its onset. Another diagnostic point is that associated signs of venous hypertension (p. 290) are invariably noted in the involved limb.

Etiologic Factors and Pathogenesis. The basis for the apparent muscle pain is not clear [7], since arterial circulation to the limb is always intact; nor has venous distention been implicated as an etiologic factor. Of interest is the finding that the symptom is noted particularly in patients in whom the deep venous system in the involved limb remains permanently occluded by the original thrombus and no recanalization has occurred.

Therapy. The only attempt to control venous claudication consists of valvoplasty of incompetent valves in the femoral vein, a procedure which has been reported to relieve the symptom [6].

Swelling

Signs. An early manifestation of chronic venous hypertension is the reappearance of swelling in the involved limb (fig. 15/1a). This may be minimal on arising in the morning, but it always increases in amount during the course of the day. If left untreated, the quantity of edema fluid accumulating in the limb continues to increase until eventually an 8-hour period of bedrest has little effect upon reducing it. Under such circumstances, the pitting character of the condition is generally replaced by a brawny, nonpitting lymphedema, the extravasated protein in the edema fluid causing a dermal and subcutaneous fibrosis which results in mechanical obstruction of lymphatic channels. (For a discussion of the factors involved in the pathogenesis of the edema of postphlebitic syndrome, see p. 240.)

Therapy. Management of swelling of the involved limb consists of the continuation of the program initiated in the hospital during the episode of acute iliofemoral thrombophlebitis and continued afterward (p. 277), including elevation of the foot of the bed (p. 281) and wearing a fabricated elastic stocking with a built-in gradient of pressure. Time spent in the standing or sitting position with the feet in dependency is reduced as much as possible. If such measures are not sufficient to control the swelling, then the patient should be placed at complete bedrest with the foot of the bed elevated and given a diet low in salt. At the beginning he should receive a single dose of parenteral furosemide (Lasix), 20 mg, to mobilize the fluid, followed by oral administration of the drug until the swelling has subsided. Then he is cautiously placed on an ambulation program using a heavy one-way stretch elastic stocking as a temporary measure. Later the firm compressive effect of the latter is no longer needed and a two-way stretch fabricated stocking with a built-in gradient of pressure is substituted, provided that the edema is controlled.

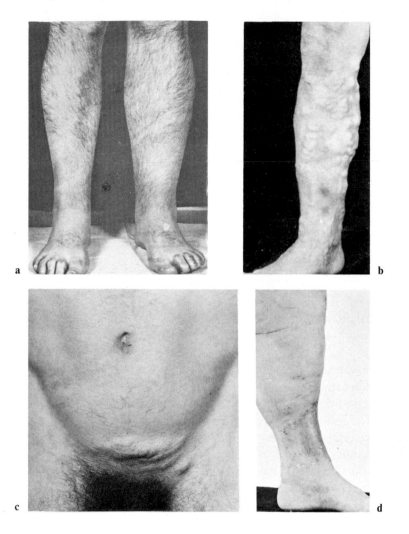

Fig. 15/1. Postphlebitic syndrome following iliofemoral thrombophlebitis. **a** Chronic edema of left leg. **b** Marked secondary varicosities of left leg; pigmentation also noted. **c** Development of suprapubic venous collateral vessels following left iliofemoral thrombophlebitis. **d** Chronic indurated cellulitis of lower portion of leg causing a fibrotic reaction and adhesion of skin to subcutaneous tissue. Reproduced from ref. [1] with permission.

Secondary Varicosities and Dilated Veins

Signs. A common abnormality associated with the postphlebitic syndrome is the appearance of dilated superficial veins, many of which demonstrate regurgitant flow (secondary varicosities) (fig. 15/1b). The latter resemble primary varicosities (p. 232) and involve the great and small saphenous systems, as well as the veins located in the suprapubic region (fig. 15/1c). (For a discussion of the etiologic factors involved in secondary varicosities, see p. 234.)

Besides secondary varicosities, large dilated subcutaneous veins frequently appear on the outer aspect of the thigh, extending onto the flank and lower portion of the lateral abdominal wall. Others are found on the medial aspect of the thigh and the anterior surface of the lower portion of the abdominal wall (see fig. 11/2).

Etiologic Factors and Pathogenesis. The basis for the appearance of secondary varicosities is the existing venous hypertension in the deep venous system. The latter, in turn, is the result of one of two mechanisms, depending upon the outcome of the processes occurring at the level of the original thrombus in the iliofemoral vein. If the occlusion remains, eventually there is a build-up of pressure in the deep venous system distal to the obstruction, the level frequently rising to the point of forcing the valves in the communicating veins to become incompetent. Under such circumstances, blood from the deep venous system now flows into the superficial veins in a retrograde fashion, overdistending them and causing the valves in them to become functionally incompetent. As a result, secondary superficial varicosities develop.

If, on the other hand, the clot in the iliofemoral vein becomes recanalized, in the process of which the valves locally are destroyed, the vessel is now patent but incompetent. As a consequence, the normal movement of blood from the deep venous system into the inferior vena cava does not take place in an efficient manner, again resulting in a build-up of local venous pressure due to the stasis present in the lower segment of the deep venous tree. This initiates a sequence of events similar to that already described above for the impatent vein. Under both situations, then, the final result is the appearance of secondary varicosities.

The dilated prominent veins which develop on the lateral and medial aspects of the thigh and extend onto the abdominal wall do not demonstrate regurgitant flow, in contrast to the secondary varicosities. They represent a portion of the collateral venous system which has developed in response to the need for removal of blood from the affected limb, in light of the pathologic changes in the deep veins that prevent these vessels from performing this function.

Therapy. Active treatment for secondary varicosities is relatively ineffective. Instead, efforts should be made to prevent their appearance or, if already present, to minimize their growth. This is accomplished by the use of the approach described for the control of edema (p. 290), which has for a goal the shunting of blood from the superficial veins into those deep vessels which are still patent. At the same time, such a measure encourages development of collateral channels in the deeper structures, where the vessels are better supported by surrounding tissues and exposed to a greater pumping action supplied by the neighboring muscles. As a consequence, blood flow through superficial veins is reduced, thus causing a lowering of pressure in these vessels. This helps to decrease distention in them and facilitates return of normal function of their valves.

If prominent secondary varicosities exist, the question of how to deal with them has not been fully answered. One view is that secondary, as well as primary, varicosities should be surgically treated since they are inefficient in the removal of blood from a limb. In practice, however, such a heroic measure is rarely carried out except possibly in the case of a conservative treatment-resistant venous stasis ulcer (p. 300) or an area of chronic indurated cellulitis (p. 295). The reason for such a view is that in the presence of already-existing abnormalities in the deep venous system, stripping of the superficial veins could very well have a significant adverse effect on the mechanism of removal of blood from a lower limb. For, under such circumstances, very few venous channels would be available and hence venous hypertension would become even more severe. Also, there is no good proof that all dilated or incompetent veins serve no function. It is possible that they are compensatory and hence still useful in the removal of blood from the lower limb.

Pigmentation
Venous hypertension, if present for any period of time, will be responsible for the development of brownish pigmentation on the lower portion of the leg, particularly above the internal malleolus (fig. 15/1b). The cause is not known, although the view has been proposed that the change may be due to rupture of delicate venules and capillaries as a result of the persistently high venous and capillary pressures to which they have been sub-

jected. Following the development of minute subcutaneous hemorrhages, the breakdown products of blood pigment are then deposited in the skin. Another possibility is that hemosiderin forms and accumulates in the skin for reasons not known at present. Deposition of pigment predisposes the affected area to much more serious complications, such as stasis dermatitis and stasis ulceration.

Once the process develops, there are no therapeutic means available for its management other than surgical removal of the skin so involved. Medical treatment has for its goal prevention of the deposits or, if already present, steps to slow down or eliminate the condition by controlling venous hypertension.

Chronic Indurated Cellulitis

Symptoms and Signs. With persistence of venous hypertension, an area of chronic indurated cellulitis may form on the inner surface of the lower portion of the leg, generally in a site of pigmentation. Usually the lesion has a brawny appearance, with no signs of activity; however, at times the process flares up, the area becoming painful, red, and hot, with a hard, scalloped inflamed border. Following therapy or spontaneously, the acute lesion then recedes into a chronic stage. After a number of such episodes, the area of involvement is infiltrated by fibrous tissue which may eventually encircle the entire circumference of the limb at the level of the initial lesion, to form a tight constricting band (fig. 15/1d). Roentgenographic examination of the mass in two planes generally reveals calcification in the subcutaneous tissue, at times to the degree of disseminated calcinosis, phleboliths, and calcification of the walls of the superficial veins.

Etiologic Factors and Pathogenesis. The cause of chronic indurated cellulitis is persistence of venous hypertension, venous stasis, and edema, these abnormalities being responsible for pooling of poorly oxygenated venous blood and for impaired arteriolar flow in the lower third of the leg. As the tissues in the involved site continue to be deprived of oxygen and nutrients, they become more susceptible to low-grade infections and superficial thrombophlebitis, eventually developing the syndrome of chronic indurated cellulitis.

Therapy. In every instance, chronic indurated cellulitis should first be given a trial of conservative therapy, involving a period of complete bedrest with the foot of the bed elevated, hot, wet soaks to the area (provided local arterial circulation is intact), and the administration of a wide-spectrum antibiotic. Cultures and sensitivity studies cannot be performed since secretion from the lesion is generally not present.

If medical therapy is ineffective, then surgical treatment is indicated. This includes removal of all abnormal structures in the site, followed by a split-thickness skin graft applied to well-vascularized muscle. Any incompetent communicating veins encountered during the course of the operation are ligated. If secondary varicosities coexist, then the great saphenous vein is stripped to just below the level of the knee and the femoral vein is ligated below the junction with the deep femoral vein. However, as already mentioned (p. 293), such a therapeutic procedure carries with it certain risks and, hence, a preliminary step must be taken to demonstrate that a significant rise in deep venous pressure will not occur after completion of the surgery. This involves temporarily ligating the great saphenous and common femoral veins and determining the effect on the level of venous pressure.

Stasis Dermatitis
Stasis dermatitis is one of the more serious manifestations of postphlebitic syndrome.

Symptoms and Signs. The condition is characterized by the presence of a weeping eczematous dermatitis (fig. 15/2a), found in the lower third of the leg in patients who have suffered from venous hypertension and stasis for a protracted period of time. Occasionally, it takes the form of an erysipeloid type of inflammation. Invariably there is intense itching (probably due to irritation of cutaneous sensory nerve endings), the condition being aggravated by the resulting persistent scratching. Generally, the lesion demonstrates superficial oozing of serum, or it may be covered by scaly cornified skin surrounded by an area of inflammation or brown pigmentation.

Etiologic Factors and Pathogenesis. The underlying mechanism responsible for the development of stasis dermatitis is the persistent rise in capillary filtration pressure, a reflection of the elevated venous pressure. At the same time, there is an increase in capillary permeability due to the partial state of ischemia originating in venous stasis and in interference with movement of blood through the arterioles into the capillary bed. As a consequence of both factors, there is a greater than normal transudation of protein-rich fluid through the capillary wall into the tissue spaces.

Therapy. There is no question that the management of stasis dermatitis requires complete bedrest and elevation of the foot of the bed, together with local measures applied to the lesion. Ambulatory treatment of the stasis dermatitis rarely results in healing or even improvement of the condition. The initial step is to attempt to harden the skin locally by the continuous application of either Burow's solution (1:20 concentration) or of a dilute solution of silver nitrate (15 ml of a 10% solution in 1 liter of *distilled* water). The medication is poured onto several layers of gauze covering the affected site and the gauze is kept wet by repeated applications of the solution during the daytime. To prevent evaporation, a piece of oiled silk or plastic is placed over the wet gauze. At night a dry dressing is applied to the lesion. Steps are also taken to eradicate any fungus infection between the toes, since this condition may act as a portal of entry for bacteria. All scaly material and necrotic tissue must be removed by debridement. With such a program, most episodes of stasis dermatitis are generally controlled in 2–3 weeks, provided that complete bedrest is continued all during this period.

Venous Stasis Ulceration

Symptoms and Signs. Stasis ulceration, the most serious manifestation of postphlebitic syndrome, is usually located on the medial aspect of the ankle, in the area drained by the great saphenous venous system (fig. 15/2b–f); less often, it is found on the lateral side and, rarely, on the upper portion of the leg. Initially there may be necrosis and separation of the superficial layers of skin, or a portion of the wall of a superficial vein may slough away, together with the overlying skin. When fully developed, the ulcer generally penetrates the tissues to reach the sheath of underlying muscle (fig. 15/2f). It is irregularly shaped, varying in size from somewhat larger than a pinhead to one involving a considerable portion of the lower segment of leg (fig. 15/2f). An infected dirty exudate, from which a foul odor emanates, usually covers the base and walls of the ulcer. The tissues at the periphery of the lesion invariably demonstrate signs of inflammation, swelling, induration, scaliness, and pigmentation.

Local pain is commonly present. Although not as severe as that associated with an ischemic ulcer (p. 42), it is described as a burning, throbbing, or aching sensation which, in most instances, becomes much more intense when the patient sits, stands, or walks. Occasionally, the symptom may be so marked as to be disabling, in this respect, resembling the pain found in major causalgia (p. 327). The cause is probably irritation of the sensory components of local peripheral nerves by the inflammatory process.

a   b   c

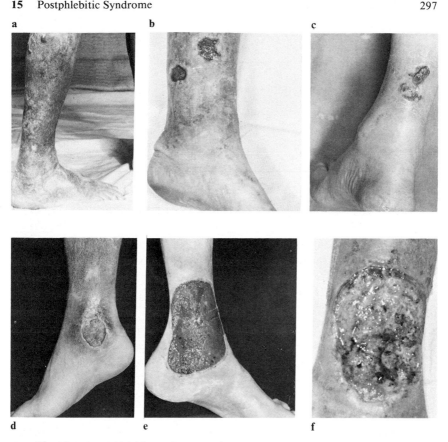

d   e   f

Fig. 15/2. Postphlebitic stasis dermatitis and ulceration. **a** Eczematous dermatitis involving lower part of leg. **b, c** Ulcerations of superficial tissues. **d-f** More extensive ulcerations, including deep tissues. Reproduced from ref. [2] with permission.

A valuable differential point between a venous stasis ulcer and an ischemic ulcer is that in the former, elevation of the involved limb will frequently decrease the severity of the pain and dependency will accentuate it, whereas the opposite types of response are noted with an ischemic ulceration. Another differentiation is the presence of other signs of venous stasis and no manifestations of arterial insufficiency in the case of a stasis ulcer and the reverse for the ischemic lesion. The location of the stasis ulcer in the vicinity of the internal malleolus is also of significance, since rarely are ulcers of arterial origin found in this location (except following injury), with most of them being located on the toes and the heels, sites where venous stasis ulcers are not noted.

Etiologic Factors and Pathogenesis. As in the case of the other manifestations of postphlebitic syndrome, the venous stasis ulcer is also the result of persistent pooling of blood in the distal venous tree of the lower limb. The associated venous hypertension is transmitted back into the microcirculation as a rise in capillary filtration pressure which, in turn, causes a greater transudation of fluid into the tissue spaces. The resulting waterlogging of the various structures locally is followed by anoxia, impaired nutrition, and accumulation of toxic waste products of metabolism. All of these factors tend to reduce the resistance of the skin and subcutaneous tissue, so that even a minor abrasion, bruise, or infection may be responsible for the development of the ulcer. In fact, it may even appear to form spontaneously.

The predilection for ulcers to develop in the vicinity of the internal malleolus is due to the fact that in this site the protective padding is scanty and the possibility of injury is considerable. Also, there appears to be a greater vulnerability of the tissues around the internal malleolus to any type of infection than exists elsewhere. Another reason is that several poorly supported communicating veins are located here and, in the presence of incompetency of the deep venous system and an increase in venous pressure that follows, a regurgitant flow occurs in these vessels as their valves become functionally incompetent. Consequently, the tissues of the ankle are continuously bathed by poorly oxygenated venous blood.

Therapy. The one disconcerting and discouraging factor in the treatment of venous stasis ulceration is the propensity for recurrences which this condition manifests even after an excellent therapeutic result has been achieved. In any event, the initial treatment program should be medically oriented and directed toward control of venous stasis and local infection and introduction of steps to stimulate growth of granulation tissue and epithelialization.

The most effective means to minimize or eliminate venous stasis is complete bedrest, with no bathroom privileges, and elevation of the foot of the bed. When this is not financially feasible, then other less effective measures have to be utilized which permit the patient to be ambulatory. Among these is the application of pure gum rubber bandages, well-fitting elastic bandages, compression leggings, the vasopneumatic apparatus, and the nonelastic support (Unna boot). On occasion an ordinary elastic bandage is used, together with a piece of sterile sponge rubber cut slightly larger than the general outline and depth of the ulcer; the latter is placed over the base of the ulcer and held in position with the elastic bandage. The compression legging applies a uniform pressure over the entire limb through the use of a rubber bladder incorporated in an outer duck casing and inflated by means of a bicycle pump. The pressure generally used is about 35 mm Hg.

The Unna boot, which consists of bandages impregnated with a mixture of gelatin, glycerine, and zinc oxide, is commercially available. The bandages are applied to the limb to form a boot and are left on for 1 or 2 weeks, provided the patient does not complain of itching or burning locally. If such symptoms are experienced, the boot must be immediately removed; otherwise, denudation around the lesion may occur. Furthermore, if the segment of the boot overlying the ulcer becomes soft due to secretion, this is also an indication for removal of the appliance, since it is no longer performing its function of applying pressure and controlling venous stasis locally. If there are definite signs of healing following the use of the first boot, then a second one is applied to the limb, this step being repeated until the ulcer is fully epithelialized.

To control the infection which almost invariably exists in the ulcer and the surrounding tissues, bedrest is essential in order to carry out the proper measures. First, to obtain accurate information regarding the agent or agents responsible for the inflammatory state, the following steps are carefully adhered to: All loose necrotic tissue is removed by debridement, the area is cleansed with a mild antiseptic, and then it is covered with sterile gauze which is left in place for 24 h. At the end of this period, the gauze is removed under aseptic conditions and the secretion at the base of the ulcer is cultured and sensitivity studies are performed. From the derived information, the proper antibiotic is administered. This measure is generally effective in controlling the infection since the existing local arterial blood supply is normal and hence a high concentration of the antibiotic can be built up in the surrounding tissue.

Together with the above therapeutic approach, the lesion must be kept clean by means of daily whirlpool treatments, followed by debridement of devitalized tissue and accumulated secretion. Also, during the course of the day, hot, wet gauze pads should be applied to the lesion for 3-hour intervals (alternating with 1-hour periods during which the limb is uncovered), with the temperature of the dressings being maintained at approximately 32 °C (90 °F) by means of a heat cradle. Naturally, this measure can only be utilized if a normal arterial circulation is present. At night, the lesion is covered with an antibiotic ointment, such as Neosporin ointment, primarily to prevent the gauze bandage from sticking to the ulcer.

After about 2 weeks or less of the outlined treatment program, the involved area should be clean and devoid of all necrotic tissue. Local infection should also be controlled, as indicated by disappearance of all signs of inflammation in the skin surrounding the lesion. Under such circumstances, the ulcer may show signs of healing spontaneously, with granulation tissue covering the base and growing upward toward the level of the skin. Epithelialization may be noticed around the periphery of the lesion. At this point, it is necessary to decrease the frequency of dressing the ulcer so as to reduce the possibility of inadvertently damaging delicate granulation tissue and epithelial cells that are developing.

If improvement is slow, epithelialization may be accelerated by the use of stimulating ointments, such as 5% crude coal tar ointment applied locally every 24 h. However, it is necessary to point out that patients suffering from chronic recurrent venous stasis ulcers may have become sensitized to such a substance, and hence certain precautions must be taken when it is used. For example, it should first be applied early in the day, so that any untoward responses to the medication, such as itching, burning, or pain, are quickly recognized. If they do develop, the coal tar must immediately be removed and the treatment discontinued. If no symptoms are experienced, daily applications should be performed for a period of approximately 10 days, but not much longer.

Attempts to increase local blood flow may also facilitate healing of the stasis ulcer. Of value in this regard is the oral administration of alpha-receptor blocking agents, such as phenoxybenzamine hydrochloride (Dibenzyline), 10 mg, 3 times a day (p. 147). Very effective in augmenting local blood flow in the presence of a venous stasis ulceration is histamine by ion transfer [3]. Following a series of treatments with the method, rapid clinical improvement may be expected, due to the marked increase in local cutaneous blood flow that quickly occurs. The vascular reaction is responsible for a more efficient removal of products of metabolism locally and a better nutritional climate in the region of the lesion. As a result, granulation tissue buildup and epithelialization are accelerated, followed by healing of the ulcer. (For the technique of application of histamine by ion transfer, see p. 203.)

In the absence of healing of the stasis ulcer by conservative means, it may be necessary to resort to a surgical approach to accomplish this goal. However, before any of the procedures available for this purpose are to be utilized, it is essential first to control medically the edema, the inflammation of surrounding tissues, and the local infection; otherwise, the surgical

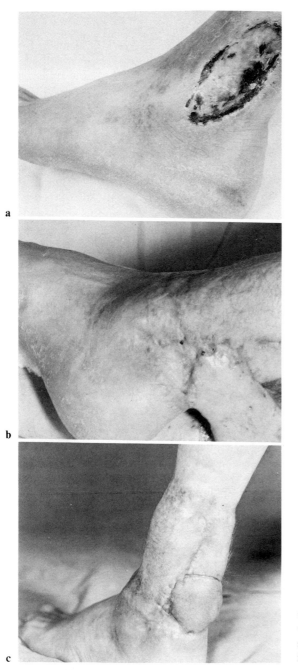

Fig. 15/3. Surgical means of treating nonhealing indolent venous stasis ulcer. **a** Ulcer site. **b** Use of pedicle skin grafting, with healing of lesion in **c**.

approach has no possibility of being successful. Among the procedures which have been advocated for the treatment-resistant, indolent venous stasis ulcers is wide excision of the lesion and surrounding indurated skin and subcutaneous tissue down to the deep fascia, followed by split-thickness skin graft or dermal overgrafting (fig. 15/3) [8]. At the same time, all incompetent ankle perforators are ligated to correct the venous stasis. Another approach is ligating the common femoral vein and stripping of the great and small saphenous veins, together with removal of a portion of the vein underlying the lesion. As already pointed out, the latter procedure is associated with some risks (pp. 293, 295).

Other more recently proposed surgical measures for the control of venous stasis are transposition of the great saphenous vein to bypass segmental obliteration of the iliofemoral vein [4, 5], a cross-pubis saphenous vein bypass procedure, and surgical repair (valvoplasty) of an incompetent femoral vein valve [6]. None of these approaches, however, has been exposed to sufficient clinical trial to be able to evaluate properly its usefulness in stasis ulceration.

References

1   Abramson, D.I.: Diagnosis and treatment of peripheral vascular disorders (Hoeber-Harper, New York 1954).
2   Abramson, D.I.: Circulatory diseases of the limbs: a primer (Grune & Stratton, New York 1978).
3   Abramson, D.I.; Tuck, S., Jr.; Chu, L.S.W.; Buso, E.: Physiologic and clinical basis for histamine by ion transfer. Archs Phys. Med. Rehabil. *48:* 583 (1967).
4   Frileux, C.; Pillot-Bienayme, P.; Gillot, C.: Bypass of segmental obliterations of iliofemoral venous axis by transposition of saphenous vein. J. cardiovasc. Surg. *13:* 409 (1972).
5   Husni, E.A.: Venous reconstruction in postphlebitic disease. Circulation *43:* suppl. 1, p. 147 (1971).
6   Kistner, R.L.: Surgical repair of the incompetent femoral vein valve. Archs Surg., Chicago *110:* 1336 (1975).
7   Negus, D.: Calf pain in the post-thrombotic syndrome. Br. med. J. *ii:* 156 (1968).
8   Thompson, N.; Ell, P.J.: Dermal overgrafting in treatment of venous stasis ulcers. Plastic reconstr. Surg. *54:* 290 (1974).

III Trauma- and Treatment-Related Vascular Disorders

16 Vascular Complications of Trauma to the Lower Limbs

Trauma to a lower limb may be responsible not only for damage to skin, nervous elements, and musculoskeletal structures, but also to the local blood supply. When critical arteries or veins are so affected, the clinical entities resulting therefrom frequently fall into the category of acute emergencies, requiring immediate diagnosis and surgical intervention. Other types of vascular injury affecting major blood vessels, although delayed in their appearance, must subsequently likewise be treated by operative means to reestablish local circulation. To a lesser extent, trauma to terminal portions of the vascular tree may also necessitate immediate management, primarily because of the seriousness of some of the associated complications. Finally, trauma may involve peripheral nervous elements or soft tissue, such a situation, in turn, initiating abnormal reflex arcs responsible for the development of severe degrees of vasospasm and pain. The present chapter deals with all these types of vascular entities due to trauma.

Vascular Entities Resulting from Trauma to Major Blood Vessels

Etiologic Factors
Injury to large blood vessels in the lower limbs can be produced by a variety of agents. Some cause direct penetrating wounds which result in severance, laceration, perforation, contusion, compression by a hematoma, or disruption of the intima of the vessels. Others inflict nonpenetrating or blunt trauma which may be responsible for contusion of arteries, followed by thrombosis and intramural hemorrhage or disruption of the intima. The increasing use of diagnostic and therapeutic procedures requiring puncture of the arterial and venous trees in the lower limbs is also responsible for vascular injuries. The femoral artery, for example, is frequently entered to

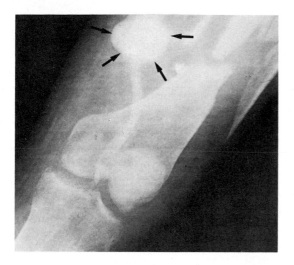

Fig. 16/1. Fracture of lower portion of femur producing injury to the superficial femoral artery, with the production of a false arterial aneurysm, as indicated by arrows. Lesion visualized by means of contrast arteriography.

carry out such measures as heart catheterization, angiography, and monitoring of blood gas levels and blood pressure. As a result, this vessel may become the site of a false aneurysm, an acquired arteriovenous fistula, severe spasm followed by thrombosis, or dissection and laceration of the arterial wall.

Common Locations for Large Blood Vessel Trauma

Fractures of long bones, a common cause of trauma to major arteries, will have the greatest effect on a deep, relatively fixed vessel, such as the popliteal artery, which is firmly attached at the upper end of the popliteal space by the tendinous arch of the adductor magnus muscle and distally, by the soleus and gastrocnemius arches. The deep femoral artery and the accompanying vein may be damaged by fracture of the shaft and intertrochanteric of the femur. If the bony injury is in the lower end of the femur, then the superficial femoral or the popliteal artery may be so affected (fig. 16/1). A fibular fracture may be associated with trauma to the posterior tibial, the anterior tibial, or the peroneal artery. The distal segment of the posterior tibial artery and the accompanying veins may be endangered by a fracture of the ankle.

Role of Diagnostic Laboratory Procedures in Large Blood Vessel Trauma

Angiography. There is still some question as to when this test is indicated as a means of determining the state of the main arteries in a traumatized lower limb. Certainly, in the case of clear-cut evidence of vascular injury, such as in the presence of severe ischemia and absent pulses in the foot, there is no need to lose precious time performing such a procedure and, instead, immediate surgical exploration is imperative, so as to institute steps for the reestablishment of local circulation. The same approach applies to a situation in which profuse hemorrhage or a pulsating hematoma already exists. Furthermore, there is no need for angiography if the injury is some distance removed from the usual location of a critical artery and pulsations are present in the foot, or if local hemorrhage is readily controlled and signs of ischemia of the foot are minimal or absent. Under such conditions, the possibility of injury to important vascular structures is very slight, and hence angiography and a surgical approach are not indicated.

Angiography is primarily useful as a diagnostic aid when the physical signs are equivocal, as for example, when manifestations of ischemia are minimal but pulses are absent in the foot and there is difficulty in determining the extent of the hemorrhage or in ascertaining whether the trauma could conceivably have injured a main artery. In such situations, the procedure may supply valuable information upon which a decision can be made regarding the need for surgical intervention. The films visualizing the arterial tree are also helpful in defining the exact location and extent of the vascular injury and in deciding upon the proper operative approach to the problem. Likewise of great importance is the fact that angiography can distinguish a hematoma or a false aneurysm from soft tissue swelling (fig. 16/1). It is necessary to point out, however, that in the case of some lesions, as for example, a severely contused or lacerated but still intact artery, the information derived from the arteriogram may be misleading. For, under such circumstances, an apparently normal vessel will be visualized, despite the fact that the existing lesion may lead to a potentially dangerous state of arterial thrombosis. Because of such a possibility, a negative result does not necessarily rule out the need for surgical intervention.

Venography. Since the accompanying vein may also be injured at the time of arterial damage, a study of the main venous system by contrast venography may be indicated. The procedure should likewise be performed if the possibility exists that a main collecting vein is the sole vessel affected by the trauma. If such a situation is identified, steps can then be immediately taken to prevent loss of a significant quantity of blood.

Types of Vascular Entities Produced by Large and Small Blood Vessel Trauma

Laceration or Severance of a Main Artery. Such a condition is generally followed by a very severe degree of hemorrhage and ischemia of the foot and leg. The response is most marked in the case of partial severance of the vessel, since, under these circumstances, the persistence of a small intact bridge of vascular tissue prevents contraction of the proximal segment of the cut vessel and normal retraction into the surrounding structures. The usual causes of laceration or severance of a main artery are sharp objects, such as a razor, a knife, or an ice pick; fragments of fractured bone; blunt instruments; and high velocity missiles. The most commonly involved vessel in the lower limb is the superficial femoral artery because of its location close to the skin and because of poor protection by bony structures.

The type of bleeding encountered depends upon whether the skin has been penetrated by the etiologic agent. If it has, then external hemorrhage will occur, a massive loss of blood being associated with hypovolemic shock. If not, a hematoma will develop locally, the lesion, in turn, acting to compress the traumatized vessel as the pressure builds up within the mass; as a result, further bleeding is inhibited or prevented, and, hence, the fall in blood pressure is less marked. The hematoma may subsequently develop into a false aneurysm (p. 309).

Another factor which may influence the clinical picture is the previous role of the involved artery in supplying circulation to the limb. In those instances in which a critical vessel, such as the femoral or popliteal artery, is traumatized, the local signs and symptoms of ischemia are very apparent.

Pain is usually severe, being located primarily in the toes. There are associated signs of absent blood flow, including a low cutaneous temperature which begins at approximately the level of the arterial lesion and extends distally to involve the remainder of the limb. The skin becomes cadaveric in appearance, with cyanotic mottling observed in some areas. The ischemic state is also responsible for neurologic manifestations, in the form of foot drop, paralysis of the small muscles of the foot, and a stocking-glove type of anesthesia or hypesthesia. Pulses in the feet are absent and oscillometric readings are not obtainable.

Acute Vascular Spasm (Traumatic Vasospasm). This condition is usually produced either by a blunt blow to the limb, a fracture of a long bone, manipulation of an artery during a surgical procedure, a crushing injury, or a gunshot wound in proximity to a vessel but not directly injuring it. The mechanism responsible for the clinical manifestations is active contraction of the circular muscle fibers in the vessel wall, causing transient complete obliteration of the lumen and cessation of blood flow to distal tissues.

Two types of arteriospasm may occur: neurogenic and myogenic. In neurogenic vasospasm, the peripheral sympathetic nervous system supplies the efferent limb of an abnormal reflex, the trigger mechanism which initiates the response being the irritated segment of vessel. Hence, there is an increase in the number and intensity of the vasconstrictor impulses reaching the neuroeffector organs in the blood vessel wall, resulting in persistent, strong contractions of the vascular muscle.

In the case of myogenic vasospasm, the precipitating factors are the same as in neurogenic vasospasm except that the sympathetic nervous system is not involved. The exact mechanism which causes the vascular circular muscle fibers to go into continuous and marked spasm is not known.

The early local clinical manifestations of both acute neurogenic and acute myogenic arteriospasm resemble those described above for laceration and severance of a main artery – symptoms and signs of severe ischemia of distal tissues. The subsequent course will depend upon whether the marked vasospastic state can be released before irreversible changes in the structures of the foot take place. If this occurs, then there is an almost immediate return to a normal state as circulation is reestablished at its previous state of efficiency. If not, arterial thrombosis invariably occurs, followed by necrosis of distal structures if the affected vessel is a critical source of blood supply. (For steps to differentiate neurogenic from myogenic vasospasm, see p. 317.)

Traumatic Arterial Thrombosis. This clinical entity may be noted in a previously normal or an abnormal artery after local trauma by such etiologic agents as a fracture, a blunt blow, shell fragments, or a bullet. As a result, the artery is directly contused, so that rupture or rolling up of the intima and possibly of the media follows. This type of change acts as a nidus for adherence of platelets and debris from the blood in the injured site until complete obliteration of the lumen occurs.

Another mechanism responsible for traumatic arterial thrombosis is moderate and indirect pressure to the exterior of the artery, applied intermittently and for short intervals over a protracted period of time. As a consequence, there is injury of the intima and a gradual growth of thrombus on the involved site until the entire lumen is obliterated. Such a situation may be found close to a joint or between bone and the tendinous insertion of a muscle.

Of the different vessels in which traumatic arterial thrombosis may occur, the popliteal artery is especially vulnerable to such a pathologic state. This is so because of the possibility of direct vascular trauma from dislocation of the knee joint and fracture of the long bones of the lower limb. Also, repeated contractions of surrounding muscles may damage the vessel in its course through the fibromuscular canal, at the level of the upper border of the femoral condyles. Another vessel susceptible to traumatic thrombosis is the segment of the superficial femoral artery that passes through the adductor canal, where it is exposed to repeated compression by contractions of neighboring muscles.

The clinical manifestations of traumatic arterial thrombosis depend upon how rapidly the process occurs and upon whether preexisting collaterals are available. If the etiologic agent is a strong blow or a fracture, causing severe trauma to a previously normal artery, with rapid and complete occlusion of the vessel, then the local clinical picture will be the same as that described above for laceration or severance of a critical artery. If, on the other hand, arterial thrombosis occurs as a result of repeated mild trauma to an artery, producing a delayed buildup of a thrombus, the symptoms and signs will probably resemble those observed with a slowly developing spontaneous thrombosis of an artery, as in the case of a chronic occlusive arterial disorder (p. 101). If the thrombotic process forms very slowly, there may be sufficient time for the development of an adequate collateral circulation. As a result, when complete occlusion occurs, very few symptoms and signs may be noted to indicate that this has taken place except the absence of pulsations in peripheral arteries in which there was previously a reduction in amplitude of the pulse wave.

Traumatic Arterial Aneurysm. This condition, also termed false aneurysm or pulsating hematoma, results from trauma to an arterial wall, with perforation of all three coats and bleeding into the surrounding tissues and the development of a hematoma (p. 307). Then the clotted material is covered by a wall of fibrin, the interior of the sac thus formed communicating with the artery through the original site of rupture (fig. 16/2a–d). Such a lesion may be caused by sharp penetrating missiles, certain surgical procedures, hypodermic needles, and fracture of long bones (fig. 16/1). Although the false aneurysm is the usual type of response to vascular trauma, at times a true aneurysm develops following injury to the outer layer of the vessel, but leaving the media and intima intact. However, the resulting weakness, thinning, and eventual stretching of the muscular coat causes dilatation of the involved segment of artery and production of the lesion.

In the lower limbs, the femoral artery is a relatively frequent site for the development of a traumatic arterial aneurysm (fig. 16/2a). However, the other main vessels are so situated that they also may be similarly affected (fig. 16/2b, c).

Ordinarily a fully developed traumatic arterial aneurysm, if the original loss of blood locally had not been excessive, may be associated with very few clear-cut complaints. Only if the lesion rapidly enlarges will pain be experienced, due to compression of nervous components by the expanding mass. The patient may also become aware of a pulsatile lesion following an injury to the limb. If the difficulty is located in a confined space, such as the popliteal fossa (fig. 16/2b), symptoms may be more severe.

On examination, a pulsating mass may be noted in an area of injury; associated thrills and systolic bruits are present only when the aneurysmal sac is not filled with clot. Signs of impairment of circulation in the distal segment of limb are minimal or absent, with oscillometric readings and arterial pulsations being normal. This is so because once the lesion is developed and the blood flow at the site of involvement is reestablished, the previous level of efficiency of circulation returns.

Since the traumatic arterial aneurysm is generally associated with so few obvious clinical findings, it is essential to examine all areas of previous trauma very carefully by palpation and auscultation to determine whether the lesion exists. Otherwise, it may remain undetected, a situation fraught with danger for the patient because of the serious complications which may follow such a condition. These include liberation of pieces of clot from the cavity of the sac with occlusion of distal arteries, thrombosis of the aneurysm and segment of vessel from which it arises, occlusion of the accompanying vein due to compression by the mass, pressure on the neighboring peripheral mixed nerves, and internal or external hemorrhage from disruption of the wall of the aneurysmal sac.

Acquired Arteriovenous Fistula. In this condition, both the artery and its accompanying vein have been simultaneously perforated as a result of trauma, thus causing the development of an abnormal communication

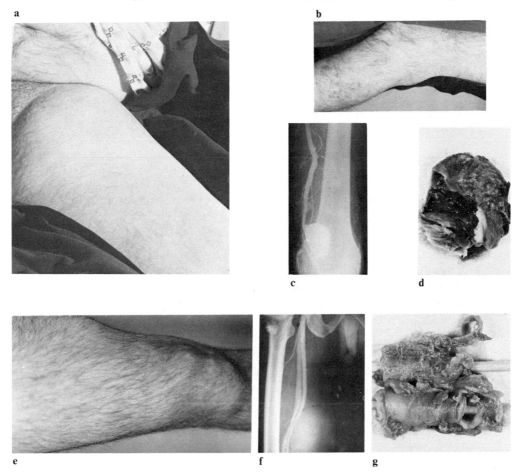

Fig. 16/2. Later complications of vascular injury. **a–d** Arterial aneurysms. **a** Lesion located in femoral artery. **b** Lesion located in popliteal artery. **c** Visualization of a popliteal arterial aneurysm by contrast arteriography. **d** Arterial aneurysmal sac removed at surgery. **e–g** Arteriovenous fistulas. **e** Lesion located in femoral artery. **f** Visualization of fistula by contrast arteriography. Contrast material injected into femoral artery in the groin, with visualization of artery, fistula, and collecting vein. **g** Arteriovenous fistula removed at surgery. Probes inserted in femoral artery and superficial femoral vein. Both segments of vessels are firmly attached to each other with a communication between them.

between them (fig.16/2e, f). The latter may take the form of either a simple direct channel (fig. 16/2g), an aneurysmal dilatation between the two vessels, an aneurysmal sac arising from the artery which, in turn, is joined to the corresponding vein at approximately the same level, or entrance of both vessels into an aneurysmal sac through a single opening. Fracture of a long bone is a common etiologic agent, although other types of trauma, like high-velocity missiles, may also be responsible for the production of the lesion.

As in the case of a congenital arteriovenous fistula (p. 362), the acquired type produces abnormal hemodynamic changes, the severity of which depends upon the caliber of the lumen of the communication and the quantity of arterial blood passing through it to enter the venous circulation. As a consequence, two systemic circulations exist, the one including the fistulous tract having no physiologic function, at the same time that it places a significant load on the heart due to the resulting augmentation in venous return. To accommodate both circulations, there is a large increase in circulating blood volume.

An acquired arteriovenous fistula is associated with several obvious abnormal clinical manifestations. These include a pulsating mass in a site of injury, over which a definite thrill is felt and a continuous bruit, with systolic accentuation, is heard. The latter response is due to the movement of blood through the fistulous tract both during systole and diastole of the heart. However, the greater pressure during the ejection phase causes the more marked intensity of sound during this period of the cardiac cycle. The skin at and above the level of the lesion has a higher than normal temperature because of the increased cutaneous circulation through dilated and varicose superficial veins draining blood from the fistula. The blood pressure in these vessels is almost as high as that in the feeding arterial system, as is the O_2 pressure in the venous blood. The skin temperature of the foot is lower than normal and the arterial pulsations at this site are reduced or absent because most of the blood reaching the limb enters the fistulous tract, since this represents an area of reduced peripheral resistance, and then passes into the superficial venous system. Momentary digital occlusion of the proximal segment of the artery feeding the fistula causes a rise in systemic blood pressure and a reduction in pulse rate (positive Branham's bradycardiac sign), the degree of change reflecting the quantity of blood passing through the open fistulous tract. If the lesion is not treated surgically, eventually congestive heart failure will develop, especially in the older patient.

Compartmental Syndromes of Lower Limbs. These clinical entities all develop as a result of the sudden onset of a severely compromised circulation to structures confined within a closed fascial space. As a consequence of the anatomic barrier, such a situation is responsible for an abrupt rise in local tissue pressure.

The most common entity in this category is *anterior tibial compartmental syndrome,* in which the soft-tissue structures in the anterior tibial compartment in the leg (fig. 16/3) are subjected to the elevated tissue pressure. The chamber is formed by the tibia, the interosseous membrane, the wall of the lateral compartment, and the anterior crural fascia, each structure contributing an unyielding partition. Enclosed in the compartment are the extensor hallucis longus, the extensor digitorum longus, and the tibialis anterior muscles, the anterior tibial artery, its venae comites, and the anterior tibial nerve. The tibialis anterior muscle receives its blood supply only from the anterior tibial artery, whereas the others in the compartment have several sources of circulation.

Trauma to the lower limb is a frequent cause of the anterior tibial compartmental syndrome. Thrombosis or laceration of the superficial femoral artery, of the proximal segment of anterior tibial artery, or of the muscle branches of the latter may all be responsible for the appearance of the syndrome. Unaccustomed severe or, at times, minor physical exercise involving the muscles of the lower limb has also been reported as an etiologic agent [3, 4].

As a result of cessation of blood flow to the soft tissues of the anterior tibial compartment, due to trauma to proximal supplying arteries, swelling of various enclosed structures develops. The resulting increase in tissue pressure further accentuates the existing ischemia which, in turn, causes greater permeability of the capillary wall and a more marked rate of edema formation. The cumulative effect of all these factors leads to loss of viability of the structures in the compartment. Another mechanism which aggravates the situation is superimposed arterial spasm.

The clinical symptoms and signs of anterior tibial compartmental syndrome generally manifest their presence abruptly. An early complaint is sudden severe pain over the muscle mass in the compartment, associated with the appearance of reddish-purple discoloration of the overlying skin and of a rise in the local cutaneous temperature. If the pathologic process continues, the skin becomes glossy and then necrotic and the involved muscles become edematous, hard, and tender on palpation. Plantar flexion of the foot causes an increase in pain. An early finding is loss of pulsations in the lower segment of the anterior tibial artery and in the dorsal pedal artery in the foot, with pulsations in the posterior tibial artery at the ankle remaining unaffected or perhaps somewhat reduced. At the same time, the tissues of the foot continue to appear normal in all regards despite the fact that signs of necrosis are apparent in the structures of the anterior tibial compartment and in the overlying skin. Neurologic findings are common, consisting of weakness of the muscles in the compartment and finally foot drop due to paralysis of the anterior tibial, extensor hallucis longus, and extensor digitorum longus muscles. Inability to dorsiflex the toes is also a common finding. An associated sign is a sensory deficit in the form of anesthesia in the cutaneous distribution of the anterior and deep peroneal nerves.

Besides the anterior tibial compartmental syndrome, pathologic changes in the other compartments of the lower limb may also be noted clinically, but much less frequently. In the case of the *lateral compartmental syndrome,* necrosis of the peroneus longus and peroneus brevis muscles may follow a direct blow to the upper fibular area (fig. 16/3), producing destruction of the nutrient vessels to the muscles. The clinical manifestations of the condition are similar to those of the anterior tibial compartmental syndrome except that they are located on the upper portion of the lateral aspect of the leg and are generally less severe [6].

In the case of the *superficial posterior compartmental syndrome*, the etiologic agent may be either a dissecting popliteal cyst, rupture of a popliteal arterial aneurysm, or a direct blow to the calf muscles. The symptoms and signs, which also resemble those of a mild form of anterior tibial compartmental syndrome, are located on the posterior surface of the leg (fig. 16/3). If there is a marked response, the posterior tibial artery may go into spasm, with loss of pulsations at the ankle. The resulting ischemia may cause secondary contracture of intrinsic plantar musculature of the foot. Direct trauma to the gastrocnemius and soleus muscles, found in the superficial posterior compartment, may be followed by equinus deformities due to contracture of these structures.

Finally, in the case of the *deep posterior compartmental syndrome,* which is rarely observed alone, the etiologic agent is most commonly fracture of the tibia and fibula, usually at the middle or distal third, levels at which nutrient branches to the tibia arise from the posterior tibial artery. Other less frequent causative factors are trauma to soft tissues in the compartment (fig. 16/3), major vein occlusion, injuries about the knee, and fracture of the tibial plateau, ankle, calcaneus, or talus. The most common

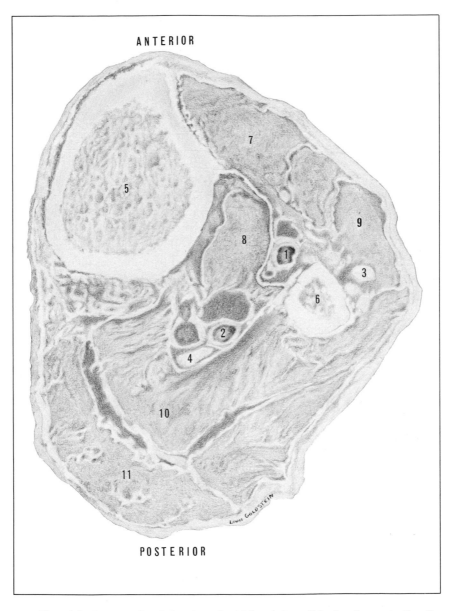

Fig. 16/3. Cross-sectional drawing of middle portion of the leg demonstrating the anatomic relationship of the different compartments to other structures. 1 = Anterior tibial artery; 2 = posterior tibial artery; 3 = peroneal nerve; 4 = tibial nerve; 5 = tibia; 6 = fibula; 7= tibialis anterior muscle; 8 = tibialis posterior muscle; 9 = peroneus longus muscle; 10 = soleus muscle; 11 = gastrocnemius muscle. Reproduced from ref. [2] with permission.

symptom of the syndrome is severe pain locally, with the cardinal signs being plantar hypesthesia in the distribution of the posterior tibial nerve, weakness of toe flexion, pain on passive toe extension, and tenseness of the tissues in the area between the tibia and triceps surae muscle in the distal medial part of the calf [5].

Injury to Major Veins. In about 10% of cases of trauma to main arteries, there is likewise an associated injury to the accompanying veins. Also, at times, a main collecting vein may be damaged whereas the corresponding artery is spared. Although destruction or occlusion of venous components does not have the serious connotation attributed to arterial injuries, still the consequences of such a difficulty may be severe enough to be responsible for loss of viability of a limb with a chronic precarious arterial circulation if there is marked distention of tissues by edema fluid. Ligation of a main vein to control bleeding will frequently be followed by a clinical picture which resembles postphlebitic syndrome with all its disabling manifestations (p. 287). This is particularly true in the case of the popliteal vein [7].

Principles of Therapy for Trauma to Blood Vessels

When injury to main arterial or venous channels in the lower limbs coexists with damage to a skeletal structure, particularly a fracture of a long bone, the question arises as to which abnormality takes precedence in the therapeutic program. One group of workers believes that, because of the relatively great seriousness of allowing a limb to remain in an acute state of ischemia for any period of time without control of the circulatory involvement, this is the initial and chief therapeutic consideration, followed by treatment of the musculoskeletal difficulty. Others, however, are of the opinion that early management of the fracture, as by some type of internal fixation to achieve stabilization, and then institution of a procedure to reestablish local circulation are the proper treatment course. Unfortunately, both approaches have inherent weakness and disadvantages. For example, if the musculoskeletal difficulty is dealt with first, this adds to the period of ischemia of distal tissues which may therefore be critically prolonged, producing irreversible changes in the foot, particularly in nervous elements. At the same time, the orthopedic procedure may contribute to further soft tissue disruption and venous stasis, both of which have serious consequences even to the point of loss of tissue viability. On the other hand, if initially vascular surgery is performed, the subsequent attempt to deal with the musculoskeletal damage must be carried out with the utmost care so as to prevent a second injury to the involved vessel or even disruption of the reconstructive procedure. The only alternative approach which minimizes the above disadvantages is the utilization of a simultaneous cooperative endeavor by two surgical teams, each attacking the problem for which it possesses expertise. Of course, such an ideal situation is rarely practical or feasible because of the complex logistics involved in carrying it out. In any event, before attempting to resolve the major deficits, it is necessary to remove traumatized soft tissues by debridement, control bleeding, and treat hypovolemic shock or hypotension.

Laceration or Severance of Large Vessels. Under these circumstances, it is essential to reestablish local circulation in order to maintain viability of the involved limb. Generally a graft procedure is required for this purpose. If the companion vein is also traumatized, it should be repaired at the same time. Grafts to bridge venous defects are not advisable, since the vessel will usually not remain patent.

Arterial Spasm and Traumatic Arterial Thrombosis. In the case of arterial spasm, the first therapeutic approach is temporary paralysis of vasomotor control over the peripheral artery by means of repeated paravertebral sympathetic blocks. This measure is very effective in removing neurogenic vasospasm, but it has no beneficial action on myogenic vasospasm. For the latter, it is necessary to expose the segment of involved artery surgically and bathe it in myovascular relaxants, such as a warm 2.5% solution of papaverine sulfate or a warm 1% solution of procaine sulfate. If relaxation of the artery does not occur in 10–15 min, the wound should be loosely closed, leaving a fine polyethylene tube in contact with the artery for installations of a 1% solution of papaverine at intervals until circulation is restored. In some instances, the adventitia of the involved artery is stripped (periarterial sympathectomy) if local therapy is ineffective, followed by forcibly stretching the lumen of the vessel with warm saline injected under pressure after the constricted portion is temporarily isolated between bulldog clamps. If none of these procedures is successful in restoring circulation, then transection of the contracted segment of artery should be carried out, after which an end-to-end anastomosis or insertion of a venous graft is performed. The same surgical approach is applicable to traumatic arterial thrombosis, since thrombectomy is almost inevitably followed by re-thrombosis.

Traumatic Arterial Aneurysm and Arteriovenous Fistula. In both these conditions, the lesion should be treated surgically as quickly as is practical, in order to prevent the serious complication associated with them. However, the urgency that exists in regard to the other aforementioned difficulties to bring about normal blood flow immediately does not apply to these two entities. In the case of arterial aneurysm, the usual approach is excision of the lesion (fig. 16/2d) and reestablishment of local circulation either by end-to-end anastomosis or insertion of a segment of venous graft. For the treatment of an acquired arteriovenous fistula, the lesion is also excised (fig. 16/2g) and arterial flow is restored by inserting an autogenous venous graft. End-to-end anastomosis is not attempted because of the high incidence of thrombosis associated with such a procedure. Usually no attempt is made to reestablish venous flow and instead the cut ends of the vein are ligated.

Different Types of Compartmental Syndromes. Therapy for all these conditions is immediate fasciotomy of the entire involved structure to reduce tissue pressure and thus prevent paralysis and necrosis of the affected muscles. Extensive incisions must be made so as to expose the whole compartment, for short ones will generally only result in herniation of the muscles through them, producing strangulation of these structures. Complete decompression of the compartment may be followed by significant return of local circulation. In the case of the anterior tibial compartmental syndrome, if this does not occur, it is then necessary to remove all of the devitalized tissue up to the interosseous membrane and cover the defect with a skin graft. If necrosis of soft tissue is extensive, an above-knee amputation may have to be carried out. In the treatment of the lateral compartmental syndrome, besides early decompression of the compartment, fibulectomy may have to be carried out in some instances.

Vascular Entities Resulting from Trauma to Terminal Blood Vessels

Common Frostbite
Exposure of the lower limbs to low environmental temperatures for protracted periods of time is responsible for the development of several types of cold injuries: common frostbite, high altitude frostbite, trench foot, immersion foot, and acute and chronic chilblains (acute and chronic per-

nio). Since the entity observed most often in a podiatric practice is common frostbite, the present section is devoted solely to a discussion of this clinical disorder.

Etiologic Factors. Common frostbite is a thermal injury which is produced by ambient temperatures that are much below freezing (–17.8°C or less; 1°F or less). The presence of wind velocity tends to exaggerate loss of body heat and to magnify the detrimental effect of the cold. Impairment of local circulation (p. 138) also contributes to more rapid development of the cold injury, as well as poor nutrition and physical inactivity.

Pathogenesis. The first effect of exposure of the skin of the lower limbs to extreme cold is marked and protracted vasoconstriction of the cutaneous vessels and, to a lesser extent, of those in deeper tissues. The resulting persistent local ischemia is further aggravated by the cessation of oxygen exchange which occurs at a low temperature. In the presence of extreme falls in environmental temperature, actual solidification of fluid and tissues will occur, with formation of intracellular ice crystals. If the involved limb is now exposed to a physiologic environmental temperature, thawing of tissues will take place, the intense vasoconstriction being replaced by dilatation of the cutaneous arterioles and capillaries resulting from paralysis of the peripheral vasoconstrictor sympathetic fibers (hyperemic stage). As a consequence of the extreme state of ischemia existing in the tissues, due to the absence of arterial inflow into the dilated microcirculation, damage occurs to the capillary endothelium; the resulting greater permeability allows for an increased transudation of fluid and red blood cells into the tissue spaces and the production of swelling of affected structures. The concentration of formed elements in the blood which follows causes sludging in the capillary bed and the development of thrombi formed of agglutinated red blood cells. With cessation of blood flow in the microcirculation, gangrene of tissue ensues (fig. 16/4). Large arteries are also affected by the severe cold, the changes taking the form of early swelling of their walls, vacuolization of the intimal cells, and proliferative alterations.

Clinical Manifestations. The symptoms and signs of common frostbite vary, depending upon the stage of the disease present at the time of the examination. The acute phase, which generally lasts for several weeks after exposure, comprises first the initial period of freezing of tissues, followed by thawing, exudation, and finally necrosis. Very early in the disorder the

patient experiences a sense of numbness, occasionally preceded by a prickling sensation.

Examination of the limb soon after exposure reveals the skin of the foot
and leg to be waxy white and very cold. Then, as thawing occurs and the
hyperemic state develops, the skin becomes red, warm, and swollen, and
blebs and blisters filled with yellow or blood-tinged fluid form. Hemorrhages are noted under the toenails, giving them a black appearance; subsequently many of them so affected will be shed. Arterial pulsations at levels
proximal to the affected segment of limb may be bounding; those in the foot
are generally absent. Necrosis of the skin of the toes may be present, the
depth of involvement depending on the severity of the existing ischemia.
With more protracted exposure to low ambient temperatures, the entire
foot may manifest signs of gangrene affecting deep tissues.

In the subacute stage, demarcation occurs between viable and necrotic
structures (fig. 16/4g) and, during this period, the hyperemic state is
replaced by a return of increased sympathetic tone, as reflected by coldness,
cyanosis or pallor, and hyperhidrosis of the skin of the foot. There may be
some neurologic findings, such as stocking-glove type of sensory loss and
reduction in light touch and fine temperature discrimination in the toes.

In the subacute stage, also, trophic changes become prominent. The
skin appears atrophic and sclerotic, particularly that of the toes. The digital
pulp pads become thinned, the nails develop thickening and irregularities,
and the normal wrinkling over interphalangeal joints is lost, due to firm
adherence of the skin to the underlying tissues. Another common finding is
epiphysial destruction in the distal and middle phalanges, with shortening
of the involved bone.

The findings in the final or chronic stage consist primarily of rigidity of
the foot, ankylosis of the phalangeal joints, and progression of the abnormal
processes already present in the toes. Necrotic tissue is no longer present,
having been previously removed by debridement or surgery. Signs of vasospasm are less or may no longer be present. Raynaud's syndrome may now
appear on exposure to cold, and there may be an increased sensitivity of the
toes to cold or other noxious stimuli. Also, there may be pain originating in
the areas of scarring, as well as in the leg.

Therapy. Considerable controversy exists regarding the treatment program for the early stage of common frostbite. In general terms, it can be
stated that at no time should the limb be overheated in order to bring about
thawing, the highest level of water temperature for immersion of the foot

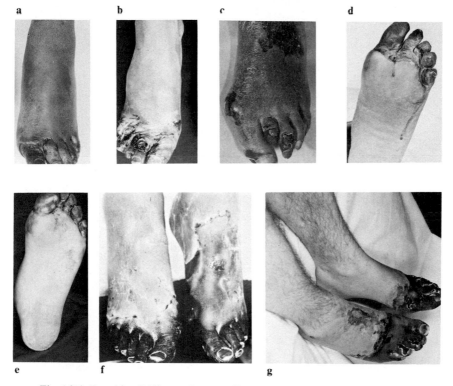

Fig. 16/4. Frostbite. Different degrees of involvement of the toes and foot proper.

being less than or equal to body temperature. Rapid rewarming appears preferable, provided the pain can be controlled with narcotics. The value of attempts to remove increased vasomotor tone by means of sympathetic blocking agents, lumbar paravertebral sympathetic blocks or, on occasion, even lumbar sympathectomy, has not as yet been unequivocally determined. Nor has the early intravenous administration of heparin, for the purpose of preventing agglutinative thrombi from forming in the capillary bed, been accepted.

Regardless of the means used to cause thawing of exposed tissues, in every case the limb should be carefully cleansed with a mild antiseptic, cotton pledges should be placed between the toes to absorb fluid from ruptured blebs or blisters, and then the limb should be covered with sterile dressings and placed in some type of cradle so as to prevent the bedclothes from resting on the foot. Tetanus-toxoid booster or tetanus antitoxin is administered. To prevent local infection, a course of wide-spectrum antibiotic is given. Most importantly, early institution of a rehabilitative program is imperative in order to control rapidly forming ankylosis and contracture of the ankle and foot and atrophy of small muscles. This is initiated even in the presence of bleb formation and necrotic tissue, conditions which would ordinarily be considered a contraindication to such a therapeutic approach. Each joint should be placed through a full range of motion a number of times every hour during the entire day, the exercises being carefully supervised.

In most instances surgical removal of necrotic structures should be delayed until clear-cut demarcation has occurred; otherwise, deeply located viable structures, covered by superficial necrotic tissue, may also be inadvertently removed in the process. Once debridement has been completed and healing is occurring in the operative sites, the rehabilitative program is intensified. Ambulation is increased, with emphasis being placed on a proper stance and gait.

Fat Embolism

Although fat embolism may be a complication of a variety of unrelated medical conditions, its primary etiologic agent is trauma, particularly to the long bones of a limb. Because of the associated high morbidity and mortality, it may untowardly influence the prognosis of the underlying primary difficulty. For this reason, it is essential to be alerted to such a possibility at all times, so as to be in a favorable position to institute immediate therapy for its control. The present section deals primarily with fat embolism which is the result of trauma.

Incidence. Fat embolism is most commonly found in persons in the second and third decades of life, when long-bone fractures are frequent, and in the sixth and seventh decades, when the incidence of fractures of the hip is high.

Pathogenesis. Two major theories have been proposed to explain the mechanism responsible for liberation of fat particles into the blood stream. In one, the *mechanical concept,* it is postulated that fat in the bone marrow of a fractured long bone is subjected to disruption of its cellular envelope by the grinding action of bony spicules and trabeculae. As a consequence, the free particles enter the tissue spaces and then the lumen of injured local veins. The fact that the latter vessels in the haversian canal of bone are prevented from collapsing by the surrounding osseous tissue facilitates movement of fat emboli into them and then into the systemic venous system. By this means, the particulate matter reaches the pulmonary vascular tree, where it is trapped in the capillary bed, thus causing mechanical blockage of the microcirculation. As a result, resistance to pulmonary blood flow is increased and pulmonary artery pressure rises, the latter response causing dilatation and strain on the right ventricle. With persistence of the abnormal situation in lung capillaries, lipase present in the pulmonary tissues produces hydrolysis of the neutral fat particles into glycerol and free fatty acid, substances which have an injurious action on the bronchial and bronchiolar tissues. Moreover, they are responsible for disruption of alveolar-capillary membranes. As a consequence of these effects, curtailment of surfactant activity, edema formation, hemorrhage, and alveolar collapse follow. Also contributing to a reduction in pulmonary function is adhesion of large numbers of platelets to the fat emboli. The aggregations then break down, with release of serotonin, a substance which has vasoconstrictor and bronchoconstrictor properties.

If liberation of the fat particles is extensive and if the ability of the pulmonary bed to contain them is surpassed, systemic embolization will follow. The resulting marked rise in pulmonary artery pressure elongates the pliable fat particles and forces them through the capillaries and venules into pulmonary veins and then into the systemic arterial circulation. There they are again arrested in terminal capillary beds, but this time in the brain, kidneys, liver, and skin, with the development of local ischemia in the involved organs.

The second view regarding the pathogenesis of fat embolism, the *physiochemical concept,* has relevance mainly to the type associated with some form of medical condition, with trauma playing no role as an etiologic agent. The hypothesis is based on the assumption that certain metabolic changes develop, mediated through physiochemical means, which cause alteration of the normal lipids in blood by a yet unexplained mechanism. As a result, there is an increased tendency for the small emulsified chylomicra to coalesce and form fat droplets large enough to block the pulmonary capillary bed.

Clinical Manifestations. Symptoms and signs of fat embolism generally develop within a few hours after an injury, although in some instances they may be delayed for as long as 4 days. The usual sequence of events consists of a period of early lucidity following the accident and then the appearance of clinical manifestations, the seriousness of which may vary markedly. In the fulminating type, associated with multiple injuries, the diagnosis of fat embolism is frequently made only after a postmortem examination. In the case of a mild episode, this possibility may not even be considered because the clinical pattern may be unclear. Moreover, the character of the symptoms and signs is also significantly influenced by the organ or organs affected.

The onset of fat embolism usually begins suddenly with a rise in temperature between 38.5 and 39°C (101.3 and 102.2°F), a rapid heart rate to as high as 140 bpm, and increased respirations to 30–50 per min. Central venous pressure generally is elevated, whereas systemic blood pressure may be unchanged or even reduced.

If the pulmonary vascular bed is the sole site of embolization, such respiratory responses as stertorous breathing, dyspnea, cough, wheezes, and rales at the bases of the lungs may be present, the physical findings being similar to those observed in pulmonary embolism (p. 265).

With entrance of fat emboli into the systemic arterial system, the clinical manifestations (besides those due to pulmonary pathology) will now include symptoms and signs originating in the involved peripheral organ or organs. In most instances cerebral changes predominate, the patient developing disorientation, drowsiness, obstreperousness, confusion, and, less often, delirium, coma, and decerebrate rigidity. Associated with such findings may be abnormal pupillary reflexes, spasticity, incontinence, and convulsions. If death occurs, it is usually due to a state of irreversible shock. The clinical manifestations of cerebral fat embolism may, in part, be due to inadequate oxygenation of the blood in the blocked pulmonary vascular bed and, in part, to the local hypoxia which is a consequence of fat embolization to the cerebral capillary bed.

Besides the cerebral vascular tree, involvement of the capillary beds in the kidneys and liver may also produce significant manifestations. Although the renal glomeruli are frequently the site of extensive embolization, rarely is this type of change sufficient to cause early clinical renal failure. Nevertheless, in the patients who have recovered from the disorder, evidence of impaired kidney function may be noted.

A brown petechial rash is a common diagnostic finding in fat embolism, the change being observed on the second or third day after the trauma is sustained. The lesions may be as small as 1 mm in diameter and are frequently overlooked. They are found primarily in the skin on the upper part of the body, and, less often, the flanks, extending onto the thighs. The rash is transient, with the lesions fading rapidly, to be replaced by new crops appearing elsewhere. The response is probably due to a form of thrombocytopenic purpura and not to mechanical obstruction of cutaneous capillaries by fat emboli.

Diagnostic Procedures. Certain laboratory tests are helpful in making the diagnosis of fat embolism. For example, there is a significant decrease in the blood hemoglobin level early in the disease. Also, in half the cases, fat is noted in the urine. Arterial blood gases (PO_2 and PCO_2) are useful in determining the degree of existing hypoxia. The electrocardiogram may show signs of acute right heart strain, and X-ray findings in the chest may consist of patchy, fluffy infiltrates of various degrees of severity. Fundoscopic examination may reveal refractile bodies within retinal vessels, due to local fat embolism.

Differential Diagnosis. In the differentiation of fat embolism, such possibilities as intracranial bleeding, chronic alcoholism, cardiac injury, and pulmonary embolism must be considered and eliminated. If a lucid, detailed clinical history is available, this is of considerable value in arriving at the proper diagnosis. The tests listed above are also very helpful in this regard.

Therapy. The first approach to the treatment of fat embolism is its prevention. This involves care and minimum manipulation of the fracture, splinting of the limb if transportation is being considered, and definitive reduction and immobilization of the fracture as soon as feasible. Other proposed prophylactic measures are intravenous administration of hypertonic glucose solution, of dextrose-alcohol mixtures, and of heparin.

Active therapy for fat embolism consists of general measures, such as maintenance of an airway, resuscitation from shock, and the parenteral administration of fluids. Oxygen therapy should be given aggressively, using either a mask, an endotracheal or cuffed tracheotomy tube, or assisted respiration, in order to attempt to control the severe arterial hypoxia. Dextran 40 has also been proposed as therapy since this medication has a beneficial effect upon the rate of perfusion through the microcirculation, at the same time that it reduces intravascular aggregation of red blood cells. Finally, when other programs have failed, high dose steroid administration should be utilized, but only in the case of the severely ill patient.

Vascular Entities Resulting from Trauma to Nonvascular Structures

Included in the category of functional vascular entities initiated by trauma to a lower limb is a group of conditions designated as post-traumatic painful vascular disorders. As the term implies, these diseases are typified by the presence of pain as the predominant finding, overshadowing other symptoms and signs of sympathetic nervous system imbalance. This section is limited to a discussion of the two most common of these conditions: major causalgia and post-traumatic vasomotor disorders. In both conditions, the precipitating factor is trauma to soft tissues and not directly to vascular structures.

Major Causalgia

Major causalgia is a vasospastic disorder typified by agonizing, burning pain and extensive trophic changes in the involved limb. It is found in about 2% of patients with injury to, but not total transection of, peripheral nervous elements, such as the popliteal and posterior tibial nerves in the case of the lower limbs.

Etiologic Factors. In most instances, the disorder develops following penetrating wounds, although a fracture, crush injury, contusion, or subcutaneous or intramuscular injection of a drug may also be the precipitating agent.

Pathogenesis. The actual mechanism responsible for the manifestations of major causalgia is not fully understood. The theory which has received experimental and clinical support presupposes that there is a short-circuiting effect in the region of the injured segment of peripheral nerve which permits direct stimulation of sensory components in the nerve by the continuous flow of sympathetic discharges. As a result, the sensory afferent impulses initiated by the process are transmitted to the thalamus where they are interpreted as pain. Another view is that the artificial synapse located at the site of the injury sets up impulses which travel to the distal segment of involved limbs where they cause liberation of neurokinin, responsible for the burning pain characteristic of the disease. It has also been proposed that infection in the wound or an irritable focus triggered by the trauma initiates and perpetuates an exaggerated state of activity in the spinal cord. There is no question that the superimposed state of disuse of the involved limb, resulting from fear that its movement would markedly increase pain, also contributes to the physical findings. It has been suggested that an underlying personality trait may exist, which makes some individuals more likely candidates for the disorder.

Clinical Manifestations. The findings associated with major causalgia may develop several days after the patient has sustained an injury to a limb or, on occasion, there may be a delay of weeks or even months. As already indicated, the most typical finding in this disorder is the continuous burning, violent pain in the foot, particularly the toes or sole. Emotional excitation may provoke exacerbations of the symptom, as well as changes in environmental conditions and cutaneous contact with such objects as the bedclothes or drafts of air. The pain generally begins in the site of injury and spreads over the entire limb. To minimize the symptom, the patient assumes a protective habitus in regard to the affected extremity. If no attempt is made to encourage movement of the limb, the skin becomes shiny, red, thin, and glossy, with normal wrinkling disappearing as firm adherence to underlying tissues occurs. The muscles become atrophied and immovable and the joints become ankylosed. Changes take place in the density of the bones in the involved limb, in the form of slight generalized loss of constituents or of the characteristic moth-eaten appearance of advanced osteoporosis. In the later stage, signs of increased sympathetic tone are noted, including low skin temperature, increased responsiveness to cold, cyanosis of the toes, and hyperhidrosis. Finally, with prolonged maintenance of the limb in dependency, edema develops. In many patients, the stage of exaggerated sympathetic tone is preceded by a vasodilator phase, during which the limb is temporarily warm and well colored, indicating that local blood flow is increased. It is in this period, that the typical burning pain first develops.

Therapy. Prophylaxis is the first approach to the management of major causalgia. This involves immediate treatment of any local injury which could possibly act as a precursor to the development of the condition and its perpetuation. In this regard, the wound should be debrided, foreign bodies removed, injured soft tissue structures repaired, hematomas evacuated, and fractures reduced and immobilized. In the presence of an acute strain, it may be necessary to infiltrate any existing hematoma with procaine or even to perform a regional block to control the pain. Injured peripheral nerves should be exposed surgically and a neurolysis performed after removing all traumatized soft tissues. These steps should then be followed by excision of the damaged section of nerve and end-to-end suture performed. Fear and anxiety should be allayed by reassurance and explanation of the various measures carried out.

Once major causalgia has developed, the initial therapeutic program consists of instituting a series of exercises for the involved limb. However, before this can be accomplished, it is necessary to control the severe pain present even at rest. This goal may require the administration of large doses of narcotics, steroids, or anti-inflammatory drugs as a preliminary step. Repeated electric stimulation of the large A-delta fibers running in the injured peripheral nerve proximal to the site of injury is frequently effective in blocking afferent pain impulses. The procedure is performed for periods of 2–3 min and may give relief for several hours. Also of value is perineural infusion of the trigger areas with lidocaine (Xylocaine). This is carried out by passing a large-bore needle through surgically prepared anesthetic skin, inserting a flexible catheter through it, removing the needle, and leaving the catheter in place. Then the area is exposed to injections of 0.5 ml of 0.5% lidocaine with ephedrine or epinephrine every 3 h for several weeks. The procedure anesthetizes only the sensory fibers in the peripheral nerve. Blocking of the tibial and/or deep or common peroneal nerves with a local anesthetic has also been found to be effective in controlling the pain.

If swelling is present in the affected limb, this must be eliminated before the exercise program is initiated. The patient is placed at complete bedrest with the foot of the bed elevated until the edema disappears and then he is given some type of elastic support provided he is able to tolerate the application of pressure to the limb. As adjunctive therapy, he is placed on a salt-poor diet and given a diuretic (furosemide [Lasix]). Splinting of the foot while the patient is at bedrest has also been utilized.

With control of the pain and the swelling, the next step is initiation of the physical therapeutic program. This involves primarily attempts to make the patient ambulatory, first with crutches and canes, but discarding them as soon as feasible. Weight bearing on the involved limb is encouraged, as well as the assumption of a proper gait, with distribution of body weight equally between the two lower limbs. Early ambulation can also be initiated in a pool, since the buoyancy of the water tends to reduce the load placed on the affected lower extremity and, hence, the severity of the pain produced by walking.

Since vasospasm is almost invariably present in the later stage of acute major causalgia, it is advisable to attempt to control and eliminate this state by means of repeated lumbar paravertebral sympathetic blocks. A sign of the beneficial effect of this measure is a progressively increasing duration of relief from pain with each subsequent injection, lasting longer than the anticipated period of sympathetic ganglionic anesthesia. If such a response occurs, there is a good possibility that a series of daily injections may result in permanent destruction of the existing abnormal reflex arc and hence recovery from the condition. On the other hand, if after a week of daily paravertebral sympathetic blocks, there are no signs of alleviation of symptoms, the procedure should be terminated. Other means for the removal of abnormal vasomotor tone are the use of alpha-receptor blocking agents, such as phenoxybenzamine (Dibenzyline) and, on occasion, lumbar sympathectomy.

Post-Traumatic Vasomotor Disorders
(Sudeck's Atrophy; Reflex Sympathetic Dystrophy)

Post-traumatic vasomotor disorders, also termed Sudeck's atrophy, reflex sympathetic dystrophy, acute atrophy of bone, and post-traumatic edema, among others, can be described as a reflex condition initiated by local tissue damage. Its development may first be noted weeks after the precipitating tissue injury was sustained, at a time when subsidence of symptoms arising from the latter would be expected.

Etiologic Factors. No one type of agent causing the initial tissue damage is responsible for the subsequent development of the post-traumatic vasomotor disorder. In fact, the appearance of the latter is unrelated to the extent and nature of the original injury and to whether it was treated properly. The condition may follow such a variety of etiologic agents as soft tissue wounds, sprains, crushing injuries, simple or compound fractures of small or large bones, or infection.

Pathogenesis. It is generally accepted that the mechanism responsible for the initiation of the condition is a reflex arc (triggered by the original local tissue damage), consisting of components of the peripheral sympathetic nervous system as its efferent limb. Following trauma, there is evidently overactivation of the central nervous system cell stations, resulting in hyperactivity of a sympathetic nervous system reflex arc. As a consequence, bombardment of impulses sets up a vicious cycle of reflexes which spread in all directions over the spinal cord, a constant circling of activity across the synapses perpetuating the various reflexes. Because of involvement of sympathetic motor neuron cells in the lateral horn of the cord, vasospasm develops, this state being responsible for vascular spasm of the microcirculation. The resulting increase in filtration pressure in this portion of the vascular tree causes the formation of local edema (fig. 16/5a), aided by raised capillary permeability due to capillary wall ischemia. Other impulses initiated by the reflex arc ascend the thalamic tract in the cord, causing an increase in severity of the pain.

Clinical Manifestations. Usually the condition is ushered in by the sudden development of severe throbbing or burning, unrelenting pain in the involved foot, primarily present during weight bearing or other types of physical exertion. In addition, there may be local tenderness and hyperesthesia. At times the onset may be insidious, with the pain being dull, aching, and diffuse in its distribution.

In the early phase of post-traumatic vasomotor disorders, a stage of reactive hyperemia is present, with the skin being red, hot, and dry. Pulses are bounding and oscillometric readings are high. This is then replaced by a state of vasospasm, reflected in reduced amplitude of pulsations, decreased oscillometric readings, low cutaneous temperature, cyanotic rubor of the skin, and hyperhidrosis. Atrophy of skin, subcutaneous tissue, underlying muscles, joint structures, and bones then appears, together with the development of edema, a constant early finding (fig. 16/5a). Ridges are noted on the toenails.

As in the case of major causalgia (p. 327), the patient first assumes a guarded rigidity of the affected limb for fear of eliciting pain on movement, with the result that atrophy of structures due to disuse is also introduced into the clinical picture. Later, after trophic changes have developed, mechanical alterations in the joints permanently prevent return of function.

A characteristic finding in post-traumatic vasomotor disorders is the early appearance of extensive changes in bone density as determined by radiographic examination. These consist of spotty and cystic decalcification (patchy bone atrophy, osteoporosis) in the foot and ankle, associated with local pain. Later, a more diffuse process supervenes, resembling the generalized ground-glass appearance of disuse. Once the changes develop in bone, return to a normal state may be markedly delayed, despite adequate therapy for the return of function to the limb.

Therapy. For the most part, the physical therapeutic program described for major causalgia (p. 327) applies equally well as treatment for post-

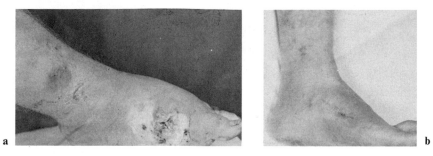

a   b

Fig. 16/5. Post-traumatic vasomotor disorders. **a** Massive edema of left foot and ulceration at site of soft tissue injury, resistant to conservative therapy. **b** Same limb following lumbar sympathectomy. Reproduced from ref. [1] with permission.

traumatic vasomotor disorders. The most important step is early institution of measures to restore normal function to the affected lower extremity. At times, a lumbar sympathectomy is required for the treatment of an indolent lesion (fig. 16/5b). As a general rule, improvement with therapy occurs slowly, and, hence, it is advisable for the patient to be made aware of such a possibility.

References

1   Abramson, D.I.: Diagnosis and treatment of peripheral vascular disorders (Hoeber-Harper, New York 1954).

2   Abramson, D.I.; Miller, D.S.: Vascular problems in musculoskeletal disorders of the limbs (Springer, Berlin 1981).

3   Carter, A.B.; Richards, R.L.; Zachary, R.B.: The anterior tibial syndrome. Lancet *ii:* 928 (1949).

4   Kennedy, J.C.; Roth, J.H: Major tibial compartment syndromes following minor athletic trauma. Am. J. Sports Med. *7:* 201 (1979).

5   Matsen, F.A.; Clawson, D.K.: The deep posterior compartmental syndrome of the leg. J. Bone Jt Surg. *57A:* 34 (1975).

6   Reszel, P.A.; Janes, J.M.; Spittell, J.A., Jr.: Ischemic necrosis of the peroneal musculature, a lateral compartment syndrome: report of case. Proc. Staff Meet. Mayo Clin. *38:* 130 (1963).

7   Sullivan, W.G.; Thornton, F.H.; Baker, L.H.; et al.: Early influence of popliteal vein repair in the treatment of popliteal vessel injuries. Am. J. Surg. *122:* 528 (1971).

17 Treatment-Related Vascular and Nonvascular Complications

Metabolic and Cardiovascular Effects of Prolonged Bed Rest and of Immobilization of a Limb

Although a protracted period of bed rest or of immobilization of a limb in a plaster cast is frequently an essential part of a therapeutic program, it is necessary to point out that both measures may at the same time be responsible for the development of serious adverse systemic reactions and abnormal changes in the tissues of the lower limbs, as well as elsewhere. This section deals with such consequences.

Deconditioning

The anatomic, chemical, physiologic, and psychologic changes in the body elicited by prolonged and strict bed rest or, to a lesser extent, by immobilization of a limb have been studied from several different aspects. The conclusions reached support the view that there is unquestionably a resultant deleterious response to such a situation, as reflected in extensive alterations in a number of vital processes. The different untoward effects, noted in virtually all organs of the body, have collectively been termed deconditioning. This state can be explained in the light of the concept that the functional capacity of any living tissue is related, within physiologic limits, to the intensity and frequency of its activity, with a decline in vital processes following physical and mental inactivity.

Changes in Metabolic Processes. It has been conclusively shown that prolonged bed rest produces cellular damage and abnormal alterations in metabolism. Within several days after development of such a state, a negative nitrogen balance develops, indicating that catabolism or endogenous tissue breakdown has been accelerated, despite maintenance of an adequate protein intake. In a normal subject experimentally placed on strict bed rest, there are losses of from 1 to 3.5 g of nitrogen per day, with a subsequent period of 7 weeks of physical activity required to regain the amount of nitrogen excreted during a similar interval of physical inactivity. In a patient with an abnormality requiring therapeutic bed rest, the loss of protein from the body during such a period is even greater. The site in both normal and abnormal individuals primarily depleted of nitrogen is voluntary muscle (p. 336). Of interest in this regard is the reported pronounced reduction in oxygen uptake during maximal physical stress noted in the deconditioned individual [31].

Among other metabolic abnormalities elicited by prolonged bed rest is a negative sodium balance, indicating involvement of the extracellular fluid. Potassium content of the body remains fairly stable. (For systemic and local changes in calcium and phosphorus contents elicited by immobilization of a limb or by bed rest, see p. 335.)

Changes in Cardiovascular Mechanisms

The most striking cardiovascular effect of complete bed rest is a pronounced decrease in stroke volume and cardiac output during upright and supine exercise [31]. The increase in heart rate under such circumstances is also significantly greater than that found in the control period. Such alterations indicate a progressive deterioration in cardiovascular performance. Even at rest, a similar type of change is noted. For example, the basal pulse rate shows a rise which averages approximately 0.5 beats/day of bed rest, and the heart demonstrates a 17% reduction in volume and a 7% decrease in transverse diameter developing over a relatively short period of bed rest.

A striking change with best rest is also observed in the vasomotor response to standing (as tested on the tilt table), which is a reflection of impairment of the autonomic (mainly sympathetic) control of the peripheral circulation in the lower limbs and splanchnic region. The marked reduction in vasomotor tone becomes manifest in the form of extensive pooling of blood, particularly in the relaxed superficial veins, with the result that venous return to the heart and systolic discharge are significantly reduced. Hence, there is a decreased cerebral blood flow responsible for the development of cerebral ischemia, not infrequently producing fainting when the patient first attempts to stand upright. Contributing to the development of such an unphysiologic state (orthostatic hypotension) are poor tone in the musculature of the lower limbs and malnutrition causing a decrease in elasticity of the different tissues. All of these factors tend to reduce the efficiency of those mechanisms which normally operate to move blood proximally out of the veins in the lower limbs against hydrostatic pressure.

Because of the resulting reduction in venous return to the heart in the deconditioned person, placing him on a tilt table at an angle of 68° will cause an average increase in pulse rate of 38 bpm over that observed in the supine position. This is in contrast to a rise of only 13 bpm obtained from the same individual before deconditioning was initiated. At the same time, the average systolic blood pressure reading obtained from him in the upright position falls an average of 14 mm Hg below that of the supine value, compared with no change observed under similar circumstances in the previous control period.

Changes in Nervous System and Mental Processes

As a result of limitation of activity during a period of bed rest, there is a significant alteration in sensory input, especially proprioceptive impulses which are responsible for regulating neuromuscular performance. Hence, when the individual first begins to ambulate, he may find that he is unsteady on his lower limbs.

Lack of mental stimulation, a state commonly present during periods of bed rest, has, as a consequence, progressively decreasing cerebration. However, such a situation can be counteracted by planned intellectual stimulation. Whether emotional responses develop will depend upon the personality of the subject at bed rest and the degree of sensory deprivation. Some individuals may become depressed, anxious, insecure, and dependent, whereas others may manifest aggressive behavior and hostility. Complaints of discomfort without basis and changes in sleep patterns may also develop. Some individuals, on the other hand, have no difficulty accepting the uncomfortable and unpleasant situation philosophically. As a general rule, the severity of the symptoms has a direct relationship to the length of bed rest.

Changes in Joints and Associated Structures.

With bed rest, significant reduction in range of motion may quickly develop in the joints of the lower extremities. Normally, connective tissue binds the cells and organs together in a structural relationship which is then temporarily altered by the stresses associated with body motion. However, during a period of bed rest, the stresses and strains of body motion are markedly reduced and, as a consequence, the opposing action of the connective tissue is practically in balance with these forces, so that little deformation of the structural relationship develops.

When physical activity is limited, impairment of mobility and flexibility of the connective tissue of the joints of the limbs rapidly results. Dense connective tissue replaces the loose meshwork of randomly oriented areolar fibers found around joint capsules, in the subcutaneous tissue, and in the muscular planes. As a result, there is a loss of motion of the joints within a few days. The response is particularly marked in those of the lower limbs, which are adversely affected by the strong muscles and heavy connective tissue in close proximity.

Changes in Immobilized Limb. Comparable vascular changes have been reported during experimental immobilization of a limb in animals. For example, within 2 weeks after application of a cast, the synovial tissue is found to be distinctly paler than that on the control side [23]. Following a longer period, the microcirculation demonstrates a generalized reduction in caliber of vessels, with a decrease in the number of capillary plexuses in the innervated synovial tissue layer.

Changes in Bone Minerals (Disuse Osteoporosis; Immobilization Osteoporosis). Immobilization of a lower limb of a human subject, as by a cast, may produce extensive chemical changes in the constituents of affected bones, especially those that are weight-bearing. Also responsible for such abnormalities, but to a lesser degree, is a prolonged period of complete bed rest. Under both sets of conditions, urinary calcium excretion becomes elevated, fecal excretion of calcium increases, and mean calcium balances become negative. In fact, the measured calcium loss during a protracted period of bed rest may average 4.2% of the estimated total body calcium [10]. The changes in phosphorus excretion and in phosphorus balance patterns are similar to those observed in the case of calcium. Urinary hydroxyproline and pyrophosphate are mildly elevated. The large loss of osseous mineral is identified using gamma ray transmission scanning [10]. In the case of the os calcis, there may be a decreased mass in the central portion of the bone which ranges from 25 to 45%. All of the described alterations appear to be reversible after initiation of an ambulation program.

The changes observed in bone with complete bed rest cannot be readily explained, for the cause may be multiple. Loss of the beneficial response to stress on standing may certainly contribute to resorption of bone. Poor appetite, frequently associated with prolonged bed rest, may result in deficient dietary calcium intake [8] and thus also play a significant role. Or there may be gastrointestinal absorptive mechanisms which become defective under such conditions. As a result, bone resorption must supply the necessary calcium to maintain body balance.

In the case of immobilization of a lower limb in a cast for a protracted period, there is no question that the loss of stress on the bone from the weight of the body or from the pull of contracting muscles is responsible, in great part, for the chemical changes that follow. Because the various stimulating mechanisms are not operating, there is a decrease in activity of osteoblasts, leading to an increase in bone resorption and production of a negative calcium balance [20] (see above) and the development of the typical findings of disuse osteoporosis.

In animals, immobilization osteoporosis has been found to develop only when the parathyroid and thyroid glands are intact. Prior removal of one or both of these structures prevents bone loss in the limb immobilized in a plaster cast [6]. Such results suggest that a local factor produced by disuse may increase the sensitivity of bone to normal circulating levels of thyroid and parathyroid hormones in the blood [6]. When the limbs of normal animals are immobilized, bone resorption or increased bone turnover causes a change in blood metabolites as evidenced by a rise in PCO_2 and a fall in pH of bone blood. Also, inactivated limbs demonstrate proliferation of osseous tissue and hypervascularization and, at the same time, bone atrophy is present [12].

Immobilization osteoporosis is generally most marked in sites distal to a fracture. The more prolonged the immobilization, the more prominent do the body changes become. The rate of development of the abnormality is more rapid than is the case for the postmenopausal or the senile type of osteoporosis. At first there are changes in calcium and phosphorus in the serum, but later these no longer occur.

Difficulty is encountered in making an early roentgenographic diagnosis of osteoporosis because of the fact that a minimum of 25% and a maximum of 50% of the calcium have to be lost from the bone before this state can be identified on the X-ray film. The typical findings of disuse osteoporosis are a reduction of density, blurring of trabeculae, and thinning of bone cortex.

Changes in Muscle Bulk (Disuse Muscle Atrophy). There is no question that prolonged bed rest or immobilization of a limb produces wasting of muscles in the lower extremities. The rate of change is almost as great as that which follows nerve denervation. The most marked effect is noted in the muscles maintained in the shortened position, as compared with those in the stretched or extended state.

With regard to the vascular responses elicited by immobilization of a limb, however, reported results vary. For example, in one study on animals using microangiography, no changes were noted in the circulation to the muscles of a limb enclosed in a cast for 2 weeks [17]. On the other hand, another investigation demonstrated that blood flow measured with a flow-meter increased under similar circumstances [19]. Comparable results were reported in cats following tenotomy, which produced atrophy of the gastrocnemius, the degree of vascular change being in proportion to the developing muscle atrophy [15]. In man, immobilization of a limb was found to result in the production of less heat locally (as determined by calorimetry) than was noted in the opposite untreated extremity. Such a finding in the treated limb was attributed to a reduction in the formation of vasodilator substances normally produced by muscle activity [16]. From the above, it is apparent that more experimental data must become available before the vascular responses associated with disuse muscle atrophy can be clearly elucidated.

Measures for Prevention of Deconditioning. In patients requiring prolonged bed rest because of a medical condition or the need to recover from an operative procedure, early institution of a rehabilitative program is essential in combatting deconditioning. They should routinely exercise the uninvolved parts of the body to minimize or prevent joint contractures, as well as to inhibit the development of systemic deconditioning. The hips should not be allowed to remain in partial flexion, a position which is often assumed when the patient lies on a soft mattress or is semireclining or sitting. Pillows should never be placed under the knees, since this step causes undesired flexion of such joints and also of the hips. Elevation of the foot of the bed for prolonged periods of time should be discouraged, especially in the elderly patient who may also be suffering from threshold or actual impaired arterial circulation to the lower limbs.

The period of bed rest should be kept to a minimum, and the patient should be permitted out of bed and into a chair and then placed on a graduated ambulation program as soon as feasible. Standing for intervals is useful in establishing the normal stresses on the long bones of the lower limbs and thus help prevent further bony changes observed with bed rest (p. 335). Attempts should be made to counteract the abnormal metabolic changes by placing the patient on a nourishing diet including a large percentage of protein, and his appetite must be psychologically stimulated. Anemia, if present, should be treated.

Decubitus Ischemic Ulcers or Gangrene of the Feet

Even when a normal arterial circulation exists in the lower limbs, persistent bed rest leading to sustained and prolonged pressure over such bony prominences as the two malleoli in the ankle, the lateral border of the foot, and the heel (fig. 17/1a) may lead to ulceration or gangrene at their points of contact with the mattress. In the presence of chronic local arterial insufficiency in patients unable to move independently, this tendency is strikingly increased, with the result that in them, even short periods of compression of the tissues may lead to extensive ulcerations. These are frequently indolent and unresponsive to conservative or surgical management and may eventually require a major amputation. If the patient is fortunate to escape such an outcome, the presence of the lesion may still be responsible for a prolonged period of hospitalization and its associated financial drain, increasing severity of the state of deconditioning and debility, and interference with a necessary rehabilitative ambulation program. In the case of the patient with a spinal cord injury, ischemic ulcerations may even contribute to his death. Many factors have been implicated as etiologic agents in the development of decubitus ischemic ulcer or gangrene of the feet and other portions of the body, but only the three most widely accepted views will be discussed below.

Mechanical Factor. The fact that the usual bony sites for the development of a decubitus ulcer or gangrene in the lower limbs (particularly the feet) are covered only by skin and a small amount of subcutaneous tissue and muscle (or by an almost avascular fat pad, as in the case of the heel) significantly contributes to their greater vulnerability to the formation of such a lesion. The initiating force may be one or more of a number of different agents, including the weight of the limb transmitted to a portion of the foot in direct contact with the mattress or compression of a local segment of skin by a tight cast, a compression bandage, or a brace. Continuous pressure exerted by a contracted lower limb crossed over the other may also be responsible for the development of an ischemic lesion.

The most common and primary etiologic factor rendering a patient susceptible to a decubitus ulcer or gangrene on the lower limb is therefore some type of mechanical force. In all cases, regardless of the precipitating

a b

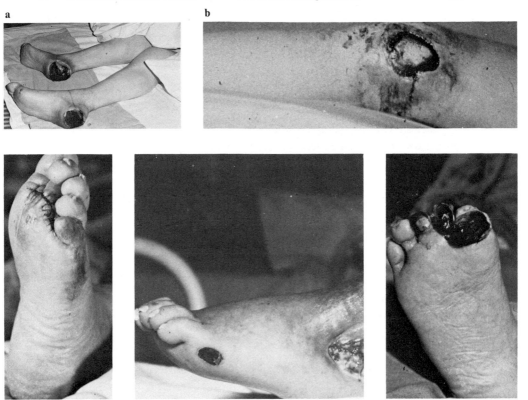

c d e

Fig. 17/1. Nutritional changes produced by various types of mechanical agents. **a** Gangrene of the heels following persistent and prolonged pressure against the mattress in a patient at complete bed rest, unable to move independently. **b** Pressure necrosis and ulceration over the patella due to application of a tight cast to a limb of a 19-year-old female patient with a previously normal local circulation. **c** Necrosis of fifth toe and adjoining portion of the foot following the tight application of an elastic bandage in a patient operated on for removal of a neuroma. **d** Development of a local area of gangrene on the lateral border of the foot following the tight application of an elastic bandage in a patient with a normal local circulation. **e** Gangrene of the great toe and second toe following the subcutaneous injection of a relatively large quantity of procaine as a preliminary step to an operative procedure. Reproduced from ref. [1] with permission.

agent, obliteration of the cutaneous and subcutaneous microcirculations occurs at the point of contact, with the result that the affected tissues begin to suffer from temporary but severe, acute ischemia during the period of application of the compression. Under such circumstances, a minor crack or abrasion of the skin, perhaps initiated by destructive enzymes produced by surface bacteria, will continue to enlarge because of perpetuation of the local ischemic state and the almost inevitable introduction of a superimposed infection, the denuded site acting as a portal of entry for bacteria.

Other contributing factors are friction against the skin supplied by wrinkled or wet bed sheets or coarse linen fibers and the macerating action of sweat, urine, and feces. Also important in this regard are the shearing forces, produced by the sliding of a tissue layer upon one below, as occurs when the patient rubs his feet against the sheets or when he is pulled, pushed, or forcibly moved across the bed. The effect of such movements may be to bend or kink the deeper arteries to the skin, eventually initiating thrombosis in them and necrosis of the overlying skin. All of these mechanisms cannot, by themselves or in combination, cause pressure ulcers, but they do make the patient more vulnerable to the mechanical factor. (For a discussion of the production of ischemic ulceration by the application of rigid casts or tight elastic bandages, see p. 344.)

In support of the above mechanical concept of decubitus ulcer formation is the experimental finding that external pressures of 50–60 mm Hg applied to the skin are enough to arrest all capillary flow, and higher levels (a mean arterial pressure of 100 mm Hg), if prolonged, can cause irreversible damage. Capillaries demonstrate marked instability with application of external pressure. Complete cessation of blood flow into the normal human forearm has been reported with the application of external pressures that were 70 mm Hg less than the subject's mean arterial blood pressure [7]. In this regard, it must be kept in mind that capillary blood pressure varies between 16 and 33 mm Hg [24] and that complete tissue ischemia may be produced by pressures which are greater than these figures if applied to the skin of the feet. Experimental studies have also demonstrated that intense pressure of short duration are at least as injurious to tissues as lower pressures applied for longer periods of time [21].

Neurotrophic Factor. Absence of afferent pain impulses from the foot, as in the case of peripheral neuropathy (p. 120), contributes to the development of decubitus ischemic ulceration. For, under such circumstances, the patient continues to be unaware of the fact that ischemia of tissues is present (because of lack of pain) until his attention is called to this abnormal situation by the appearance of ulcers on the foot or elsewhere. Not only is pain sensation lost but also the normal adaptive cutaneous vascular responses to external pressure, such as axon reflexes which initiate periods of local reactive hyperemia in the skin. Both factors are responsible for prolongation of the ischemic state resulting from mechanical compression of the skin. However, neurotrophic mechanisms only play a secondary role in the development of decubitus ulcers and frequently are absent when they exist.

Metabolic Factor. There is no question that the debilitated patient is much more susceptible to the formation of decubitus ulcers than is the well-nourished individual. As has already been emphasized, bed rest is associated with extensive abnormal changes in the chemistry of the body, including a negative nitrogen, calcium, and phosphorus balance (p. 332), contributing to osteoporosis, wasting of tissues, loss of weight, avitaminosis, and electrolyte imbalance. All of these alterations may play a secondary role in the development of the ischemic lesion, as does anemia, a factor in determining whether cellular hypoxia and necrosis will occur. It is therefore apparent that well-nourished tissue can better tolerate the destructive effects of local mechanical compression leading to ischemia than can tissues of the debilitated patient.

Treatment. The conservative therapeutic management of decubitus ischemic ulcers or gangrene of the lower limbs, for the most part, involves measures to prevent the initiation of such lesions. All of the etiologic factors mentioned above should be controlled or eliminated if possible, especially continuous pressure on weight-bearing sites. If bed rest is required, diligent and meticulous nursing attention in routinely repositioning contact of the lower limbs with the mattress and body care are imperative. Great effort should be made to protect the heel from bearing the weight of the limb and the leg and foot should be prevented from remaining in the everted position for any period of time. Anemia should be corrected and the albumin/globulin ratio in the blood should be maintained at a normal level by a high protein diet or administration of albumin or plasma, together with vitamin supplements.

To compensate for inadequate nursing staff, many substitutes have been offered. These include the use of water beds, special foam mattresses, and viscoelastic devices designed to distribute body weight uniformly and thus reduce or eliminate excessive pressure on bony prominences. Sheep-skin (natural or synthetic) or synthetic gel pads placed on the conventional mattress have also been proposed as protective mechanisms against undue pressure on the surface of the body. Means should likewise be introduced to maintain the skin of the feet and legs in a firm condition and hence more resistant to the deleterious effects of prolonged pressure. The practice of using nylon or rubber sheets over the mattress should be discouraged.

Once an ulcer has developed, it becomes even more important to remove all compression on the skin in the vicinity of the lesion. The actual treatment of the involved area is no different from the approach utilized in the management of other ischemic ulcers or gangrene (p. 145). A recent innovation is the CO_2 laser beam, which vaporizes the necrotic material in an infected decubitus ulcer, leaving a sterile base that can then be covered with a skin graft.

Local Edema Associated with Limb-Cast Application

Swelling of a lower limb is not an uncommon concomitant of a tight or improperly applied limb cast. The response may be noted either during the time the compression exists or immediately afterward, in most instances slowly disappearing on resumption of normal physical activity.

Pathogenesis of Edema Formation. The limb swelling can be attributed to a number of different factors acting singly or in conjunction with each other. One of these is the prolonged period of dependency of the lower limb, eventually producing paralysis or loss of vascular tone in the cutaneous and subcutaneous arterioles, capillaries, and venules. Another is the continuous compression of these vessels by the pressure exerted on the skin by the cast, which has the same effect. The reduction in muscle tone due to the long period of muscle inactivity may also contribute to edema formation by permitting a buildup of local venous hypertension which, in turn, is reflected back into the microcirculation as an elevated capillary filtration pressure. The atrophy of disuse of subcutaneous tissue and voluntary muscle may be responsible for some loss of support for the superficial veins, which likewise allows for a rise to occur in venous pressure. All these forces facilitate the transudation of fluid through the capillary wall into the tissue spaces and the production of edema. An adjunctive mechanism is the increased capillary wall permeability due to a relative state of local ischemia of all tissues, including vascular endothelium, resulting from the compressive action of the cast. Moreover, removal of this force at the end of the treatment period may be responsible for flooding of the paralyzed capillary bed by a large quantity of blood, thus also contributing to a rise in capillary filtration pressure and an acceleration of movement of fluid into the intercellular spaces.

Aside from the compressive effects of the cast on the microcirculation and superficial veins, destruction of thin-walled lymphatics of the limb by the original local trauma may result in the development of hard, nonpitting swelling, generally present around the ankle and on the dorsum of the foot.

It is important, also, to note that there are some patients with an underlying congenital lymphatic deficiency but with no clinical manifestations who may for the first time develop definite lymphedema after a sprain, a strain, or a fracture. This may occur because simultaneous injury of local lymph channels and the casting required for the primary difficulty may collectively produce an overload of the underlying inadequate lymphatic system and hence may now be responsible for the development of clinical lymphedema.

Differential Diagnosis. It is very important to differentiate the edema produced by the mechanisms discussed above from that due to occlusion of a collecting vein, such as the popliteal or iliofemoral vein (p. 260), for the therapeutic approach is entirely different for the two states. Contributing to the problem is the possibility that the original trauma responsible for the need to apply a cast could at the same time have injured the main deep vein. Or the prolonged period of immobilization could have initiated intravascular clotting in such a vessel.

A significant differential point is that if a popliteal or iliofemoral thrombophlebitis develops while the cast is still applied, the buildup of tension in the tissues due to the formation of the edema will cause pain severe enough to require immediate removal of the constriction. Moreover, if edema forms at the time the cast is removed at the prescribed time, the type produced by occlusion of a main collecting vein slowly disappears (in a period of 2 or 3 weeks) and only if proper therapy is immediately instituted (p. 277). On the other hand, the swelling due solely to mechanical forces supplied by compression of tissues by the cast becomes significantly less soon after normal ambulation is resumed. Systemic responses are not noted with its appearance, wherease these are invariably present in the case of popliteal or iliofemoral thrombophlebitis (p. 260).

Iatrogenic Vascular Disorders

Vascular Complications of Foot and Ankle Surgery

Conventional podiatric surgical procedures have not infrequently been responsible for the development of serious vascular complications, including gangrene necessitating major amputation of a lower limb, at times due to inadequate attention to pertinent technical measures. Currently, the incidence of such adverse responses has significantly increased, mainly because of failure to recognize the existence of arterial insufficiency in the foot being subjected to an operation or because of utilization of more heroic measures than warranted or advisable in a limb with normal circulation.

Moreover, there has been a definite trend toward relying heavily upon a recently inserted vascular bypass to deliver an adequate blood flow to a limb with arteriosclerosis obliterans so that a podiatric procedure could presumably now be performed with impunity. The great risk associated with such reasoning is that if the graft should occlude in the immediate postoperative period, there is no possibility for healing of the podiatric-incurred wound. As a result, gangrene will invariably develop in this site, followed by amputation of the limb. Hence, it is imperative to delay the second (podiatric) operation until there is no question that the vascular prosthesis is functioning efficiently and that it will continue to do so for the foreseeable future. Another factor which evidently contributes significantly to the incidence of iatrogenic vascular complications of foot and ankle surgery is that there are a greater number of complex and complicated surgical techniques being attempted at present. (For the various measures and approaches that may help reduce untoward vascular responses to podiatric operative procedures, see p. 356.)

Vascular Trauma following Conservative Therapy or Diagnostic Procedures

Certain nonsurgical therapeutic or diagnostic measures may also be responsible for the development of ischemic ulcerations or gangrene, even in the limb with normal circulation. In the absence of an adequate blood flow, this possibility is markedly exaggerated.

Complications of a Rigid Cast (Tight-Cast Syndrome) or Elastic Bandage. Nutritional lesions may develop on the leg and foot, despite an underlying normal arterial circulation, if a rigid cast or a tight elastic bandage is applied in such a manner as to exert unnecessary and protracted pressure, particularly on skin and subcutaneous tissue overlying bony prominences. Eventually, the resulting persistent ischemia of the structures subjected to such compression is followed by necrosis and the production of an ulcer or an area of gangrene (fig. 17/1 b–d). In the presence of an underlying compromised arterial circulation, the lesion may become so extensive that it can only be treated by major amputation.

Adverse Reactions to Intraarterial and Intravenous Puncture. In an era distinguished by a significant increase in the number of invasive diagnostic procedures carried out on patients in hospitals, there has also been a corresponding rise in the incidence of iatrogenic vascular trauma. Such techniques as angiography and cardiac catheterization may be followed by contusion, laceration, severance, hemorrhage, dissection, spasm, and even thrombosis of the artery utilized in the test. If the injury is extensive, an arterial aneurysm may subsequently develop or an arteriovenous fistula may form if the associated vein is also affected by the trauma.

Among the vessels most often damaged in the course of performing diagnostic procedures is the femoral artery in the groin, since it is superficial and readily accessible. Extravasation of radiopaque material into the tissues of the dorsum of the foot, in the process of carrying out a percutaneous contrast venogram, may result in necrosis of involved tissues, especially if an underlying local arterial insufficiency exists. Such a procedure may also be responsible for extensive venous thrombosis if the contrast material is not adequately washed out of the vessels after termination of the test. A similar response may be noted following the intravenous administration of sclerosing or hypertonic solution. Injection into a superficial vein of powerful vasoconstricting agents, such as norepinephrine (Levophed), for the treatment of shock may also cause marked spasm of all neighboring vessels, with the result that local necrosis of skin may follow.

Inadvertent puncture of arteries in the lower limbs when attempting intravenous administration of drugs may produce almost immediate vascular spasm, thrombosis, and necrosis of the foot. Among those medications reported to produce massive gangrene when accidentally given intraarterially are amphetamine sulfate (Benzedrine sulfate), amobarbital (Amytal), secobarbital, pentobarbital (Nembutal), meperidine hydrochloride (Demerol), chlorpromazine hydrochloride (Sparine), ether, and propoxyphene hydrochloride (Darvon).

The mechanism by which necrosis results from the intraarterial injection of the above medications is not clear. One possibility is that the high concentration of the material elicits chemical injury of small arteries, arterioles, and capillaries, followed by thrombosis of these vessels, ischemia and tissue death. When given intravenously the drugs have no deleterious effect because there is thorough mixing with and dilution by venous blood before they reach the peripheral arterial tree.

Complications of Subcutaneous Administration of Drugs. The local injection of fairly large quantities of anesthetic drugs in high concentrations into the foot to control the pain of surgery may be associated with the development of necrosis of the overlying skin (Fig. 17/1 e). This is especially true if the solution also contains a vasoconstrictor and if the local circulation is precarious. The cause of the nutritional difficulty is evidently marked stretching of the overlying tissues and mechanical obstruction of the microcirculation to the skin and subcutaneous tissue produced by the large amount of fluid injected.

Volkmann's Ischemic Contracture

Volkmann's ischemic contracture, although generally observed in the upper limb, may also be found in the lower extremity following injury to soft tissues or a fracture in the vicinity of the knee. It may also develop after improper use of orthopedic or podiatric appliances, such as the application of tight plaster of Paris casts and constricting bandages.

Pathogenesis. The condition develops when a main artery to the limb is organically obstructed or remains in a state of severe spasm for a considerable period of time. Associated with cessation of blood flow in main channels is the spasm of those vessels on which the collateral circulation depends. Another etiologic agent is direct injury to bellies of muscles in the lower limbs, causing local swelling of these structures within their confining sheaths. As a consequence, tissue pressure will rise rapidly, thus contributing to obstruction to arteriolar inflow and venous drainage and anoxemia of local tissues.

Clinical Manifestations. The symptoms and signs of Volkmann's ischemic contracture appear 2–6 h after the tissues have sustained an injury either locally or to their blood supply. The clinical picture consists of: a deep boring pain in the central calf region which responds poorly to drug treatment, tenderness in the muscles in which infarcts have developed, a sense of numbness in the foot, including the toes, a stocking-glove type of anesthesia, and a gradual swelling of the foot and leg. The local skin becomes cold and pale or cyanotic and arterial pulsations in the foot slowly disappear. Frequently there is paralysis of the deeper muscles of the leg, particularly the flexor hallucis longus. The common finding of nerve damage is due to ischemia and not to compression by fibrosis, the posterior tibial nerve being often so affected.

Treatment. Management of Volkmann's ischemic contracture consists of excision of all irreparably damaged muscle and nerve, followed by such reconstructive procedures as may be required to minimize the deficiencies [32]. However, it is advisable to wait at least 3 or even 6 months for evidence of spontaneous recovery before attempting heroic treatment of the condition. During such a period, the limb should be splinted to minimize contracture, joints should be frequently exercised through a range of motion, and electrical stimulation of muscles should be carried out. A point to consider when treating Volkmann's ischemic contracture is that voluntary muscle fibers affected by necrosis have the power of regeneration, the prognosis depending on the extent and reversibility of the damage.

Tourniquet Injuries
Pneumatic tourniquets are frequently used to provide a bloodless field in which to perform an operative procedure on the foot [4]. However, such an approach is not without risk, for persistent paralysis, acute arterial occlusion, and even loss of a limb have been reported following the use of this simple instrument. Not infrequently, the cause for the appearance of complications following its application has been incorrect pressure-sensing devices in the pressure gauge, resulting in the utilization of much higher than required pressures to achieve the desired effect [13].

Pathogenesis. The basis for the adverse reactions to the application of a tourniquet has not been clearly defined. With regard to the etiology of the post-tourniquet paralysis syndrome producing functional neuromuscular impairment, several views have been advanced. One offers the possibility that the clinical manifestations are the result of direct crushing of peripheral nerves by forces developed by the application of the tourniquet [3, 25, 29]. *Ochoa* et al. [27], in an anatomic study on baboons, found that the segment of nerve compressed by the tourniquet edge pressure demonstrated complete obliteration of the nodal gap and rupture of Schwann cells and organelle. However, it is necessary to point out that the pressures used by these investigators were 2 to 3 times greater than those utilized clinically on patients. Of further interest is the work of *Rudge* [29], who noted that the site of the nerve lesion coincided exactly with the previous location of the tourniquet.

Another view regarding the etiology of tourniquet complications is that the damage to the tissues, including muscles, is caused by indirect metabolic changes stemming from the existing ischemia in the portion of limb distal to the application of the tourniquet [9. 28, 33]. In this regard, there is no question that temporary cessation of arterial blood flow into an extremity is associated with extensive histologic [26], chemical, metabolic, and biochemical alterations. For example, as the period of ischemia is prolonged, tissue PCO_2 continues to rise, the result contributing to a lowering of pH and the production of respiratory acidosis [2]. Such a situation may be responsible for the development of muscle fatigue and a hypocoagulable state [30] leading to postoperative hematoma formation. The associated rapid fall in PO_2 in the limb to below 10 mm Hg causes increased capillary permeability to plasma and protein, thus permitting transudation of fluid into the tissue spaces and the development of edema [35]. Which factor or combination of factors is responsible for the neuromuscular damage has not been determined as yet, although prolonged vascular occlusion with subsequent thrombus formation [22], possibly in vasa nervorum (arterioles supplying peripheral nerves), has been advanced as an etiologic mechanism [28]. Opposed to such a concept, however, is the finding of hypocoagulability during periods of ischemia [30].

That maintenance of a tourniquet pressure for a period of time produces histologic changes in the affected tissues is supported by experimental studies in the rat [18]. Following the application of pressures as low as 100 mm Hg for 1 h, significant histologic alterations were observed in the ischemic muscles about 24 h later. They consisted of cellular infiltration, interstitial capillary hemorrhages, and various stages of cellular degeneration. Gross changes were not noted after periods of application of 100 mm Hg.

Clinical Manifestations. The signs and symptoms of the tourniquet paralysis syndrome [25], one of the most common complications of the use of a tourniquet, result from injury sustained by both sensory and motor fibers in the peripheral mixed nerve. In the milder cases, the motor involvement may manifest itself in the form of difficulty in moving a part. With greater damage to the mixed nerve, frank paralysis may be present, associated with sensory impairment, in the form of absence of position sense, deep pressure, vibration sense, and light touch sensation. Rarely is pain sensation lost and, in fact, hyperalgesia is not uncommon. Generally, the sympathetic fibers in the peripheral mixed nerve are not involved, so that skin color, skin temperature, and sweat and oil gland secretion are normal. With passage of time, there may be some return of motor function and sensation, provided the damage to the peripheral nerve was not too extensive.

Preventive Measures. Obviously, management of tourniquet complications is primarily prophylactic in nature. Of importance in this regard are the positioning of the pressure cuff and protection of the skin which it encompasses. For this purpose, several layers of sheet wadding are wrapped around the circumference of the limb in a smooth and wrinkle-free manner and then the tourniquet is applied over them. As a consequence, the possibility of pinching the skin is minimized.

As a general rule, the compressing cuff is wrapped around the limb at a level of maximum circumference so as to have the greatest amount of soft tissue intervening between the pressure source and the underlying vulnerable neurovascular structures [2]. In the case of the lower extremity, the ideal location is the proximal portion of the thigh which, infortunately, has the disadvantage of eliciting definite pain, especially in nervous subjects. However, the symptom can be controlled by adequate premedication. Preliminary facilitation of venous drainage by application of an expressing bandage has been suggested as a means of raising the pain threshold [11]. When local anesthesia or local intravenous sedation is being used, ankle tourniquets may be employed since they are more readily tolerated by the patient.

At no time should a tourniquet be placed so that pressure is applied directly over the common peroneal nerve in its subcutaneous course or around the upper part of the leg in the vicinity of the calf which is made up of closed fascial spaces (see fig. 16/3).

The question of the optimal safe pressure to apply by means of the tourniquet to achieve a bloodless field has not been satisfactorily answered. Although levels of 500 mm Hg would unquestionably prevent arterial inflow, there is no real need to expose the tissues to such abnormal forces. Since blood pressure tends to rise during the course of an operation, taking this fact into consideration, it has been suggested that an adequate tourniquet pressure would be the sum of the average of the preoperative systolic blood pressure readings and 70 mm Hg (an arbitrary but reasonable figure) [2, 14], with minor changes being made for muscle mass at the site of application [2, 14]. Other suggested figures are one hundred mm Hg greater than the systolic pressure at the ankle (as determined by the Doppler ultrasonic flowmeter) and 200 mm Hg over the systolic pressure at the thigh. The pneumatic tourniquet, with its precise adjustment capability, contributes to the attainment of the optimal pressure.

Not only is too high a pressure inadvisable and potentially dangerous, but one that is too low to prevent all arterial inflow can likewise have adverse effects. Under such circumstances, blood continues to enter the limb during the operation, but venous outflow is interfered with. As a result, venous hypertension is produced, causing marked congestion of all tissues, including nervous elements, which if prolonged may have a permanent deleterious effect.

Another matter about which there is no unanimity is the duration of the application of the tourniquet pressure. According to *Bunnell* [5], the pressure can be applied for 1.5 h, followed by a 10-min release of pressure, which then allows the tourniquet to be reapplied for another 1.5 h with impunity. However, others have suggested that there is no specific length of time during which a tourniquet may be safely used. *Spira* et al. [34] have reported that even a period of 3 h of continuous application of a tourniquet has resulted in no ill effects being observed. These workers suggested that absence of adverse responses to such a long period of ischemia could be attributed to persistence of blood flow to the constricted area through the osseous nutrient artery which enters the bone above the level of application of the tourniquet. On the other hand, the view has also been proposed that a maximum safe period of application of a tourniquet to the lower limb is 60 min, thus avoiding ischemic lesions of nerves. If a longer period is required to complete the operation, the safest approach is to continue the procedure without the use of a tourniquet. It has also been suggested to deflate the cuff after 60–90 min and delay a second period of inflation for 15 or 20 min.

There are several other factors which have been proposed to make the use of a tourniquet safer and still of value in facilitating the operative procedure. First, it is essential to check the accuracy of the pressure gauge before each application of the tourniquet in order to be certain that the level of pressure that will be used is the desired one. Secondly, the limb should initially be elevated for 3 min at a 60° angle to permit venous drainage before applying the cuff pressure in order to minimize the amount of venous blood in the limb. Also very important is rapid inflation of the pressure cuff so as to halt all arterial inflow almost instantaneously, thus preventing pooling of blood in the venous tree. Deflation of the cuff should also be carried out quickly for the same reason.

References

1   Abramson, D.I.; Miller, D.S.: Vascular problems in musculoskeletal disorders of the limbs (Springer, Berlin 1981).
2   Arenson, D.J.; Weil, L.S.: The uses and abuses of tourniquets in bloodless field foot surgery. J. Am. Podiat. Ass. *66:* 854 (1976).
3   Brown, D.; Brenner, C.: Paralysis of nerve induced by direct pressure and by tourniquet. Archs Neurol. Psychol. *51:* 1 (1974).
4   Brunner, J.M.: Safety factors in the use of the pneumatic tourniquet for hemostasis in surgery of the hand. J. Bone Jt Surg. *33A:* 221 (1951).
5   Bunnel, S.: Surgery of the hand; 2nd ed., p. 96 (Lippincott, Philadelphia 1949).
6   Burkhart, J.M.; Jowsey, J.: Parathyroid and thyroid hormones in the development of immobilization osteoporosis. Endocrinology *81:* 1053 (1967).
7   Burton, A.C.; Yamada, S.: Relation between blood pressure and flow in the human forearm. J. appl. Physiol. *4:* 329 (1951).
8   Dallas, I.; Nordin, B.E.C.: Calcium intake and osteoporosis. Am. J. clin. Nutr. *11:* 263 (1962).
9   Dery, R.; Pelletier, J.; Jaques, A.; et al.: Metabolic changes induced in the limb during tourniquet ischemia. Com. Anaesth. Soc. J.*12:* 376 (1965).
10 Donaldson, C.L.; Hulley, S.B.; Vogel, J.M.; et al.: Effect of prolonged bed rest on bone mineral. Metabolism *19:* 1071 (1970).
11 Dushoff, I.M.: Hand surgery under wrist block and local infiltration anesthesia using an upper arm tourniquet. Plastic reconstr. Surg. *51:* 685 (1973).
12 Geiser, M.; Trueta, J.: Muscle action, bone rarefaction and bone formation: an experimental study. J.Bone Jt Surg. *40B:* 282 (1958).
13 Hamilton, W.K.; Sokoll, M.D.: Tourniquet paralysis. J. Am. med. Ass. *199:* 95 (1967).
14 Hinman, F.: The rational use of tourniquets. Surgery Gynec. Obstet. *81:* 357 (1945).
15 Hudlická, O.; Hnik, P.; Stulcová, B.: Changes in blood circulation in skeletal muscle undergoing atrophy. Physiologist, Wash. *7:* 163 (1964).
16 Hultén, O.: The influence of a fixation bandage on the peripheral blood vessels and the circulation. Acta chir. scand. *101:* 150 (1951).
17 Hulth, A.; Olerud, S.: Disuse of extremities. II. A microangiographic study in the rabbit. Acta chir. scand. *12:* 388 (1961).
18 Husain, T.: Experimental study of some pressure effects on tissues, with reference to bed-sore problem. J. Path. Bact. *66:* 347 (1953).
19 Imig, C.J.; Randall, B.F.; Hines, H.M.: Effect of immobilization on muscular atrophy and blood flow. Archs phys. Med. Rehabil. *34:* 296 (1953).

20 Jowsey, J.; Phil, D.; Kelly, P.J.; et al: Quantitative microradiographic studies of normal and osteoporotic bone. J. Bone Jt Surg. *47A:* 785 (1965).
21 Kosiak, M.: Etiology and pathology of ischemic ulcers. Archs phys. med. Rehabil. *40:* 62 (1959).
22 Kroese, A.J.; Stiris, G.: Does pre-operative pneumatic tourniquet cause thrombosis? A venographic study. J. Oslo City Hosp. *24:* 69 (1974).
23 Lindström, J.: Microvascular anatomy of synovial tissue. Acta rheum. scand. *7:* suppl., 1 (1963).
24 McLennan, C.E.; McLennan, M.T.; Landis, E.M.: Effect of external pressure on vascular volume of the forearm and its relation to capillary blood pressure and venous pressure. J. clin. Invest. *21:* 319 (1942).
25 Moldaver, J.: Tourniquet paralysis syndrome. Archs Surg., Lond. *68:* 136 (1954).
26 Nitz, A.J.; Matulionis, D.H.: Ultrastructural changes in rat peripheral nerve following pneumatic tourniquet compression. J. Neurosurg. *57:* 666 (1982).
27 Ochoa, J.; Fowler, T.J.; Gilliatt, R.W.: Anatomical changes in peripheral nerves compressed by a pneumatic tourniquet. J. Anat. *113:* 433 (1972).
28 Paletta, F.X.; Willman, V.; Ship, A.G.: Prolonged tourniquet ischemia of extremities: an experimental study on dogs. J. Bone Jt Surg. *42A:* 945 (1960).
29 Rudge, P.: Tourniquet paralysis with prolonged conduction block: an electrophysiological study. J. Bone Jt Surg. *56B:* 716 (1974).
30 Rutherford, R.B.; West, R.L.; Hardaway, R.M.: Coagulation changes during experimental hemorrhagic shock. Ann. Surg. *164:* 203 (1966).
31 Saltin, B.; Blomqvist, G.; Mitchell, J.H.; et al.: Response to exercise after bed rest and after training. Circulation *38:* suppl. 7, p. 1 (1968).
32 Seddon, H.J.: Volkmann's contracture: treatment by excision of the infarct. J. Bone Jt Surg. *38B:* 152 (1956).
33 Solonen, K.A.; Tarkkanen, L.; Narvanen, S.; et al.: Metabolic changes in the upper limb during tourniquet ischemia: a clinical study. Acta orthop. scand. *39:* 20 (1968).
34 Spira, E.; Katznelson, A.; Czerniak, P.; et al.: Osseous blood circulation in the lower limb: animal and clinical experiments. Israel J. med. Scis *1:* 573 (1965).
35 Webb, W.R.: Biologic foundations of surgery. Surg. Clins N. Am. *45:* 267 (1965).

18 Medicolegal Aspects of Vascular Complications of Treatment of Foot and Ankle Problems

General Considerations

Currently, the practicing podiatrist, as well as other dispensers of health care, must contend with an increasing tendency of the general public to resort to the courts for redress, in the form of financial compensation, for what is interpreted, justifiably or not, as an incorrect diagnosis of a medical problem or an unsuccessful or poor therapeutic result following a surgical procedure. Because there exists a fairly large group of trial attorneys interested in initiating malpractice suits and because the decisions handed down by juries have frequently been very generous in favor of the plaintiff, this practice has grown tremendously. Another factor which has helped to exacerbate the problem with regard to both frequency and size of malpractice claims is the pro-plaintiff changes in the law. The latter include substituting statewide or national standards for local ones as the normal practice and setting more vigorous standards for the responsibility of podiatrists and physicians to inform patients of potential risks of treatment. Such alterations in legal doctrine have increased the incentive to sue, raised compensable damages, extended the scope of liability, and reduced the plaintiff's cost of proving negligence by shifting some of the burden of proof to the defendants.

As a consequence of the above actions, a somewhat defensive attitude has developed among the various members of the health disciplines, resulting in a marked increase in the use of expensive and frequently unnecessary diagnostic procedures and consultations so as to be prepared for any contingency that might arise.

Unfortunately, the malpractice crisis is not over and may not even have peaked. Hence, malpractice insurance premiums can be expected to continue rising. Moreover, professional liability claims are still not settled any faster, the usual period of time at present being 42 months. It can therefore be anticipated that for the podiatrist involved in a malpractice suit, the time lost from practice in giving depositions and appearing in court will not be lessened in the near future. Moreover, it is necessary to note that, aside from the economic aspects, a malpractice suit may lead to a chronically stressful situation, resulting in insomnia, appetite change, irritability, headache, and a host of other symptoms characteristic of a disturbed mental state. Such psychologic responses may negatively affect the ability of the podiatrist to practice his specialty, particularly with regard to the doctor-patient relationship and the exercise of proper clinical judgment. For all these reasons, attention should be centered upon those measures which tend to reduce or minimize the possibility of development of a malpractice suit. In this chapter, these are discussed in detail in the hope that information thus obtained will contribute to the achievement of the desired goal.

Steps to Minimize Malpractice Suits

Establishment of a Proper Working Relationship with the Patient

One of the most common causes for the initiation of malpractice suits is a misunderstanding on the part of the patient regarding the improvement expected from the contemplated elective medical or surgical therapy. This stems, in great part, from inadequate communication or rapport between him and the podiatrist or possibly from an attitude assumed by the latter of talking down to, rather than with, the patient. The limitations of, and possibility of risks and complications associated with, a specific diagnostic procedure or an operation should be openly and frankly discussed with him and not denied, neglected, or dismissed from mind. The patient should also be made fully aware of the amount of pain that can generally be expected with the procedure. At the same time, of course, the realistic benefits and the achievable goals should be emphasized, with consideration of the relative value of alternative measures. However, at no time should any statements be made that could conceivably be construed by the patient as a guarantee of a good result from the contemplated procedure. Nor should a specific or definite period of time for complete recovery from the operation be advanced, since a target date of this type is dependent upon many variables, including the presence or absence of complications. Through such a detailed discussion, false expectations are prevented from developing in the patient's mind and the possibility of disappointment in the outcome minimized. At the same time, the patient should be impressed by the concern and interest in his physical difficulty which has been manifested by the podiatrist during the session.

Record Keeping

General Considerations. Contemporaneous and comprehensive, legibly written or typed accounts of all pertinent positive and negative findings relating to the patient's condition and progress are of inestimable value if a malpractice suit has been filed. Attention must be called to the fact that if the notes are in a form which presents difficulty in deciphering and if the signature of the podiatrist writing the report is illegible (which unfortunately is not infrequently the case), the contained information becomes of little or no value in the settlement of the claim. The ready availability of pertinent data may significantly influence the judge or jury to reach a conclusion in favor of the defendant, whereas failure to have adequate documentation of clinical findings may result in a negligence verdict against a podiatrist even when the care was proper. At no time should the medical records on the chart show any signs of tampering, alterations, or extensive corrections, since such changes raise questions in the mind of the examiner regarding their authenticity.

Another point which may become the basis for a malpractice suit is ordering medications from the pharmacist by telephone during an office visit. Because 10–15% of the names of proprietary drugs sound very similar, the podiatrist must be very careful to prevent an improper drug from being prescribed for his patient by error. A record of the matter should be made in the patient's office chart. Also of great importance is that if a prescription is filled out, it should be written legibly, lettered, or typed to prevent mistakes by the pharmacist in dispensing the drugs.

Recording of Conversations with the Patient. All appropriate discussions with the patient concerning possible risks, untoward responses, and realistic goals for achievement should be carefully documented in the patient's office chart and later in the hospital record if hospitalization is required. In the case of the latter, the conversation should be summarized by the attending podiatrist himself and not by a member of the house-staff. Also included in the chart should be a statement to the effect that the patient is willing to accept the possible risks associated with the procedure and has indicated this by signing the necessary permission and release forms in the presence of disinterested witnesses.

Pre- and Postoperative Progress Notes. Of great importance is the inclusion in the hospital records of a comprehensive initial history, physical findings, and pertinent results of clinical and laboratory testing. Progress notes relating to the patient's general physical state and appearance of the operative foot, especially immediately postoperatively, should be clearly and concisely presented. Such an approach should be continued on a daily basis until the patient is ready for discharge from the hospital. Also part of the hospital record should be a listing of all the precautionary steps that were taken. If a complication like infection develops, all measures to control the condition should be carefully described in the progress notes. Although time-consuming, such attention to detailed charting may prove very useful if the need to justify a specific procedure should ever arise.

Preoperative Measures

In order to minimize complications of an operation, it is necessary first to consider the precautionary steps to be taken in the pre-surgery stage, either in the office or after the patient is already in the hospital.

Determination of Coexisting Systemic Disorders. There is a tendency for some podiatrists to concentrate their interests and concern, understandably, on abnormalities in the foot which require medical or surgical therapy, without giving much attention to or considering the patient as a whole. Such an attitude, however, may at times have disastrous consequences, even following the institution of minor treatment programs, if certain systemic disorders coexist. Included in this group of conditions are diabetes mellitus (p. 357), cardiopulmonary diseases, severe anemia, and hypertension, among others. Besides the adverse effects of hypertension itself, it is important for the anesthesiologist in the event that a surgical procedure is to be performed, to be aware of the treatment program the patient is following to control this condition. Also to be kept in mind is the fact that when hypertension and diabetes are both present in a patient, the risk of vascular complications is significantly increased. For under such circumstances, there is an acceleration of small vessel disease due to a doubling of the rate of formation of exudates common to diabetes. Whatever steps are essential and feasible to minimize or control the untoward effects of the above disorders should be instituted without delay. Naturally, if the operative procedure is to be performed under regional or local anesthesia or if only medical therapy is being contemplated, the role that such conditions might play in the outcome becomes less significant but not eliminated.

State of Local Circulation. As has already been emphasized throughout this volume, a complete and meticulous evaluation of the state of the local arterial, venous, and lymphatic circulations must always be performed on both lower limbs before attempting a surgical podiatric procedure on a foot or ankle. In the presence of clinically significant local arterial impairment, such an approach is foolhardy and has great potential for initiating a malpractice suit. For it is generally accepted that most, if not all, podiatric procedures are elective in nature, a factor which markedly complicates the problem in the event of a poor or unsuccessful therapeutic result requiring the need for an amputation. (For the potential danger associated with performing a podiatric surgical procedure immediately after insertion of a vascular prosthesis, see p. 344.)

When venous insufficiency exists, in the form of pitting or nonpitting edema, pigmentation, stasis dermatitis or ulceration, varicosities, or chronic indurated cellulitis, no podiatric operations should be attempted unless the complications of venous hypertension can be controlled. Otherwise, there is a good possibility that the healing process will be greatly prolonged or that a nonhealing, treatment-resistant lesion may develop in the operative site. In the presence of irreversible changes like fibroedema or elephantiasis, podiatric procedures are contraindicated, since there is very little possibility of proper healing.

When lymphedema (acquired or congenital) of the foot and leg is present, any type of local surgery can again be expected to result in either poor or no healing of the operative site. Moreover, trauma to the lymphatic channels, which inevitably follows even minor operative procedures on the foot, may exaggerate the already existing swelling and lead to a greater accumulation of lymphedematous fluid in the tissues, a situation which also hinders wound repair. Moreover, lymph fluid may continue to drain from cut lymphatics for relatively long periods of time.

Role of Diabetes Mellitus in Prognosis. As has already been emphasized (p. 117), the presence of diabetes mellitus profoundly untowardly affects healing ability of tissues and significantly increases the risk of local infection in the operative site. Furthermore, its existence predisposes to early onset of a more rapidly progressing state of arteriosclerosis obliterans which results in a reduced local arterial circulation. Compounding the seriousness of such a condition is the fact that diabetes itself is responsible for occlusive disease in small terminal arteries and in the microcirculation (microangiopathy). As a consequence of all these factors, elective surgery in the foot of a diabetic should be held to a minimum, particularly since the degree of arterial insufficiency can be expected to be most severe in this site, the most distal portion of the limb. Because of such reasons, it is advisable not to attempt to debride an ulcerative lesion in the foot of a diabetic; instead a vascular consultant should be called in to perform this precarious chore.

One must not be satisfied with relying solely upon the results of a single fasting blood sugar to rule out the presence of diabetes. Such an approach may be misleading since a normal figure can still be obtained in a mild diabetic. The least that should be attempted is to perform a 2-hour post-prandial blood glucose test.

Steps Minimizing Risks Associated with Laboratory Study of Local Circulation. Since some of the laboratory techniques essential for the collection of pertinent vascular data are invasive and associated with discomfort and even risk, attempts should be made to prevent or minimize such possibilities. For example, if a drug is to be injected intravenously or intra-arterially for diagnostic purposes, as in the case of contrast venography or arteriography, preliminary testing with a small quantity of the material should always be done before injecting large quantities, in order to minimize some type of sensitivity reaction from developing. Also of importance in this regard is to ascertain whether there is any history of allergies or of previous adverse responses to medications or diagnostic procedures, in order to be prepared to carry out any necessary emergency treatment.

Because the patient may still develop side reactions despite the above precautions, it is essential to have certain medications readily available in the angiography room so as to be able to cope with most situations which might arise under such circumstances. These include: epinephrine, 1:1,000; diphenhydramine hydrochloride (Benadryl); intravenous pentobarbital sodium (Nembutal); isoproterenol hydrochloride (Isuprel Hydrochloride); calcium gluconate, and caffeine sodium benzoate.

Renal function tests should be performed on all patients suspected of having kidney disease if they are being considered for angiography. Those with significant renal impairment should not be subjected to the procedure unless the information thus derived is essential and cannot be obtained by any other means. Other prophylactic measures for very ill patients are avoidance of fluid restriction and the administration of intravenous mannitol infusion before and during angiography.

Measures in the Operative Period
All surgical procedures should, of course, be carried out with celerity, scrupulous care, and minimum sacrifice of viable tissue. Meticulous hemostasis should be obtained and attempts should be made to prevent trauma

to tissues in the vicinity of large veins. Rigid casts and tight elastic bandages should be applied with the latter precaution in mind. Also, every effort should be made to reduce the pressure exerted by a constrictive appliance on vulnerable areas in the vicinity of bony prominences by the use of adequate padding. This measure is particularly important in the case of the elderly patient who is prone to local arterial insufficiency due to arteriosclerosis obliterans. Such an approach may help prevent localized ischemic ulceration and gangrene (p. 344).

Post-Test or Postoperative Precautions

Local Routine Steps. Aside from recording the immediate systemic responses to the test or the operation, the arterial and venous circulations in the affected limb should be closely inspected, first twice daily and then every day. Of great importance in the examination are the cutaneous temperature, color, and turgor of the toes, the patient's ability to move them, and the presence or absence of symptomatic or asymptomatic swelling of the foot and leg. Meticulous inspection of the site of performance of the diagnostic procedure or of the operative wound should be routinely carried out.

Complications. If these arise following a therapeutic program, they should immediately be treated. With the appearance of signs and symptoms of acutely impaired arterial circulation, it is essential to seek consultation with a vascular surgeon, who may find it necessary to institute emergency steps to increase local blood flow. If signs of acute venous insufficiency due to deep venous thrombosis develop, the expertise of an internist knowledgeable in the field of vascular disorders should be called upon for initiation and supervision of the treatment regimen. With regard to this aspect of treatment, as a general rule, it is advisable for the podiatrist to acquiesce immediately to a request by the patient or a member of his family to call in a medical or surgical consultant on the case. Failure to do so may result in severely damaging testimony at the trial.

In the presence of infection in the operative field, a meaningful culture and sensitivity study should be carried out, as outlined on page 299, and the appropriate antibacterial agents administered. If no benefit is observed in a period of several days, it is essential to repeat the culture and sensitivity study, since a change in the bacterial flora may have occurred. In this regard, it is common practice for the plaintiff's lawyer to test the podiatrist's or physician's expertise and knowledge of the field by asking him or her how many times a culture and a sensitivity study were performed. Testimony indicating that only one had been done throughout the period of treatment of a postoperative infection is a telling point in support of the malpractice suit, since such a situation may be interpreted as negligence. This is especially true if the infection had not been controlled by antibiotics and more heroic treatment, such as an amputation, had to be carried out because of the development of systemic responses to absorption from the operative site.

Hospital Discharge Measures. Before the patient leaves the hospital, an appointment should be made for his appearance in the office for a follow-up visit, to determine the degree of healing in the operative site. At the same time he should receive a list of directions for home treatment of the foot. Some time should be spent with him discussing the rationale for the various suggested measures.

In the event that the patient does not appear at the appointed time, a certified or registered letter should be sent to him (with a copy and receipt retained in the office file) explaining the critical need for further treatment of the foot in order to facilitate total recovery. Included in the letter should be a paragraph to the effect that if there is no response to the request 2 weeks after receipt, the professional relationship will be considered terminated and the patient should seek treatment elsewhere. Such measures are necessary to prevent him from subsequently claiming that he had suffered from abandonment by the podiatrist.

IV Other Vascular Entities Observed in a Podiatric Practice

19   Clinical Entities with Circulatory Components

This chapter is devoted to capsulized descriptions of a fairly large number of unrelated clinical conditions, some which fall into the category of peripheral vascular disorders and others which demonstrate components of a circulatory nature. What they do have in common is that at some time or another, all can be expected to be encountered in a podiatric practice. A detailed and comprehensive presentation of their clinical manifestation is not practical because of lack of space and, instead, the discussion is limited to those facets of each entity which represent changes in the arterial, venous, or lymphatic system in the lower limbs.

Congenital Vascular Disorders of the Lower Limbs

There are a number of congenital conditions found in the lower limbs which manifest clear-cut physical signs of involvement of arteries, veins, or lymphatics, or a combination of such components. The more important clinical entities of this type are discussed below.

Congenital Arteriovenous Fistula
Etiologic Factors. A congenital arteriovenous fistula consists of multiple vascular communications of small caliber between the arterial and venous systems locally, with no intervening capillary bed. Antecedent trauma plays no role in its development, as contrasted with an acquired arteriovenous fistula (p. 310), and instead the condition represents a persistence of connections which exist at the beginning of the process of differentiation of arteries and veins from a common embryologic anlage.

Symptoms and Signs. A congenital arteriovenous fistula may be present for many years before complaints develop, these resulting from a progressive increase in the size of the fistulous communications. Even then, the patient may only experience a sense of discomfort. In later life, there are frequently symptoms of cardiac strain and then failure occurs as the load on the heart becomes greater with aging and this organ becomes less able to cope with the persistently high venous return from the contribution of the volume of blood passing through the secondary circulation.

On examination, variable-sized vascular masses are noted under the skin. These are dilated venous channels (secondary varicosities) which are receiving blood directly from the arterial tree via the abnormal communications. Far less frequently than in the case of the acquired arteriovenous fistula, a continuous bruit can be heard and a thrill palpated. Of great importance is the finding that the involved limb is longer and larger in girth than the opposite normal one, thus indicating that the fistula was functioning before the epiphyseal centers were closed. The skin temperature of the affected limb is lower than normal in the distal portion and higher than normal in the proximal portion. There may also be increased hair growth in the latter site. Various types of hemangiomas (p. 364) may be found in conjunction with congenital arteriovenous fistulas. There may be signs of venous pooling in the lower part of the leg as a result of the existing local high venous pressure proximally. Arteriography reveals almost immediate filling of the venous tree due to rapid movement of the radiopaque material from the arteries, through the abnormal communications, into large veins.

Congenital Venous Disorders
Diffuse Dilatation of Subpapillary Venous Plexus. This condition resembles spider veins (p. 215) except that in most instances, the abnormal vessels are more extensive and not limited to the lower limbs. Since the venules are thin-walled and very close to the surface of the skin, they are vulnerable to trauma. As a result, ecchymosis is a common complication of the condition, but rarely external bleeding.

Phlebectasia. This is another congenital malformation, consisting of enlargement and fusiform dilatation of superficial venous channels in the limb (fig. 19/1a). It may be mistaken for the distended venous network observed in congenital arteriovenous fistula (see above) and in acquired arteriovenous fistula (p. 312). However, the high venous pressure found in the latter two conditions does not exist in phlebectasia and the dilated veins collapse on elevation of the limb.

Klippel-Trenaunay Syndrome. This is a congenital vascular malformation present at birth which is associated with the presence of varicose veins on one lower limb, cutaneous hemangiomas, decreased lymphatic trunks, local soft-tissue hypertrophy, and elongation of the extremity due to lengthening of the long bones. Besides the dilatation and incompetency of the superficial veins, the deep venous system demonstrates malformations in the form of compression of the popliteal or femoral vein by a fibrovascular band or complete agenesis of the collecting veins. In view of the extensive abnormalities in the deep venous system, it is essential to differentiate this condition from simple primary varicosities, for attempts to eradicate the superficial varicose veins by stripping or by other surgical means will be followed by disastrous results. Of help in making the differentiation is venography which reveals the presence of malformations in the deep venous system. Also useful is arteriography, which may identify arteriovenous fistulas at distal ends of small arterial branches opening into vascular pools.

Congenital Vascular Tumors

Hemangioma. This type of vascular tumor is probably a congenital growth of tissue in which blood channels form. The *cutaneous hemangioma* is the most common neoplasm of infancy and childhood, frequently being present at birth. The tumor may vary in size from a tiny fleck to a lesion involving a whole limb. In most instances, it grows slowly and ceases enlarging when adulthood is reached. Histologically, the tumor consists of endothelial-lined spaces of varying sizes embedded in sparse interstitial connective tissue. The amount of lipoid and fibrous tissue in the tumor determines its consistency. The clinical findings generally consist of a palpable mass, discoloration of skin overlying it, and swelling. Pain may be present locally.

There are several groups of cutaneous hemangiomas: the cutaneous capillary, the cavernous, the mixed, and the systemic. The *cutaneous capillary hemangioma* is the most common, accounting for 75% of the hemangiomas seen in children. It consists of a number of different types: the strawberry nevus, the port-wine stain (birthmark), and the sclerosing. The *cavernous hemangioma* is similar to the capillary hemangioma except that the majority of the vessels forming it are widely dilated. The *mixed hemangioma* consists of the cavernous type with an overlying capillary (strawberry or port-wine) component.

The *systemic hemangioma* is a rare congenital neoplastic tumor which usually affects a large part of an entire lower limb and may also extend onto

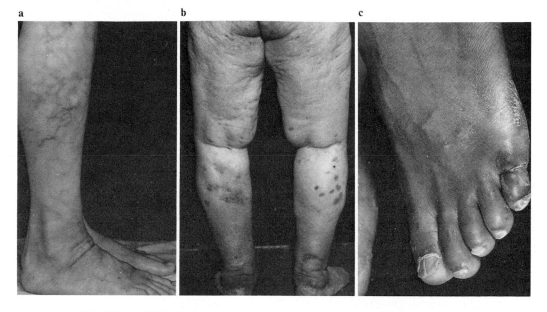

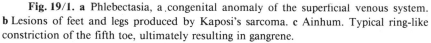

Fig. 19/1. a Phlebectasia, a congenital anomaly of the superficial venous system. **b** Lesions of feet and legs produced by Kaposi's sarcoma. **c** Ainhum. Typical ring-like constriction of the fifth toe, ultimately resulting in gangrene.

the trunk. In most instances, the surface of the tumor is marked with a port-wine stain. The involved limb is generally enlarged and discolored at birth and progressively increases in size. The lesion consists of great numbers of dilated blood sinuses, resembling varicose veins, and capillary elements which often project through the discolored area. The latter vessels are easily injured and bleed profusely. All the tissues of the limb become hypertrophied, including the long bones. Associated findings are signs of vasospasm and hyperhidrosis.

Telangiectasis. This type of tumor consists of vascular lesions of the skin and mucous membranes, characterized by dilatation or prominence of arterioles, capillaries, venules, and even small arteries in the involved sites. The condition is congenital, although an acquired similar alteration of the cutaneous microcirculation also exists, as for example in the case of simple telangiectasis associated with such disorders as acne rosacea, systemic lupus erythematosus, progressive systemic sclerosis (generalized scleroderma), syphilis, prolonged exposure of skin to wind or sun, and treatment with radium or X-ray. The possibility has been proposed that telangiectasis is a true tumor of blood vessels.

Telangiectasis has several subdivisions: cherry angioma (senile vascular nevus), spider angioma (spider nevus), hereditary hemorrhagic telangiectasis (Rendu-Osler-Weber's disease), ataxia-telangiectasis, essential progressive telangiectasis, and congenital poikiloderma. *Cherry angioma* consists of tufts of dilated capillaries, giving the appearance of bright red or purplish raised papules, varying in size from a pinhead to a pea. The condition is frequently found on the limbs of middle-aged or elderly persons. The *spider angioma* resembles the spider nevi found in patients with liver disease or in pregnant women. It consists of a central raised, dilated, pulsating arteriolar feeder vessel, communicating directly with radiating venular tributaries running parallel to the skin surface. An area of erythema surrounds the central vessel, extending beyond the visible extent of the vascular legs. *Rendu-Osler-Weber's disease* is an inherited maldevelopment of minute blood vessels, producing raised, small, pinpoint spider-like telangiectatic lesions in the skin and mucous membranes. The condition consists of dilated capillaries and venules with thin walls, covered by a thinned-out skin or mucous membrane. The lesion is rarely found in the skin of the lower limbs. *Ataxia telangiectasis* is limited to the upper part of the body and the head. *Congenital poikiloderma* is also not found in the skin of the lower limbs. Essential *progressive telangiectasis* is composed of dilated thin-walled ectatic venules located in the upper corium. It is typified by the appearance of numerous, small, enlarged blood vessels and telangiectasis in a fiery red skin, especially marked on the feet and ankles, and extending up the legs. Associated findings are burning, tingling, and numbness in the involved limb.

Kaposi's Sarcoma (Multiple Idiopathic Hemorrhagic Sarcoma of Kaposi). This disorder is a low-grade malignant tumor of blood vessel origin which is characterized by successive appearance of vascular lesions in the skin of the lower limbs and, less often, elsewhere, particularly in men after the age of 40. Nothing is known regarding its etiology, although there is some evidence to support the view that it is a dysplasia of the reticuloendothelial system. Of importance is the finding that Kaposi's sarcoma is associated with an exceptionally high frequency of some type of primary neoplasm, such as malignant lymphoma, leukemia, or a carcinoma having an entirely separate histogenesis.

The histologic picture of Kaposi's sarcoma consists initially of hemorrhage into the cutis from local dilated and engorged vessels in the dermis. Then the blood vessel endothelium proliferates, new imperfect sinuses form resembling hemangiomas (p. 364), and an increase in lymphocytes, plasma cells, and mast cells becomes prominent. In the final stage, the microscopic picture is that of an angiosarcoma or fibrosarcoma, the predominant finding being spindle-shaped fibroblasts interspersed within walled vascular spaces.

Kaposi's sarcoma displays a rather typical clinical pattern [4]. Initially the lesions are bluish-red or reddish brown, well-demarcated macules on the lower limbs, varying from a few millimeters to a few centimeters in diameter. These slowly become elevated and multiple and then coalesce to form ill-defined, slightly infiltrated bluish-black plaques or collections of firm, reddish or purple nodules (fig. 19/1b). New lesions are constantly appearing in different portions of the limb. A constant associated finding is marked nonpitting edema of the involved limb, the cause of which is not clear. Despite extensive involvement of the extremity by the pathologic process, symptoms are generally minimal, aside from some tenderness in the nodules and plaques and pruritis. After a variable course, ranging from a few months to 25 years, death results in Kaposi's sarcoma, generally from progressive cachexia, infection, or hemorrhage from a lesion.

Glomus Tumor (Subungual Tumor). This is a rare congenital vascular anomaly which is a pathologic alteration of the normal glomus (arteriovenous shunt and its afferent artery and efferent veins, together with a rich network of sympathetic nerve fibrils). It is found in the nail beds of the toes and sole of the foot, as well as in the fingers and elsewhere on the limbs. Histologically, the glomus tumor demonstrates an overgrowth of vascular spaces and of epithelioid cells normally present in the glomus. As in the latter, there is an extensive network of nonmedullated and medullated nerve fibers in the collagenous reticulum, together with many pacinian corpuscles.

The most outstanding symptom is the intense, sharp, burning pain present in the vicinity of the lesion and radiating up the entire lower limb. The precipitating agent is distention of the numerous venous channels in the tumor mass by blood, thus producing compression of the neighboring rich plexus of small nerve fibrils. The symptom may appear spontaneously or it may be initiated by exposure of the feet to extreme cold or heat, particularly the latter. Pressure from clothing or from bed clothes may also precipitate an attack of agonizing pain. Elevation of the affected lower limb or application of an arterial occlusion pressure to a proximal segment relieves the pain since both measures decrease the amount of blood in the foot and hence reduce the pressure in the tumor.

The lesion is generally found in a subungual or subcutaneous location, varying from 0.8 to 2.5 cm in diameter. It is deep red to purple or blue in color and is sharply demarcated from surrounding structures. At times it may not be visible or palpable, under which circumstances, the pin test may help identify its presence. This consists of applying pressure to the skin with the head of a pin, direct contact with the tumor eliciting excruciating pain, which may persist for hours. Deformity of the nail and phalanx may result if the subungual region is involved.

Therapy consists of surgical extirpation of the tumor since it is benign, thus producing an immediate cure. No recurrences take place if the lesion is entirely removed.

Congenital Lymphatic Tumors. Such disorders are much less common than those of blood vessels. They are divided into the simple, the cavernous, and the cystic. There is also a malignant type, the lymphangiosarcoma, which usually is found in a long-standing lymphedematous limb.

The *simple lymphatic tumor* is usually congenital and benign, consisting of small well-defined large networks of lymphatic spaces, into which lymphatic channels enter. The tumor is generally located in the skin and is slow-growing. The *cavernous type* is also congenital, appearing at birth or shortly thereafter and it grows slowly. It is considered to arise from abnormal mesodermal rests which form isolated imperfect lymph vessels. The tumor consists of numerous large, dilated lymph sinuses containing lymph and, at times, some blood. The lesions are generally located in the skin and subcutaneous tissue. Occasionally large cavernous lymphangiomas are found in the lower limbs associated with congenital lymphedema (p. 242). The last type of lymphatic tumor, the *cystic lymphangioma,* is considered to develop from embryonal rests, generally appearing during early childhood. The histologic changes resemble those of the cavernous lymphangioma. The tumor is usually found in the upper limbs and rarely in the lower.

Congenital Annular Bands
Constricting fibrous bands are congenital malformations which may be responsible for partial or complete amputation of an involved structure, particularly a digit. They may be associated with other developmental

anomalies, such as syndactyly, clubfoot, cleft palate, and harelip. Congenital annular bands may be the result of improper histogenesis, a form of congenital collagen dysplasia (Streeter's dysplasia), rather than a scar [8].

Ainhum is the name given to a congenital annular band found in the dark-skinned races, particularly the North American Black, in which the fibrous constriction is located in the digitoplantar fold of the fifth toe (fig. 19/1c). Eventually the process encircles the digit, and then, with deeper penetration, it causes a ring-like strangulation of the distal tissues, associated with pressure atrophy and resorption of the bone. Gradually, the tip of the toe becomes enlarged and bulbous, followed by spontaneous amputation. Roentgenographic examination during the period of progression of the process generally reveals narrowing of the shaft, thinning of the cortex of the phalanx, and pathologic fracture and rotation of the distal phalanx. Systemic symptoms are absent, the complaints being limited to the vicinity of the fifth toe on one or both feet. When the constricting band first develops, there is some pain; generally this becomes more marked as the process affects deeper structures. Symptoms may persist for a period of years until digital amputation is completed.

Congenital annular bands are also found elsewhere in the foot and leg, but less frequently than in the case of involvement of the fifth toe. For example, the development of such a lesion at the level of the ankle has been responsible for gangrene of the entire foot. There is no effective therapeutic approach to the management of congenital annular bands.

Popliteal Artery Entrapment Syndrome
Popliteal artery entrapment syndrome is a rare vascular disorder in which the popliteal artery assumes one of several anomalous courses. In one it runs medially to the medial head of a normal gastrocnemius muscle instead of between the two heads of this structure. In another the gastrocnemius or the plantaris has either an aberrant origin or an accessory head, or the medial head of the gastrocnemius has a lower and more lateral insertion than normal, thus separating the popliteal artery in its usual course from the popliteal vein or both vessels from the nerve.

Regardless of the type of congenital abnormality which exists, the popliteal artery suffers injury when the person walks. Either this vessel is squeezed by the contraction of the gastrocnemius muscle or it is compressed between the muscle and the bone. Consequently, insufficient blood supply reaches the muscle during physical effort and intermittent claudication

(p. 5) develops. If the condition is not surgically treated, eventually repeated vascular trauma may produce degeneration of the wall of the popliteal artery, followed either by aneurysmal dilatation, plaque formation, or thrombosis [7]. Occlusion occurs slowly, allowing for the development of a rich collateral circulation around the knee.

Diagnosis of the popliteal artery entrapment syndrome can generally be made on the basis of the physical findings, with arteriography acting as a confirmatory procedure. Because of the increase in blood flow through collateral vessels around the knee, the skin temperature in this site is significantly raised ('hot knee') [1, 2]. Palpation of the knee reveals the presence of pulsations in the large secondary vessels, particularly on the lateral and posterior aspects of the joint. If thrombosis of the popliteal artery has not as yet occurred, flexing the knee acutely by gastrocnemius action may produce paresthesias in the toes; forced plantar hyperextension or dorsiflexion of the foot will result in loss of pulsations in the distal tibial arteries [10]. Permanent complete occlusion of the popliteal artery results in absent pulsations in the tibial arteries of the foot and loss of oscillometric readings on the lower segment of the leg. Arteriography will visualize the block in the popliteal artery and the presence of an extensive collateral circulation around the knee. If the popliteal artery is not totally occluded, it may be found in an aberrant position.

Connective Tissue Disorders

The connective tissue (collagen) disorders are characterized by widespread and extensive involvement of the blood vessels, the changes in the limbs being merely incidental to much more significant and serious vascular abnormalities elsewhere. No attempt will be made below to discuss these conditions in detail and, instead, the presentation will be limited to a description of the vascular changes in the lower limbs.

Scleroderma (Progressive Systemic Sclerosis)

Scleroderma is the term loosely used to designate a number of clinical entities, each having a different prognosis. One of these is *morphea* or localized scleroderma, in which the process is limited to small areas of the skin of the limbs and elsewhere. The condition is characterized by discrete oval lesions with ivory-colored centers and violaceous halos at the periphery. There are no associated systemic responses and the outlook with regard to longevity is excellent. The second type, *diffuse* or *generalized scleroderma,* is a rare malignant form of progressive systemic sclerosis. The cutaneous process is first found on the proximal portion of the lower limbs, eventually progressing to the legs and feet. Systemic manifestations are common and severe, and the prognosis is very poor. The most frequent clinical type is *acrosclerosis,* in which the process begins in the feet and hands and extends proximally. The prognosis is much better than in the case of diffuse, generalized scleroderma.

Acrosclerosis affects women 3 times as often as men, being first noted in the fourth and fifth decades. The abnormal change responsible for the condition is replacement of subcutaneous tissue by altered connective tissue to which the skin becomes firmly adherent.

Pathology. The alterations consist of fibrinoid degeneration of the colloid bundles in the lower cutis, an increase in thickness and density of the fibers, with straightening of these structures, and compression of the cellular elements in the collagen tissue. Initially the cutis and subcutis are swollen and infiltrated with lymphocytes and mononuclear cells, but with progression of the condition, these alterations disappear, to be replaced by atrophy of sweat glands, hair follicles, and adjacent muscles.

Pathologic changes are also present in vascular elements, including degeneration of walls of small arteries, with thickening of the intima due to deposition of concentric layers of fibrous tissue. As the latter process continues, the lumen of involved vessels becomes small until there is complete obliteration, leading to focal necrosis. The microcirculation is also affected, the cutaneous and muscle capillaries becoming abnormally dilated and reduced in number. The basement membrane of these vessels is thickened and reduplicated, associated with degeneration of the endothelium.

Symptoms and Signs. In acrosclerosis, at first there is swelling of the fingers and less marked changes in the toes. This abnormality is associated with tenseness, stiffness, and difficulty in moving the digits. The next stage involves permanent alterations in the skin, which becomes thickened, smooth, and firm. Wrinkling over the small joints of the fingers and, to a lesser degree, of the toes is lost because of the firm adherence of the overlying skin to the subcutaneous tissue. Elsewhere on the distal segment of the lower limb, it is no longer possible to raise the skin in a fold. The final stage is typified by atrophy of tissues, including the digits which become shorter due to bony absorption of the tufts. Changes in the joints, which appear early in the disease, now become much more severe, this being responsible for a clawlike appearance, more prominent in the hands, but also present in the feet. Associated findings are: (1) atrophy of skeletal muscle of the lower limbs; (2) distortion, deformity, and cracking of the nails; (3) atrophy of sweat and sebaceous glands causing dryness and scaliness of the skin, and (4) absence of hair. Episodes of Raynaud's syndrome (pp. 37, 38) are common. Deposition of brown pigment and telangiectasis may be found in the skin of the lower limbs. There may be deposits of subcutaneous nodules, consisting of calcium (calcinosis), which form on pressure areas.

With progression of the sclerodermatous process, the resulting reduction in local blood flow due to mechanical factors may lead to development of such nutritional disturbances as superficial ulcerations following even very minor trauma. Especially vulnerable to such a state are the tissues on and in the region of the ankles. Necrosis of the tips of the toes may also develop. Despite the presence of serious trophic changes, arterial pulsations in the feet remain normal, the cause for the alterations being compression of the cutaneous microcirculation by the local sclerodermatous process.

Systemic (Disseminated) Lupus Erythematosus

Systemic lupus erythematosus is a widespread connective tissue disorder involving primarily the vascular system and the serous and synovial membranes.

Pathology. The predominant pathologic change is an arteritis, with degeneration of the subendothelial connective tissue in small arteries, arterioles, and capillaries, the greatest change being noted in the microcirculation. In the more severe type, supporting structures are also involved, leading to necrosis of the muscular and elastic tissue in the vessel wall. In the chronic or proliferative phase, there may be invagination of the wall into the lumen, causing plugging of the vessel. In the skin, early histologic alterations consist of swelling of the upper layer, atrophy of the epidermis, and liquefaction necrosis of the basal cell layer.

Signs. The vascular manifestations of systemic lupus erythematosus in the lower limbs are generally of a mild degree. Raynaud's syndrome is noted in 20% of patients, particularly in those who also have local joint involvement. Rarely is gangrene of toes noted, this occurring as a result of occlusion of digital arteries. At the same time, pulsations are generally present in the main arteries of the involved foot. Occasionally, chronic ulceration may develop over the malleoli. There may be some manifestations of sympathetic imbalance, in the form of mottling of the skin and rubor. Edema of the lower limbs has been reported.

Dermatomyositis

Dermatomyositis is a rare connective tissue disorder characterized by nonsuppurative inflammation and degeneration of voluntary muscles of the body, associated with dermatologic changes.

Pathology. Associated with involvement of muscle bundles, there is diffuse round cell infiltration around capillaries, arterioles, and small arteries in the skin, subcutaneous tissue, and muscle.

Symptoms and Signs. The predominant complaints are weakness and tenderness in voluntary muscles, which are soft and doughy at the beginning but later become atrophied and less painful; associated with such abnormalities is restriction of movement. Raynaud's syndrome is a fairly common finding. Pulsations in the feet are generally reduced and oscillometric readings are low. Trophic changes may be noted in the feet, as well as periungual erythema and cuticular telangiectasis. Areas of deepened skin pigmentation may alternate with depigmented sites.

Polyarteritis Nodosa

Polyarteritis nodosa is a generalized connective tissue disease which affects medium-sized arteries in particular. It appears to have a close relationship with hypersensitivity phenomena.

Pathology. The primary histologic change is acute arteritis, resulting in degeneration of the media and proliferation of the intima, followed by partial or total obstruction of the lumen of the artery. Hemorrhages or microaneurysms form, due to destruction of the vessel wall. Typically, aggregations of neutrophilic and eosinophilic leukocytes, lymphocytes, plasma cells, and histocytes are found within the wall of the artery and surrounding it. When organization takes place, there is proliferation of connective tissue in the vicinity of the affected vessel. Characteristically, inflammatory and reparative stages coexist in the same area of involvement.

Symptoms and Signs. In the lower limbs, there may be ischemic ulceration caused by thrombosis of cutaneous arterioles or small aneurysmal nodules along the course of the vessels. Because of pathologic changes in the vasa nervorum of peripheral nerves, numbness and tingling may be present in the toes, at times associated with foot drop. There may also be some impairment of vibratory sense perception and of light touch in the toes.

Rheumatoid Arthritis

Rheumatoid arthritis, which falls into the category of connective tissue disorders, is associated with some clinical manifestations of vascular insufficiency. Also, there is a possibility that prolonged steroid therapy, when given to susceptible patients with this disorder, may be responsible for the activation of an angiitis. However, most of the pathologic evidence supports the view that vascular inflammation is an integral part of the disease [11].

Pathology. The arterial changes in rheumatoid arthritis vary from slight inflammation to necrotizing arteritis [9]. Examination of biopsies of striated muscle has revealed arteritic changes in very small arteries in approximately 10% of cases [12]. Histologically, there is infiltration of the adventitia of the vessels, primarily by large mononuclear cells. Severe destruction of the arterial wall is not noted. Vasculitis may also be found in the articular tissues early in the course of the disease, associated with a significant reduction in the number of arteries supplying the region in the vicinity of a joint. There may also be inflammatory infiltrates, consisting predominantly of plasma cells. The synovial changes are related to the presence of clinically active joint disease, not specific for rheumatoid arthritis.

The histologic vascular alterations in the skin are responsible for the ulcerations observed in this location. They take the form of nodules with three distinct zones: a central layer of necrosis and fibrinous changes; an intermediate layer of palisaded histiocytes, young fibroblasts, and small round cells, and an outer layer of fibrous connective tissue in which are found numerous altered blood vessels [3]. Similar nodules are found in the subcutaneous tissue. Thrombosed vessels are usually noted in young nodules, which may be the explanation for the common finding of central necrosis in the lesions.

Vascular Signs. One of the more common vascular findings in rheumatoid arthritis is vasospasm (p. 36), although there is no apparent relationship between the location of this state and the site of the arthritic process. It is possible that disuse resulting from the presence of pain in the joints on movement may, in part, be responsible for the vasospasm. In any event, the lower extremity suffering from rheumatoid arthritis is generally cold, somewhat cyanotic, and clammy, such changes usually being limited to the distal portion of the limb, particularly the foot. Raynaud's syndrome (pp. 37, 38), involving episodic color changes in the fingers and, less often, the toes, may accompany such findings. Peripheral neuropathy may also be present, due to the inflammatory vasculitis in the peripheral nerve trunks. Purpuric spots and ecchymosis may be noted in the skin of the involved limb, probably related to the arteritis characteristic of connective tissue disorders. The administration of steroids as therapy may accelerate the occurrence of such lesions.

Subcutaneous nodules are present in about one quarter of the adult patients with rheumatoid arthritis, generally indicating a more severe form of the disease. They are located lying freely in soft tissue over bony prominences or in areas subjected to repeated periods of pressure, as in the case of the heel.

Superficial, indolent, treatment-resistant ulcerations of rheumatoid arthritis may be found over both malleoli, more often on the lateral aspect. The lesions generally demonstrate a dirty base and signs of inflammation around the periphery. Therapy utilized for venous stasis ulcers (p. 298) should be instituted but, unfortunately, rarely is it successful in causing healing. Attempts should be made to prevent mechanical ischemia resulting from persistent contact of the involved area of the limb with the mattress. At times the arteritic process in the skin and subcutaneous tissue is of such a marked degree that gangrene of toes develops. It is of interest that forefoot reconstruction (panmetatarsal head resections) in advanced cases of rheumatoid arthritis is frequently performed with excellent relief of symptoms and good healing of the operative site. However, failure to respect the existing compromised small blood vessel circulation to soft tissues has led to the loss of digits.

Miscellaneous Disorders

Paget's Disease of Bone (Osteitis Deformans)
Paget's disease of bone is found chiefly in skeletal structures possessing a rich arterial circulation and hematopoietic marrow. It is characterized by deformity of the external bony contour, the typical pathologic abnormality being primary resorption of bone.

Pathogenesis. A greatly increased local blood flow accompanies the period of bone destruction [5, 6], an apparent direct relationship existing between the magnitude of the circulatory response and the degree of resorptive activity. In line with this finding is the observation that spontaneous remissions are associated with a reduction in the osseous circulation. In the acute stage of the disease, the periosteal blood supply is particularly increased; at the same time, there is a decrease in circulation to the distal, noninvolved portion of bone. The marked vascularity of bone in Paget's disease is probably responsible for the increase in cardiac output observed in this disorder.

Vascular Symptoms and Signs. Associated with swelling or deformity of the involved long bone of a lower limb, there is a significant rise in skin temperature in the vicinity of the pathologic change. Symptoms which result from movement of the affected limb are probably related to the local inflammation and structural abnormality of the bone.

Erythema Nodosum

Erythema nodosum is a nonspecific syndrome characterized by transient appearance of cutaneous and subcutaneous nodules resembling bruises, associated with fever, malaise, and migratory arthritis. There is no single etiologic factor, the condition being found in association with a variety of infections (especially streptococcal) and also following the ingestion of sulfonamide compounds, iodides, and bromides by people sensitive to these drugs. Certain oral contraceptive medications may have the same effect. There is a tendency for the attacks to occur in the spring and autumn, women between the ages of 20 and 30 years being chiefly affected.

Pathology. Histologic examination of an active nodule reveals an infiltration of lymphocytes and polymorphonuclear leukocytes about the vascular network in the middle and lower portion of the corium and adjacent fat. The vessel walls are edematous and the capillary bed is dilated. There may also be atrophy and necrosis of the fat in the subcutaneous tissue.

Symptoms and Signs. The characteristic nodule is relatively superficial, firm, red, hot, tender, and painful. It is about 1–2 cm in diameter, with the overlying skin shiny and raised. The lesion assumes a bruised appearance as edema and erythema develop. At times ecchymosis may form in the nodule and elsewhere in the skin. Most lesions last for a few days to 6 weeks, and they stop and recede at different stages of formation. With involution, the color of the nodules changes from the original bright erythematous hue to purple, yellow, greenish gray, or brown. On occasion, the nodules may coalesce and appear fluctulant, but they do not break down or suppurate to form an ulcer or an abscess. The usual site for the nodules is the anterior surface of the legs in the pretibial region; they may also be found on the soles of the feet, the calves, knees, thighs, and occasionally elsewhere.

Frequently the appearance of the nodules is associated with arthritis of the ankles, knees, wrists, and other joints and a fever up to 38.3 °C (101 °F), thus resembling acute rheumatoid arthritis. Chest X-ray may reveal bilateral hilar lymphadenopathy, at times accompanied by diffuse pulmonary mottling. Erythema nodosum is self-limiting, with an excellent prognosis.

Weber-Christian Disease
(Relapsing Febrile, Nodular, Nonsuppurative Panniculitis)

Weber-Christian disease is a rare disorder, characterized by the appearance of single or multiple crops of subcutaneous nodules, located particularly on the legs, but also elsewhere on the body. Its cause is unknown, although a large number of etiologic agents have been proposed, including a relationship to connective tissue disorders (p. 370). The condition occurs most often in obese women between the ages of 30 and 50 years.

Pathology. The subcutaneous panniculus is the site of the abnormal changes in Weber-Christian disease. Histologic examination of a nodule generally reveals nonsuppurative necrosis of fat cells and infiltration of tissue with lymphocytes, monocytes, and polymorphonuclear leukocytes. Fibrinoid degeneration may be seen in the interlobar areas and in vessel walls.

Symptoms and Signs. In Weber-Christian disease, there are frequent bouts of fever, unassociated with a leukocytosis; in fact, a leukopenia may be present. Each attack of increased temperature may last as long as several months, with spontaneous remissions. The nodules vary in size from 0.5 to 5 cm in diameter and may or may not be tender. In the early stage of their development, the skin over the indurated masses is often red, but later a brownish discoloration forms. Multiple nodules in proximity have a tendency to coalesce and produce indurated plaques under the skin. With progression of the disease, atrophy of the subcutaneous fat occurs, resulting in deformity of the skin. Associated findings are swelling of the leg and occasionally even necrosis of, and drainage from, the nodules. The diagnosis of the condition can be made by biopsy of active subcutaneous lesions. Rarely is Weber-Christian disease a cause of death. When this occurs, however, necropsy generally reveals widespread involvement of adipose tissue.

References

1   Bouhoutsos, I.; Goulios, A.: Popliteal artery entrapment: report of a case. J. cardiovasc. Surg. *18:* 481 (1977).
2   Chavatzas, D.; Barabas, A.; Martin, P.: Popliteal artery entrapment. Lancet *ii:* 181 (1973).
3   Collins, D.H.: Subcutaneous nodule of rheumatoid arthritis. J. Path. Bact. *45:* 97 (1937).
4   Davis, J.: Kaposi's sarcoma: present concept of clinical course and treatment. N.Y. J. Med. *68:* 2067 (1968).
5   Edholm, O.G.; Howarth, S.: Studies in the peripheral circulation in osteitis deformans. Clin. Sci. *12:* 277 (1953).
6   Edholm, O.G.; Howarth, S.; McMichael, J.: Heart failure and bone blood flow in osteitis deformans. Clin. Sci. *5:* 249 (1945).
7   Insua, J.A.; Young, J.R.; Humphries, A.W.: Popliteal artery entrapment syndrome. Archs Surg., Chicago *101:* 771 (1970).
8   Raque, C.J.; Stein, K.M.; Lane, J.M., et al.: Pseudoainhum constricting bands of the extremities. Archs Derm. *105:* 434 (1972).
9   Scott, J.T.; Hourihane, D.O.; Doyle, F.H., et al.: Digital arteritis in rheumatoid disease. Ann. rheum. Dis. *20:* 224 (1961).
10 Servello, M.: Clinical syndrome of anomalous position of the popliteal artery. Differentiation from juvenile arteriopathy. Circulation *26:* 885 (1962).
11 Sockoloff, L.; Bunim, J.J.: Vascular lesions in rheumatoid arthritis. J. chron. Dis. *5:* 668 (1957).
12 Sockoloff, L.; Wilens, S.L.; Bunim, J.J.: Arteritis of striated muscle in rheumatoid arthritis. Am. J. Path. *27:* 157 (1951).

Subject Index